Biotechnology and Sports Engineering

Biotechnology and Sports Engineering

Editor

Joung Hwan Mun

MDPI • Basel • Beijing • Wuhan • Barcelona • Belgrade • Manchester • Tokyo • Cluj • Tianjin

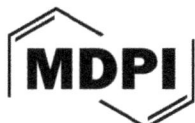

Editor
Joung Hwan Mun
Sungkyunkwan University
Korea

Editorial Office
MDPI
St. Alban-Anlage 66
4052 Basel, Switzerland

This is a reprint of articles from the Special Issue published online in the open access journal *Applied Sciences* (ISSN 2076-3417) (available at: https://www.mdpi.com/journal/applsci/special_issues/Biotechnology_and_Sports_Engineering).

For citation purposes, cite each article independently as indicated on the article page online and as indicated below:

LastName, A.A.; LastName, B.B.; LastName, C.C. Article Title. *Journal Name* **Year**, *Volume Number*, Page Range.

ISBN 978-3-0365-5205-7 (Hbk)
ISBN 978-3-0365-5206-4 (PDF)

© 2022 by the authors. Articles in this book are Open Access and distributed under the Creative Commons Attribution (CC BY) license, which allows users to download, copy and build upon published articles, as long as the author and publisher are properly credited, which ensures maximum dissemination and a wider impact of our publications.

The book as a whole is distributed by MDPI under the terms and conditions of the Creative Commons license CC BY-NC-ND.

Contents

About the Editor vii

Joung-Hwan Mun
Special Issue on Biotechnology and Sports Engineering
Reprinted from: *Appl. Sci.* **2022**, *12*, 7859, doi:10.3390/app12157859 1

Yunhee Chang, Jungsun Kang, Gyoosuk Kim, Hyunjun Shin and Sehoon Park
Intramuscular Properties of Resting Lumbar Muscles in Patients with Unilateral Lower Limb Amputation
Reprinted from: *Appl. Sci.* **2021**, *11*, 9122, doi:10.3390/app11199122 5

Jung Chul Lee, Chong Hoon Lee, Dong Wha Chung, Hee Joo Lee and Jae Yong Park
Analysis of Age-Based Bone Mineral Density in the Korean Adult Population Using Dual-Energy X-ray Absorptiometry
Reprinted from: *Appl. Sci.* **2020**, *10*, 8469, doi:10.3390/app10238469 19

Ji Yeon Hyun, Seungeon Ha, Jongmin Baek, Junghun Han, Honggi An, Sung-Hun Woo, Yoon Suk Kim, Sang Woo Lee, Sejung Yang and Sei Young Lee
Analysis of Random Dynamics of Cell Segmented by a Modified Active Contour Method
Reprinted from: *Appl. Sci.* **2020**, *10*, 6806, doi:10.3390/app10196806 29

Hyungdong Lee, Woojun Ye, Jaehyun Lee, Hyunggun Kim and Doyoung Byun
Silver Nanowire Micro-Ring Formation Using Immiscible Emulsion Droplets for Surface-Enhanced Raman Spectroscopy
Reprinted from: *Appl. Sci.* **2020**, *10*, 8018, doi:10.3390/app10228018 43

Ahnryul Choi, Seungheon Chae, Tae-Hyong Kim, Hyunwoo Jung, Sang-Sik Lee, Ki-Young Lee and Joung-Hwan Mun
A Novel Patient-to-Image Surface Registration Technique for ENT- and Neuro-Navigation Systems: Proper Point Set in Patient Space
Reprinted from: *Appl. Sci.* **2021**, *11*, 5464, doi:10.3390/app11125464 51

Jung-Hyun Park, Ho-Sang Moon, Hyunggun Kim and Sung-Taek Chung
Detection of Movement Intention for Operating Methods of Serious Games
Reprinted from: *Appl. Sci.* **2021**, *11*, 883, doi:10.3390/app11020883 65

Chang-ok Cho, Jin-Hyoung Jeong, Yun-jeong Kim, Jee Hun Jang, Sang-Sik Lee and Ki-young Lee
Comparison of Endurance Time Prediction of Biceps Brachii Using Logarithmic Parameters of a Surface Electromyogram during Low-Moderate Level Isotonic Contractions
Reprinted from: *Appl. Sci.* **2021**, *11*, 2861, doi:10.3390/app11062861 79

Woojae Hong, Soohwan Jeong, Minsung Ko, Hyun Hak Kim and Hyunggun Kim
Effect of the Location of Strut Chordae Insertion on Computational Modeling and Biomechanical Evaluation of Mitral Valve Dynamics
Reprinted from: *Appl. Sci.* **2021**, *11*, 6205, doi:10.3390/app11136205 99

Nam-Ik Kim, Sagn-Jin Kim, Jee-Hun Jang, Woon-seob Shin, Hyok-ju Eum, Buom Kim, Ahn-Ryul Choi and Sang-Sik Lee
Changes in Fatigue Recovery and Muscle Damage Enzymes after Deep-Sea Water Thalassotherapy
Reprinted from: *Appl. Sci.* **2020**, *10*, 8383, doi:10.3390/app10238383 111

Eun-Hee Park, Seung-Wook Choi and Yoon-Kwon Yang
Cold-Water Immersion Promotes Antioxidant Enzyme Activation in Elite Taekwondo Athletes
Reprinted from: *Appl. Sci.* **2021**, *11*, 2855, doi:10.3390/app11062855 123

Yichen Wu, Zuchang Ma, Huanhuan Zhao, Yibing Li and Yining Sun
Achieve Personalized Exercise Intensity through an Intelligent System and Cycling Equipment:
A Machine Learning Approach
Reprinted from: *Appl. Sci.* **2020**, *10*, 7688, doi:10.3390/app10217688 137

Lorenzo Fraccaroli and Franco Concli
Introduction of Open-Source Engineering Tools for the Structural Modeling of a Multilayer
Mountaineering Ski under Operation
Reprinted from: *Appl. Sci.* **2020**, *10*, 5310, doi:10.3390/app10155310 151

Sung-Un Park, Dong-Kyu Kim and Hyunkyun Ahn
A Predictive Model on the Intention to Accept Taekwondo Electronic Protection Devices
Reprinted from: *Appl. Sci.* **2021**, *11*, 1845, doi:10.3390/app11041845 167

Kyoung-Hyun Lee, Jin-Seok Lee, Byung-Chan Lee and Eun-Hyung Cho
Relative Weights of Physical Strength Factors in Sports Events: Focused on Similarity Sports
Events Group According to the Sports Physiological View
Reprinted from: *Appl. Sci.* **2020**, *10*, 9131, doi:10.3390/app10249131 177

Ah-Hyun Hyun and Yoo-Jeong Jeon
Effect of Mat Pilates on Body Fluid Composition, Pelvic Stabilization, and Muscle Damage
during Pregnancy
Reprinted from: *Appl. Sci.* **2020**, *10*, 9111, doi:10.3390/app10249111 187

Yoo Jeong Jeon, Seung Ku Lee and Chol Shin
Relative Hand Grip and Back Muscle Strength, but Not Mean Muscle Strength, as Risk Factors
for Incident Metabolic Syndrome and Its Metabolic Components: 16 Years of Follow-Up in a
Population-Based Cohort Study
Reprinted from: *Appl. Sci.* **2021**, *11*, 5198, doi:10.3390/app11115198 201

About the Editor

Joung Hwan Mun

Dr. Joung Hwan Mun is a tenured professor in the Department of Biomechatronic Engineering at Sungkyunkwan University, to which he returned after receiving his Ph.D. degree in biomedical engineering from the University of Iowa in 1998. His research interests include 3D human modeling, musculoskeletal injuries, sports medicine, ergonomics, biomedical electronics, and expert systems based on artificial intelligence. He is the author of over 80 SCI papers; holds 20 patents; and is leading collaborative projects with Samsung Medical Center, Korea University Medical Center, and the University of Iowa, among others. He was listed as a noteworthy engineering educator, researcher, and consultant by Marquis Who's Who in recognition of his significant contribution to biomedical engineering. He continues to serve as conference chairman of the International Conference on Biotechnology and Sports Engineering (ICON-BASE), which is held annually to share the latest trends in biotechnology and sports engineering research. He is a director at the Bio Information and Communications Technology (B-ICT) Research Center, leading a team dedicated to cutting-edge multidisciplinary research across embedded systems in healthcare, AI and IoT for medical devices, and wearable sensors and engineering analysis of human motion.

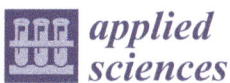

Editorial

Special Issue on Biotechnology and Sports Engineering

Joung-Hwan Mun

Department of Biomechatronic Engineering, College of Biotechnology and Bioengineering, Sungkyunkwan University, Suwon 440-746, Korea; jmun@skku.edu; Tel.: +82-31-290-7827

Citation: Mun, J.-H. Special Issue on Biotechnology and Sports Engineering. *Appl. Sci.* 2022, 12, 7859. https://doi.org/10.3390/app12157859

Received: 2 August 2022
Accepted: 3 August 2022
Published: 4 August 2022

Publisher's Note: MDPI stays neutral with regard to jurisdictional claims in published maps and institutional affiliations.

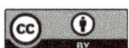

Copyright: © 2022 by the author. Licensee MDPI, Basel, Switzerland. This article is an open access article distributed under the terms and conditions of the Creative Commons Attribution (CC BY) license (https://creativecommons.org/licenses/by/4.0/).

1. Introduction

We are in the midst of the fourth industrial revolution, a time of change and innovation. The limitations to independent studies have been shown, and a multidisciplinary convergence that transcends the boundaries of academic disciplines has become indispensable. Biotechnology and sports engineering are especially intimately connected, and when they advance together, they may significantly improve the quality of human life.

The aim of this Special Issue is to share the latest research trends in biotechnology and sports engineering that explore future directions for development. In total, 40 papers were submitted, and 16 papers covering various topics of interest were accepted (i.e., a 40% acceptance rate). Here, a brief introduction to the research topics and related works is given.

2. Integration of Biotechnology and Sports Engineering

Biotechnology covers a wide range of topics that make use of living organisms and subcellular components, but its biggest concern is human health. The first paper by Chang et al. [1] presented therapeutic strategies for amputees with lower back pain associated with a lack of neural control of movement. The intramuscular characteristics of the lumbar muscle at rest were analyzed using a myotonometer with age-matched lower limb amputees and controls. Lee et al. [2] provided a valuable reference for the pathophysiology and treatment of bone diseases. This study used the commonly used method of dual-energy X-ray absorptiometry to measure the difference in Korean subjects' bone mineral density and content based on age and gender.

Today's frontiers in biotechnology include cellular and molecular systems which are incredibly complicated, making their investigation more difficult. Two studies on biomedical visualization suggested novel approaches to detect biomolecules. It is important to distinguish between different cellular types in diagnosis and treatment given their significant impact on therapeutic approach and prognosis. Hyun et al. [3] compared three different center point localization methods using the time-lapsed images of cellular dynamics. They found that modified active contours with denoising significantly reduced localization errors. To precisely detect biomolecules, Lee et al. [4] built micro/nano-scale structures composed of silver (Ag). Their ring patterned fabrication method showed enhanced intensity that can be applied to surface-enhanced Raman spectroscopy studies.

The goal of computer-aided surgery is to supplement human limitations in surgery, improve the consistency of surgical procedures, and achieve higher quality surgical operations while reducing the time they take. Choi et al. [5] proposed a unique registration process for the use of image-guided surgical navigation systems. Their strategy was to optimize the registration point cloud by applying specialized augmentation and creation steps. The new protocol exhibited improved registration accuracy in all conditions when compared with the conventional method.

Biosensors in the field of human movement study provide the advantage of detecting and interpreting the motor signals of the central nervous system. In two studies, surface electromyography was used in a non-invasive manner to measure the magnitudes and patterns of muscle activity. Park et al. [6] designed a unique balancing handle as a symmetric upper extremity training method, which allowed the quantitative evaluation of physical function and monitoring of rehabilitation therapy outcomes. Cho et al. [7] proposed logarithmic parameters to assess the potential endurance times in low-effort tasks.

Strut chordae (SC) that sustain the tunnel-shaped mitral valve (MV) have distinctive structures and functions in the inflow and outflow tracts of the heart. To better understand the complicated MV structures and implant design, Hong et al. [8] simulated how changes to the SC insertion position affect MV function and dynamics. The stress distributions and the leaflet coaptations over the whole cardiac cycle were compared, and the best design was evaluated.

Studies regarding physical recovery programs, such as fatigue recovery and muscle reparation from sports injuries, are being actively developed. Kim et al. [9] evaluated the potency of a deep-sea water thalassotherapy (DSWTT)-based exercise program on fatigue and muscle rehabilitation, with findings indicating a considerable effect on muscle recovery in particular. Park et al. [10] reported the relationship between cold-water immersion (CWI) and antioxidant enzyme activation in elite Taekwondo athletes. Blood tests revealed the increase in antioxidant enzyme concentration in the experimental group. Finding the right exercise intensity is just as important in preventing sports injuries and obtaining exercise benefits. To help individuals find/achieve the appropriate exercise intensity, Wu et al. [11] presented a novel machine-learning-based method that combined the advantages of absolute and relative intensity methods. A user's static body data and questionnaire survey could predict personalized exercise targets.

Today's sports are combined with diverse engineering technologies (e.g., finite element analysis (FEA) and internet of things (IoT)) in order to promote athletic ability, player safety, and fan engagement. FEA is a fundamental technique for reducing development costs and times. Fraccaroli and Concli [12] created a precise virtual model of ski mountaineering that used sports mechanics to simulate the behavior of actual materials. Taekwondo electronic protection devices have IoT features that automatically detect the strength of an attack and judge its validity using an advanced sensor attached to the protective equipment. Park et al. [13] investigated athletes' acceptance intention of electronic devices in Taekwondo matches using a predictive model. Their model revealed better means to regulate the sensitivity of these devices and facilitated the application of engineering technologies in sports.

Clinical exercise physiology is a field that examines how physical activity and exercise affect both short-term and long-term bodily responses. Lee et al. [14] used accumulated measurement data from local sports centers to investigate relevant physical factors in sports events. Physical fitness measurements from 16,645 subjects were used to calculate the relative weights of each factor (muscular power, muscular endurance, power, coordination capability, agility, flexibility, cardiorespiratory endurance, and balance) in four sports categories. Hyun and Jeon [15] studied the effects of 12 weeks of Pilates on pregnant women with regard to body composition, lipid metabolism, pelvic stabilization, and muscle damage. The results demonstrated that mat Pilates is a safe and effective form of exercise for pregnant women. Muscle strength is associated with health outcomes and can be a good indicator for the diagnosis of metabolic status. The 16-year cohort study of Jeon et al. [16]'s with 2538 participants verified that lower relative hand grip and back muscle strength are associated with a high risk of future metabolic abnormality.

3. Present Findings and Future Pathways

The first Special Issue entitled "Biotechnology and Sports Engineering" has successfully brought together the contributions of authors and peer reviewers across different disciplines. Knowledge building is not just a matter of linearly adding to previous information but making more synergistic and complementary effects. The continuous exchange of knowledge between disciplines must be made to facilitate the advancement of human health and wellbeing.

Funding: This research received no external funding.

Acknowledgments: I would like to take this opportunity to thank all who have contributed to this Special Issue. Without the contributions of many talented authors, dedicated reviewers, and the editorial team of *Applied Sciences*, this issue would not be possible. I hope that the readers found this Special Issue informative and useful.

Conflicts of Interest: The author declares no conflict of interest.

References

1. Chang, Y.; Kang, J.; Kim, G.; Shin, H.; Park, S. Intramuscular Properties of Resting Lumbar Muscles in Patients with Unilateral Lower Limb Amputation. *Appl. Sci.* **2021**, *11*, 9122. [CrossRef]
2. Lee, J.; Lee, C.; Chung, D.; Lee, H.; Park, J. Analysis of Age-Based Bone Mineral Density in the Korean Adult Population Using Dual-Energy X-ray Absorptiometry. *Appl. Sci.* **2020**, *10*, 8469. [CrossRef]
3. Hyun, J.; Ha, S.; Baek, J.; Han, J.; An, H.; Woo, S.; Kim, Y.; Lee, S.; Yang, S.; Lee, S. Analysis of Random Dynamics of Cell Segmented by a Modified Active Contour Method. *Appl. Sci.* **2020**, *10*, 6806. [CrossRef]
4. Lee, H.; Ye, W.; Lee, J.; Kim, H.; Byun, D. Silver Nanowire Micro-Ring Formation Using Immiscible Emulsion Droplets for Surface-Enhanced Raman Spectroscopy. *Appl. Sci.* **2020**, *10*, 8018. [CrossRef]
5. Choi, A.; Chae, S.; Kim, T.; Jung, H.; Lee, S.; Lee, K.; Mun, J. A Novel Patient-to-Image Surface Registration Technique for ENT- and Neuro-Navigation Systems: Proper Point Set in Patient Space. *Appl. Sci.* **2021**, *11*, 5464. [CrossRef]
6. Park, J.; Moon, H.; Kim, H.; Chung, S. Detection of Movement Intention for Operating Methods of Serious Games. *Appl. Sci.* **2021**, *11*, 883. [CrossRef]
7. Cho, C.; Jeong, J.; Kim, Y.; Jang, J.; Lee, S.; Lee, K. Comparison of Endurance Time Prediction of Biceps Brachii Using Logarithmic Parameters of a Surface Electromyogram during Low-Moderate Level Isotonic Contractions. *Appl. Sci.* **2021**, *11*, 2861. [CrossRef]
8. Hong, W.; Jeong, S.; Ko, M.; Kim, H.; Kim, H. Effect of the Location of Strut Chordae Insertion on Computational Modeling and Biomechanical Evaluation of Mitral Valve Dynamics. *Appl. Sci.* **2021**, *11*, 6205. [CrossRef]
9. Kim, N.; Kim, S.; Jang, J.; Shin, W.; Eum, H.; Kim, B.; Choi, A.; Lee, S. Changes in Fatigue Recovery and Muscle Damage Enzymes after Deep-Sea Water Thalassotherapy. *Appl. Sci.* **2020**, *10*, 8383. [CrossRef]
10. Park, E.; Choi, S.; Yang, Y. Cold-Water Immersion Promotes Antioxidant Enzyme Activation in Elite Taekwondo Athletes. *Appl. Sci.* **2021**, *11*, 2855. [CrossRef]
11. Wu, Y.; Ma, Z.; Zhao, H.; Li, Y.; Sun, Y. Achieve Personalized Exercise Intensity through an Intelligent System and Cycling Equipment: A Machine Learning Approach. *Appl. Sci.* **2020**, *10*, 7688. [CrossRef]
12. Fraccaroli, L.; Concli, F. Introduction of Open-Source Engineering Tools for the Structural Modeling of a Multilayer Mountaineering Ski under Operation. *Appl. Sci.* **2020**, *10*, 5310. [CrossRef]
13. Park, S.; Kim, D.; Ahn, H. A Predictive Model on the Intention to Accept Taekwondo Electronic Protection Devices. *Appl. Sci.* **2021**, *11*, 1845. [CrossRef]
14. Lee, K.; Lee, J.; Lee, B.; Cho, E. Relative Weights of Physical Strength Factors in Sports Events: Focused on Similarity Sports Events Group According to the Sports Physiological View. *Appl. Sci.* **2020**, *10*, 9131. [CrossRef]
15. Hyun, A.; Jeon, Y. Effect of Mat Pilates on Body Fluid Composition, Pelvic Stabilization, and Muscle Damage during Pregnancy. *Appl. Sci.* **2020**, *10*, 9111. [CrossRef]
16. Jeon, Y.; Lee, S.; Shin, C. Relative Hand Grip and Back Muscle Strength, but Not Mean Muscle Strength, as Risk Factors for Incident Metabolic Syndrome and Its Metabolic Components: 16 Years of Follow-Up in a Population-Based Cohort Study. *Appl. Sci.* **2021**, *11*, 5198. [CrossRef]

Article

Intramuscular Properties of Resting Lumbar Muscles in Patients with Unilateral Lower Limb Amputation

Yunhee Chang *, Jungsun Kang, Gyoosuk Kim, Hyunjun Shin and Sehoon Park

Rehabilitation Engineering Research Institute, Incheon 21417, Korea; js0670@kcomwel.or.kr (J.K.); gskim7379@kcomwel.or.kr (G.K.); hjshin@kcomwel.or.kr (H.S.); mbb1020@kcomwel.or.kr (S.P.)
* Correspondence: yhchang2@kcomwel.or.kr; Tel.: +82-32-509-5249

Featured Application: This study can assist in forming a basis for the therapeutic strategies for the prevention and treatment of low back pain in amputees.

Abstract: Lower limb amputees (LLAs) have a high incidence of low back pain (LBP), and identifying the potential risk factors in this group is key for LBP prevention. This study analyzed the intramuscular properties of the resting lumbar muscle in thirteen unilateral LLAs and age-matched controls to predict the onset of LBP. To measure the lumbar intramuscular properties, resting erector spinae muscles located in the upper and lower lumbar regions were examined using a handheld myotonometer. The dynamic stiffness, oscillation frequency, and logarithmic decrement were measured. In our results, the stiffness and frequency of the upper lumbar region were greater in the amputee group than in the control, whereas the decrement did not differ between the two groups. Additionally, the measured values in the lower lumbar region showed no significant difference. Within each group, all three factors increased at the upper lumbar region. In the LLAs, the frequency and stiffness values of the upper lumbar on the non-amputated side were significantly higher than those on the amputated side. These results indicate that the upper lumbar muscles of the amputees were less flexible than that of the control. This study can help in providing therapeutic strategies treating LBP in amputees.

Keywords: lower limb amputation; low back pain; lumbar intramuscular properties; myotonometry

1. Introduction

Low back pain (LBP) is a common musculoskeletal disorder among lower limb amputees (LLAs), where 52% of LLAs experienced persistent, severe LBP and had a greater prevalence of LBP (52–89%) than that of the non-amputees [1–3]. Identification of potential risk factors in people at high risk for LBP is critical for disease prevention and management.

Abnormal lumbar muscle activity is one of the factors affecting the LBP of LLAs. Factors contributing to left-right asymmetry include static asymmetry (i.e., leg length discrepancy, LLD) and dynamic asymmetry (i.e., asymmetrical trunk-pelvic movement) (Figure 1) [4–6].

With respect to static asymmetry, LLAs generally use prosthetic legs for walking after amputation, which are intentionally shortened to facilitate the toe clearance of the prosthesis. Many previous studies have reported the use of short prosthetic legs by LLAs [4,7], and that a LLD greater than 30 mm can affect the lumbo-pelvic kinematics [8].

When the length of the prosthesis is shortened, the pelvic inclination on the prosthetic side is lowered [8], and when exposed to this static asymmetry for a long time, the prosthetic pelvic muscle is stretched and the contralateral lumbar muscle is shortened. This characteristic causes asymmetry of the lumbar muscles, resulting in structural problems such as changes in the curvature of the spine (i.e., scoliosis) [9–11].

Dynamic asymmetry is also closely related to the amputee's gait, as LLAs excessively recruit the trunk to advance the prosthesis when walking. These characteristics increase the lateral flexion and axial rotation of the trunk towards the prosthetic leg and increase the activity of the global trunk muscle [5]. Excessive muscle activity and trunk-pelvis motion during walking increase the spinal load, and exposure to repetitive walking increases the risk of LBP [12]. A previous study reported that the trunk muscle force and spinal load in the non-amputated side (NAS) increased by 10–40% and 17–95%, respectively, compared with those in the amputated side (AS), which changed the recruitment pattern of trunk muscles [13].

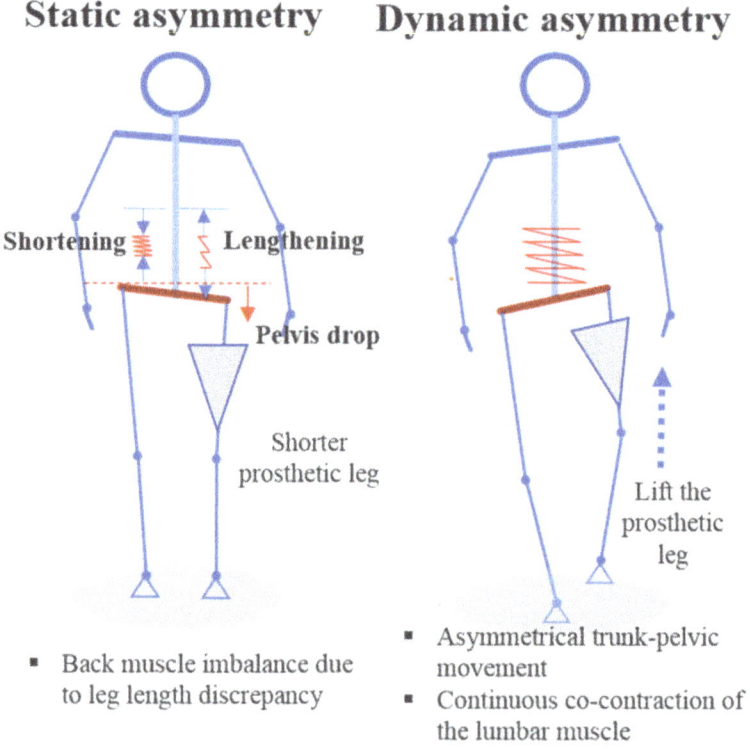

Figure 1. Schematic of static and dynamic contributing factors associated with lumbar muscle imbalance in patients with unilateral transfemoral amputation.

Lumbar muscle activity patterns during LLA's walking are similar to those in patients with LBP [14,15]. In healthy individuals, the erector spinae muscle relaxes during the double limb support and swing phases, but in patients with LBP, the activity of the erector spinae muscle is increased throughout the entire gait cycle [15–17]. The activity of erector spinae muscle in patients with chronic low back pain (CLBP) is 8 to 48% higher than in healthy individuals [14]. This is closely related to the guarding mechanisms that protect the spine from pain.

However, LLAs increase the activity of the erector spinae as a functional strategy for gait propulsion, not due to LBP [12]. In preparing the trunk for movement of the prosthetic leg, it is necessary to provide stability to the lumbar region, which increases the muscle activity of the trunk. As a result, the activity of the erector spinae muscle increases throughout the gait cycle, and the recruitment pattern of the trunk muscles may change, similar to that in patients with LBP.

As mentioned above, the asymmetry of pelvic inclination caused by LLD or trunk-pelvis asymmetry movement due to abnormal gait changes the onset or recruitment pattern of the back muscles, causing overall lumbar muscle imbalance. Abnormal patterns or excessive activation of muscles can lead to musculoskeletal problems in the long term. Therefore, it is of utmost importance to identify potential risk factors to prevent them.

Many studies have been conducted to analyze the properties of muscles in relation to LBP. In particular, analyzing the properties of resting lumbar muscles is useful to identify potential risk factors for back pain [18], and analyzing the stiffness of resting lumbar muscles enables the analysis of inherent skeletal muscle properties in a state where central nervous system (CNS) activation is excluded [19].

To identify the lumbar muscle properties, the stiffness is mainly analyzed. High muscle stiffness means high muscle tone, and prolonged exposure to these situations is interpreted as a high risk of muscle fatigue or LBP [20].

In previous studies, authors reported increased lumbar muscle tone in patients with CLBP and a 20% greater stiffness of the erector spinae muscles at rest, as compared to that in patients without LBP [21]. High stiffness of the spinal muscles indicates hypertonia due to chronic mechanical overload with or without an inflammatory response [22]. A high muscle stiffness value is a valid factor for predicting the occurrence of LBP, and relevant evidence has mainly been studied in patients with ankylosing spondylitis [23]. However, studies in LLAs with high prevalence of LBP are rare.

Intramuscular properties are measured using a variety of methods such as diagnostic ultrasound, magnetic resonance elastography, ultrasonic shear-wave elastography, and electromyography [24]. Although these methods can provide high reliability and quantified data, their high cost and operational complexity can make them difficult to use in simple clinical practice.

Several recent studies have investigated intramuscular properties using a handheld myotonometer. It is a non-invasive device that can quantify stiffness, frequency, and decrement of myofascial tissue, and real-time quantitative measurement of myofascial stiffness can support diagnostics and patient-driven interventions. Studies using a myotonometer were conducted in patients with ankylosing spondylitis [23,25], Parkinson's disease [26], and stroke [27], and the reliability was confirmed with an intraclass correlation coefficient of 0.80 or greater [28].

As mentioned above, most previous studies related to LBP in LLAs have focused on the kinematic changes such as trunk and lumbo-pelvic movement asymmetry [5,6] as well as variations in the trunk-pelvis coordination during walking [14]. Although some studies have reported asymmetry of lumbar muscle activity using surface electromyography [29], to the best of the authors' knowledge, there are few studies on the changes in the intramuscular properties of lumbar muscles in LLAs. Understanding the biomechanical characteristics (i.e., the intramuscular properties) of groups with a high prevalence of LBP will help prevent disease and provide adequate treatment by identifying the potential risk factors.

Therefore, this study aims to compare the biomechanical properties of lumbar muscles using a handheld myotonometer in LLAs and healthy controls. The results of this study will be utilized as basic data for establishing rehabilitation strategies for amputees with LBP.

2. Methods

2.1. Participants

Thirteen LLAs and thirteen age matched controls participated in this study. The general characteristics of participants are shown in Table 1.

Table 1. General characteristics of the participants (n = 26).

Amputated Level (n)	Amputee Group (n = 13)	Control Group (n = 13)	t-Value
	TFA (10)/TTA (3)	NA	NA
Amputated side (n)	Right (5)/Left (8)	NA	NA
Prosthesis use (years)	4.5 ± 1.1 *	NA	NA
Prosthesis use time per day (hours)	9.2 ± 1.8	NA	NA
Age (years)	43.2 ± 9.9	42.5 ± 5.5	0.221
Weight (kg)	70.5 ± 6.2	73.1 ± 4.7	−1.196
Height (m)	1.71 ± 4.13	1.75 ± 0.06	−1.800
BMI (kg/m^2)	23.6 ± 2.1	24.0 ± 1.9	−0.581

* Value is presented as mean ± standard deviation; TFA, transfemoral amputation; TTA, transtibial amputation; BMI, body mass index; NA, not applicable.

As a result of verifying the subjects' homogeneity using the independent sample t-test, there was no statistically significant difference between the groups in age, weight, height, and BMI ($p > 0.05$).

The inclusion criteria for amputees were as follows: male patients with unilateral transfemoral and transtibial amputation due to post traumatic injury; patients with no history of neurological symptoms except phantom and stump pains; patients without problems in daily activities (i.e., walking) and ability to walk without assistive devices; and patients without medication or physical therapy due to LBP within 3 months. In addition, the control group (CG) was selected from healthy individuals without any medications and history of LBP in the past 3 months.

In particular, those with pre-existing spinal pathology or chronic LBP prior to traumatic amputation, coexistence of spinal trauma that occurred at the time of traumatic injury, those with persistent LBP for 3 months or more due to the possibility of fatty degeneration of the spinal muscles [30], and those with a BMI greater than 30 kg/m^2 were excluded from this study to improve the reliability of quantification of intramuscular properties [31].

The purpose of the study was explained to all participants and informed consent was obtained. The study was conducted with the approval of the Research Ethics Committee of the Rehabilitation Engineering Research Institute (RERI-IRB-190114-1).

2.2. Instruments

Lumbar intramuscular properties were measured using a MyotonPro® (Myoton AS, Tallinn, Estonia); it is an objective and reliable non-invasive measurement device that can quantitatively evaluate the biomechanical properties of soft tissues such as muscles and tendons [23,28]. Figure 2 shows the actual experimental status and extracted data using MyotonPro®.

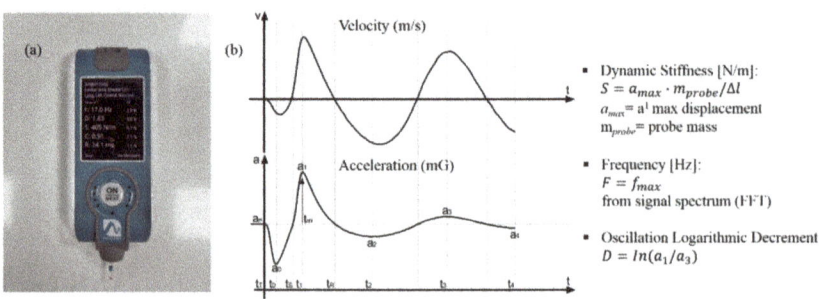

Figure 2. Myotonometer used in the experiment (a) and the extracted signal characteristics (b).

The MyotonPro® provides a controlled pre-load of 0.18 N for initial compression of the subcutaneous tissue and imposes an additional 15 ms impulse of mechanical force of 0.40 N to induce a damped or decaying natural oscillation of the tissue [32]. The peak acceleration (α_{max}) of the natural oscillation is estimated using an accelerometer. The first integral of the acceleration signal extracts velocity and the second integral extracts the displacement. The MyotonPro® quantifies dynamic stiffness (S), as defined in Equation (1)

$$S = \frac{m\alpha_{max}}{\Delta l} \quad (1)$$

where m is the mass of the probe of 18 g (0.18 N), α_{max} is the maximum amplitude of the oscillation in the acceleration signal, and Δl is the amplitude of the displacement signal after the end of the impulse time. The MyotonPro® can measure tissue stiffness within a subcutaneous depth of 2 cm [23].

2.3. Measured Variables

The measured variables include the dynamic stiffness (N/m), oscillation frequency (Hz), and logarithmic decrement. Dynamic stiffness (i.e., tone) is an intramuscular property defined as the resistance to deformation that occurs when external force is applied. Oscillation frequency (i.e., resting tension) refers to the intrinsic muscle tension in the absence of spontaneous muscle contraction.

Logarithmic decrement (i.e., elasticity) is measured as the damping ratio of the signal of acceleration as the tissue recovers after deformation. A decrease in the logarithmic decrement value indicates an increase in tissue elasticity and a decrease in tissue plasticity [18,25,32].

2.4. Experimental Procedure

Subjects were placed in a prone position on an examination table with the skin of the lumbar area exposed, and their arms were placed next to the torso for a comfortable posture.

To measure the lumbar intramuscular properties, we selected four sites around the spine: the upper (i.e., T12–L1) and lower lumbar regions (i.e., L4–L5) as shown in Figure 1. The upper lumbar region includes the erector spinae muscles, which corresponds to the inflection point of the thoracolumbar curvature, where high loads and rotational forces occur [33]. The lower lumbar region contains the multifidus muscles, which play a key role in maintaining stability of the spine [34]. Lumbar measurement levels were initially approximated in the uppermost part of the iliac crests, then the specific levels were identified the L4–L5 and T12–L1 spinous processes, and bilateral measurement sites were marked on the left and right extensor muscle bulk prominences (Figure 3) [18].

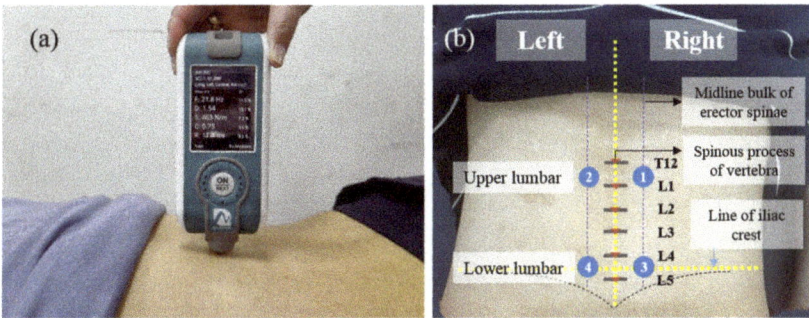

Figure 3. A photograph of the measurement using a myotonometer (**a**) and a schematic of the selection criteria for the four measurement sites of the lumbar (**b**).

Before measuring, the subjects held a relaxed position without muscle contraction for 10 min. The stiffness of the resting lumbar fascia is known to increase after 10 min from its initial state and is also a fundamental intrinsic property of the fascia [18]. After rest, the lumbar intramuscular properties of the subjects were measured while they held their breath for 5 s at the end of the inspiratory phase to minimize the effect of the intra-abdominal pressure [35]. All MyotonPro® measurements were conducted by the same skilled physical therapist to minimize measurement errors.

2.5. Statistical Analysis

Statistical analysis was performed using the Statistical Package for the Social Sciences, Statistics version 20 (IBM Corp., Armonk, NY, USA). The mean and standard deviation of all data were calculated, and the normality of the data was verified using the Kolmogorov–Smirnov test.

Within each group, the differences in the intramuscular properties between the right and left of the spine and between the upper and lower lumbar regions were compared using a paired *t*-test. In addition, the difference between the two groups in the three conditions (i.e., the AS, NAS, and CG) were compared using analysis of variance (ANOVA). Tukey's multiple comparison test was used for post-hoc analysis, and the statistical significance for all tests was set at $p < 0.05$.

3. Results

3.1. Differences in Lumbar Intramuscular Properties of the AS (or Right) and NAS (or Left)

Table 2 shows the differences in lumbar intramuscular properties of AS and NAS within the amputee group.

Table 2. Comparison of lumbar intramuscular properties between AS and NAS sides in the amputee group.

	Lumbar Part	Amputee Group (*n* = 13)		SE	t-Value
		AS	NAS		
Stiffness (N/m)	Upper	303.2 ± 51.3 §	329.1 ± 51.2	8.57	−3.026 *
	Lower	225.9 ± 51.2	237.6 ± 61.3	8.73	−1.348
	SE	16.89	17.92	-	-
	t value	4.579 ***	5.105 ***	-	-
Frequency (Hz)	Upper	16.5 ± 1.9	17.4 ± 1.5	0.30	−2.704 *
	Lower	14.0 ± 1.4	14.1 ± 1.5	0.33	−0.503
	SE	0.60	0.58	-	-
	t value	4.318 ***	5.590 ***	-	-
Decrement (Ratio)	Upper	1.25 ± 0.24	1.17 ± 0.17	0.06	1.379
	Lower	1.15 ± 0.23	1.13 ± 0.23	0.04	0.496
	SE	0.06	0.06	-	-
	t value	1.881	0.744	-	-

AS, amputated side; NAS, non-amputated side; SE, standard error; § mean ± standard deviation; * $p < 0.05$, *** $p < 0.001$.

Mean values of stiffness and frequency were greater in NAS than in the AS for both upper and lower lumbar regions; the upper and lower lumbar stiffness increased by 8.6% and 5.2%, and the upper and lower lumbar frequency increased by 5% and 1.2%, respectively (statistical significance was only in the upper lumbar). The decrement values were less in the NAS than in the AS in both upper and lower lumbar regions (decreased by 6.2% and 1.6%, respectively); however, there was no significant difference.

Table 3 shows the differences in intramuscular properties of the right and left sides within the CG.

Table 3. Comparison of lumbar intramuscular properties between the right and left sides in the control group.

	Lumbar Part	Control Group (n = 13)		SE	t Value
		Right	Left		
Stiffness (N/m)	Upper	282.1 ± 38.7 [§]	281.6 ± 39.3	5.14	0.169
	Lower	225.6 ± 47.1	227.2 ± 41.2	3.02	0.130
	SE	8.55	9.68	-	-
	t value	6.375 ***	5.580 ***	-	-
Frequency (Hz)	Upper	15.3 ± 1.3	15.8 ± 1.3	0.29	−1.807
	Lower	14.0 ± 1.5	14.3 ± 1.6	0.11	−2.432 *
	SE	0.39	0.41	-	-
	t value	3.124 **	3.023 *	-	-
Decrement (Ratio)	Upper	1.29 ± 0.34	1.13 ± 0.25	0.04	4.487 ***
	Lower	1.02 ± 0.20	1.00 ± 0.16	0.03	0.506
	SE	0.07	0.04	-	-
	t value	3.921 **	3.010 *	-	-

SE, standard error; [§] mean ± standard deviation; * $p < 0.05$, ** $p < 0.01$, *** $p < 0.001$.

The right and left stiffness values were not significantly different in either upper or lower lumbar regions. Frequency values were greater on the left side for both upper and lower lumbar regions (increased by 3.4% and 2.0%, respectively); however, statistical significance was found only in the lower lumbar region. Conversely, decrement values were greater on the right side in both upper and lower lumbar regions, with 12.4% and 1.5% increase, respectively (statistical significance was only in the upper lumbar region).

3.2. Differences in the Lumbar Intramuscular Properties of the Upper and Lower Regions

Table 2 shows the differences in the lumbar intramuscular properties of the upper and lower regions within the amputee group. Mean values of stiffness and frequency were greater in upper than in the lower lumbar region for both AS and NAS. In the upper region, the stiffness of the AS and NAS increased by 25.5% and 27.8%, and the frequency increased by 15.6% and 18.6%, respectively, all statistically significant. The decrement value was greater in the upper than in the lower lumbar region in both AS and NAS (increased by 8.3% and 3.7%, respectively); however, there was no significant difference.

Table 3 shows the differences in lumbar intramuscular properties of the upper and lower regions within the CG.

The stiffness and frequency values were greater on the upper lumbar region for both the right and left sides; in the upper region, the stiffness of the AS and NAS increased by 19.3% and 19.2%, and the frequency increased by 8% and 9.2%, respectively, all statistically significant. In addition, decrement values were greater in the upper region in both the right and left sides (21% and 11.1% increase, respectively) and there was a statistical significance.

3.3. Differences in Lumbar Intramuscular Properties between Amputees and the Control Group

Table 4 shows the differences in lumbar intramuscular properties for the three conditions (i.e., AS, NAS, CG), and the presented CG values are the mean values of the right and left sides.

Table 4. Comparison of lumbar muscle properties in AS, NAS, and CG.

	Lumbar Part	Lower Limb Amputees		CG (C)	F Value	Tukey HSD
		AS (A)	NAS (B)			
Stiffness (N/m)	Upper	303.2 ± 51.3 §	329.1 ± 51.2	281.9 ± 38.0	3.291 *	B>C
	Lower	225.9 ± 51.2	237.6 ± 61.3	226.4 ± 43.6	0.192	NS
Frequency (Hz)	Upper	16.5 ± 1.9	17.4 ± 1.5	15.5 ± 1.2	4.455 *	B>C
	Lower	14.0 ± 1.4	14.1 ± 1.5	14.2 ± 1.6	0.082	NS
Decrement (Ratio)	Upper	1.25 ± 0.24	1.17 ± 0.17	1.21 ± 0.29	0.336	NS
	Lower	1.15 ± 0.23	1.13 ± 0.23	1.01 ± 0.18	1.184	NS

AS, amputated side; NAS, non-amputated side; CG, control group; § mean ± standard deviation; * $p < 0.05$; NS, no significance.

In the upper lumbar region, the stiffness of the AS and NAS tended to be 14.4% greater than that of the CG (F value = 3.291, $p < 0.05$). In addition, the frequency of the AS and NAS tended to be 10.9% higher than that of the CG (F value = 4.455, $p < 0.05$). Especially in the NAS, there were significant differences among the three conditions. In the post-hoc analysis (Tukey's HSD), the stiffness and frequency of NAS significantly increased compared to the CG ($p < 0.05$). On the other hand, there was no statistical difference in the stiffness and frequency of the lower lumbar region.

In addition, the decrement values of the NAS were less than those of the AS or CG (decreased by 12.4% and 6.6%, respectively), but were not statistically significant.

4. Discussion

The identification of potential risk factors for LBP is crucial in terms of disease prevention and treatment. This study analyzed the properties of resting lumbar muscles using a handheld myotonometer for LLAs with a high risk of LBP to understand LBP in patients with lower limb amputation.

The most notable point in the results of this study is the significant increase in the stiffness and frequency of the upper lumbar region on the NAS of amputees. The stiffness of the NAS (329.1 N/m) increased by 8.5% and 16.9%, respectively, compared with those of the AS (303.2 N/m) and CG (281.6 N/m), and the frequency of the NAS (17.4 Hz) was increased by 5.5% and 12.3%, respectively, compared with that of the AS (16.5 Hz) and CG (15.5 Hz).

In particular, in the amputees, the difference between the AS and NAS of the upper lumbar was significantly increased more than that in the lower lumbar. However, there was no significant difference between the right and left sides of the upper lumbar in the CG. Therefore, unlike the CG, bilateral differences in stiffness and frequency can be interpreted as a potential risk factor related to LBP in the amputees.

In our study, there was no difference in the stiffness of the right and left portions in the CG. However, in a similar previous study using the portable MyotonPro, comparing the stiffness of the right and left sides of 20 young male and female adults, it was reported that males and the right side had greater stiffness than females and the left side, respectively. This was affected by the right-hand dominance (all subjects in the study had right-handed dominance) and low-level CNS activation, suggesting further study of the effect of gender difference [18]. In a study by Nair et al., the stiffness was measured a total of three times with an interval of one week, and the difference in mean values measured over 3 weeks was compared. The men who participated in the experiment showed stiffness values in the range of 231.7 N/m to 267.7 N/m, and there was little difference between the left and right mean values at week 1 (234.6 N/m vs. 236.3 N/m). However, it can be seen that the difference between the left and right increased significantly in the second (242.9 N/m vs. 257.5 N/m) and third weeks (231.7 N/m vs. 264.3 N/m). In the discussion, the authors said that the inter-individual variance increased more than the intra-individual variance during the 3 weeks of measurement. They did not specify the reason for this, and they suggested further research. However, it is not appropriate to directly compare the results of our study with that of Nair et al. because our experiment was conducted once a day and the change over time was not considered. Nevertheless, it was confirmed that the average stiffness values presented by Nair et al. were lower than those of the CG and amputees in our study. In addition, in the study of Nair et al., the average age of male subjects was 21 years, and unlike our study, the subjects were younger, and the measurement site (L3–L4) was different. Owing to these factors, it is thought that the lumbar stiffness of the CG was higher in our study. In the future, we believe that additional research on the difference in stiffness according to age and measurement site of individuals without LBP is necessary [18].

In general, the tendency of changes in stiffness and frequency values is similar because of the characteristics of the two variables (when the stiffness value increases, the frequency value also increases). Through these factors, it is possible to evaluate the muscle tone (or tension), which is an intrinsic property of the muscle. High muscle tone means high intramuscular pressure (i.e., hypertonia), which reduces blood supply and can lead to muscle fatigue [36]. Accumulated muscle fatigue can cause back pain; hence, proper management is required.

In our study, the stiffness and frequency differences between the right and left sides of amputated patients were associated with providing an asymmetric static and dynamic environment to the amputated patients.

First, one of the factors contributing to static asymmetry in amputated patients is LLD [6]. Several previous studies involving LLD have reported that the leg lengths of the amputees are asymmetrical; 85% of amputees had prostheses that were too short or too long (n = 113, 29 TFAs and 84 TTAs) [4], and 14 out of 17 amputees had prostheses that were too short [7]. It has also been reported that the LLD of the amputees with LBP is greater than that of amputees without LBP, and LLDs greater than 30 mm affect the lumbo-pelvic kinematics [8]. The anterior pelvic tilt angle of TFA increased when standing or walking compared with that of the CG [37].

Intentionally shortening the length of the prosthesis to facilitate toe clearance on the prosthetic side during TFA walking causes the problem of descent of the pelvis of the prosthesis [8]. Asymmetric pelvic oblique angles result in muscle imbalance, stretching the lumbar muscles of the short leg (the AS) and shortening the lumbar muscles of the contralateral (the NAS). These characteristics can result in a prolonged distortion of the asymmetric pelvis or fixation of the imbalance in muscle condition, resulting in scoliosis [9]. In fact, functional scoliosis due to LLD occurs frequently in LLAs [10], and scoliosis has been reported in 43% of LLAs (18 out of 42) on radiological examination [11].

Second, the asymmetry of the left and right lumbar muscles in the amputees is closely related to gait. Abnormal gait patterns in amputees cause asymmetric trunk movement, which in turn alter muscle recruitment patterns.

In general, during normal gait, the thoracic erector spinae muscle on the opposite side of the stance leg contracts concentrically before the lumbar erector spinae muscle is activated. This characteristic contributes to moving the upper trunk while reversing the curve of the spine toward the swing leg. Thereafter, the lumbar erector spinae muscle controls the trunk and supports the pelvis and swing leg elevation through eccentric contraction [38,39].

When trunk neuromuscular control is compromised by LBP, the timing of activation of trunk muscle tissue is altered as above [15,17].

For example, people with LBP had increased lumbar and thoracic erector spinae activation during the swing phase of gait, early onset and delayed offset of the lumbar erector spinae, and increased co-contraction of trunk flexors and extensors compared with those without LBP [14,15,17].

This phenomenon is a mechanism to protect the spine from LBP by increasing the stability of the spine. When LBP patients walk at a high speed, increasing the lumbar erector spinae activity during swing phase to increase the stiffness of the lumbar spine is also effective for speed-dependent perturbations [14].

Amputees also increase lateral flexion and axial rotation of the trunk toward the amputated leg when walking, and these properties increase the activity of the global trunk muscles. This is a strategy that uses the proximal (i.e., trunk) to advance the amputated limb, and excessive muscle activity and trunk-pelvic movement increase the spinal load, increasing the risk of LBP [5,13].

With regard to spinal load, Shojaei et al. found that the trunk muscle force and spinal load were 10–40% and 17–95% higher, respectively, in the stance phase (i.e., heel strike and toe-off phase) to the sound side during TFA walking compared with the AS. At the same time, increases of 6–80% and 26–60% have been reported compared to those in normal controls. This occurs because the antagonist muscles contract simultaneously during the non-amputated stance phase, and at the same time as the recruitment pattern of the trunk muscles changes, the trunk is mainly used to assist the advancement of gait. The author of this paper suggested that repeated exposure to these high loads may increase the risk of LBP given the repetitive nature of walking [13].

Moreover, in this study, decrement factors other than stiffness and frequency were analyzed. The decrement refers to the elasticity of a muscle, and as stiffness or frequency increases, the decrement decreases. Maintaining adequate elasticity enables efficient muscle activity with less mechanical energy [32], whereas a decrease in elasticity causes muscle fatigue and restricts the speed of movements [40].

As indicated by the results of this study, there were significant differences in stiffness and frequency between amputees and controls, but there was no significant difference in decrement between the two groups. On the other hand, as for the average value of decrement, the elasticity of the non-amputated upper side was the lowest, and the elasticity of the contralateral side (the AS) was higher than that of the CG. In addition, the average value of the lower lumbar decrement showed a decrease in elasticity on both sides of the amputee group compared with that in the CG.

In conclusion, there was no significant difference in the decrement factor, whereas the stiffness or frequency values of the upper lumbar in our study showed significant differences within or between groups. This means that it is difficult to identify potential risk factors for LBP using the decrement value. In addition, the fact that there was a significant difference between the left and right of the upper decrement within the CG makes it more difficult to use as an evaluation factor. This may be the reason why most previous studies have focused on stiffness to identify potential risk factors associated with back pain.

In addition, in the results of this study, significant differences in intramuscular properties were observed in the upper region of the lumbar rather than in the lower region. In both groups, the stiffness and frequency of the upper region were significantly increased compared with those in the lower region, because the muscle arrangement or properties of the upper and lower lumbar were different. This is because the upper and lower lumbar regions are composed of muscle fibers and superficial fascia, respectively [41].

As mentioned above, the erector spinae muscle measured in this study corresponds to the inflection point of the thoracolumbar curvature [42], which is a region where high loads [33] and rotational forces [43] occur even in the upper lumbar region (T12–L1). The lower lumbar region (L4–L5) contains the multifidus muscles that play an important role in maintaining spine stability. In fact, the upper stiffness value of our study tended to be higher than those of Nair et al. Although our subjects were older, the lumbar measurement level was higher than that of Nair et al. (L3–L4), which is thought to be because this area is the inflection point of the thoracolumbar curve and stress is more concentrated in this area [18].

In addition, in both groups, all three factors were significantly higher in the upper than in the lower lumbar region. The higher muscle tone and lower elasticity in the upper region than in the lower region means that muscle fatigue is more likely to occur in the upper lumbar region.

In general, relaxation of the erector spinae muscle occurs during the double limb support phase and swing phase during walking [16]. However, in patients with CLBP, the activity of the erector spinae muscle increases throughout the gait cycle [15,17].

Insufficient muscle relaxation and sustained activity of motor units contribute to muscle damage and degeneration [44].

The pattern of muscle activation during walking in LLAs is similar to that in LBP patients. The initial activity of the lumbar erector spinae prepares the trunk for movement towards the amputated leg by providing stability to the lumbar spine before the heel of the amputated leg contacts the floor. This unique neuromuscular control strategy of LLAs translates into a functional strategy for locomotion than that of LBP patients. These characteristics support the increase in the non-amputated upper stiffness in our findings. Gait strategies that require greater activation of the trunk muscles of the supporting leg to provide stability to the lumbar region for propulsion on the AS are thought to increase muscle stiffness and frequency, especially in the upper part on the NAS [12].

Continuous activation of muscles can cause musculoskeletal problems in the long term, so it should be prevented. Nevertheless, the imperative question is which strategy to apply to prevent these musculoskeletal problems. If increased lumbar muscle activity is associated with a maladaptive coping method, treatment strategy such as myofeedback may help reduce the increased lumbar muscle activity.

As the asymmetry of the left and right muscle stiffness of the amputees shown in our study is more likely to develop into LBP if it persists for a long time, it is of utmost importance to eliminate risk factors that cause asymmetric characteristic in amputated patients.

As mentioned above, LLD identified as a static risk factor should be aligned as symmetrically as possible, and pelvic descent due to leg length should be avoided. In addition, asymmetric movements of the trunk and pelvis caused by abnormal gait patterns should be improved through prosthetic gait training. In particular, proper muscle strengthening and education are required to prevent excessive trunk rotation, extension, and lateral flexion during the training process.

Therefore, it is necessary to establish a strategy to relieve LBP by regularly evaluating the lumbar muscle condition of LLAs. Furthermore, we believe that myotonometry can be useful as a simple non-invasive measurement tool for clinical evaluation. If the stiffness of the muscle is high, the muscles should be relaxed through stretching or massage. It is also necessary to improve the exercise methods and lifestyle to strengthen the back muscles through patient education.

This study has several limitations. Although voluntary muscle contraction was restricted by taking sufficient rest before the experiment, complete restriction of muscle contraction could not be confirmed by quantitatively measuring the electrical activity of the muscles. Future studies should consider concurrent electromyography to ensure the reliability of the results. In addition, it is necessary to analyze the muscle properties according to the level of amputation or the presence or absence of LBP and the increase in the number of subjects.

5. Conclusions

Regarding the high prevalence of LBP among patients with lower limb amputation, we analyzed the biomechanical and viscoelastic properties of lumbar muscles in unilateral LLAs. We found that the frequency and stiffness values of the upper lumbar muscles in LLAs were greater than those in the CG. In particular, the frequency and stiffness values of the NAS were greater than those of the AS. The decrement values were not significantly different between the two groups, and within each group, all three factors increased in a statistically significant manner in the upper region than those in the lower region.

Long-term exposure to high muscle stiffness can lead to muscle fatigue, which in turn increases the risk of developing LBP. Therefore, it is necessary to eliminate asymmetric static and dynamic risk factors, such as leg length discrepancy or abnormal prosthetic gait that can cause LBP in LLAs.

Additionally, it is necessary to provide bilateral symmetrical leg lengths and to maintain the flexibility of the upper back muscles through stretching and strengthening exercises. It is also believed that a continuous monitoring of the back muscles with a simple device such as a hand-held myotonometer will considerably contribute toward preventing LBP in LLAs.

Author Contributions: Conceptualization, methodology, visualization, writing—reviewing, editing, and investigation, Y.C.; conceptualization, methodology, formal analysis, data curation, and investigation, J.K.; supervision, investigation, G.K.; project administration, funding acquisition, H.S. and S.P. All authors have read and agreed to the published version of the manuscript.

Funding: This research was supported by the Bio and Medical Technology Development Program of the National Research Foundation (NRF) funded by the Ministry of Science and ICT (No.2017M3A9E2063255).

Institutional Review Board Statement: The study was conducted according to the guidelines of the Declaration of Helsinki, and approved by the Institutional Review Board of Rehabilitation Engineering Research Institute (RERI-IRB-190114-1).

Informed Consent Statement: Informed consent was obtained from all subjects involved in the study.

Data Availability Statement: The datasets generated during and/or analysed during the current study are available from the corresponding author on reasonable request.

Acknowledgments: We would like to thank Editage (www.editage.co.kr, accessed on 26 May 2021) for editing and reviewing this manuscript for English language.

Conflicts of Interest: The authors declare no conflict of interest.

References

1. Ehde, D.M.; Smith, D.G.; Czerniecki, J.M.; Campbell, K.M.; Malchow, D.M.; Robinson, L.R. Back pain as a secondary disability in persons with lower limb amputations. *Arch. Phys. Med. Rehabil.* **2001**, *82*, 731–734. [CrossRef]
2. Ephraim, P.L.; Wegener, S.T.; MacKenzie, E.J.; Dillingham, T.R.; Pezzin, L.E. Phantom pain, residual limb pain, and back pain in amputees: Results of a national survey. *Arch. Phys. Med. Rehabil.* **2005**, *86*, 1910–1919. [CrossRef]
3. Kušljugić, A.; Kapidžić-Duraković, S.; Kudumović, Z.; Čičkušić, A. Chronic low back pain in individuals with lower-limb amputation. *Bosn. J. Basic Med. Sci.* **2006**, *6*, 67. [CrossRef]
4. Friberg, O. Biomechanical significance of the correct length of lower limb prostheses: A clinical and radiological study. *Prosthet. Orthot. Int.* **1984**, *8*, 124–129. [CrossRef]
5. Morgenroth, D.C.; Orendurff, M.S.; Shakir, A.; Segal, A.; Shofer, J.; Czerniecki, J.M. The relationship between lumbar spine kinematics during gait and low-back pain in transfemoral amputees. *Am. J. Phys. Med. Rehabil.* **2010**, *89*, 635–643. [CrossRef]
6. Devan, H.; Hendrick, P.; Ribeiro, D.C.; Hale, L.A.; Carman, A. Asymmetrical movements of the lumbopelvic region: Is this a potential mechanism for low back pain in people with lower limb amputation? *Med Hypotheses* **2014**, *82*, 77–85. [CrossRef] [PubMed]
7. Morgenroth, D.C.; Shakir, A.; Orendurff, M.S.; Czerniecki, J.M. Low-back pain in transfemoral amputees: Is there a correlation with static or dynamic leg-length discrepancy? *Am. J. Phys. Med. Rehabil.* **2009**, *88*, 108–113. [CrossRef] [PubMed]
8. Lee, R.Y.; Turner-Smith, A. The influence of the length of lower-limb prosthesis on spinal kinematics. *Arch. Phys. Med. Rehabil.* **2003**, *84*, 1357–1362. [CrossRef]
9. Schmid, A.B.; Dyer, L.; Böni, T.; Held, U.; Brunner, F. Paraspinal muscle activity during symmetrical and asymmetrical weight training in idiopathic scoliosis. *J. Sport Rehabil.* **2010**, *19*, 315–327. [CrossRef]
10. Gailey, R.; Allen, K.; Castles, J.; Kucharik, J.; Roeder, M. Review of secondary physical conditions associated with lower-limb amputation and long-term prosthesis use. *J. Rehabil. Res. Dev.* **2008**, *45*. [CrossRef]
11. Burke, M.; Roman, V.; Wright, V. Bone and joint changes in lower limb amputees. *Ann. Rheum. Dis.* **1978**, *37*, 252–254. [CrossRef] [PubMed]
12. Butowicz, C.M.; Acasio, J.C.; Dearth, C.L.; Hendershot, B.D. Trunk muscle activation patterns during walking among persons with lower limb loss: Influences of walking speed. *J. Electromyogr. Kinesiol.* **2018**, *40*, 48–55. [CrossRef]

13. Shojaei, I.; Hendershot, B.D.; Wolf, E.J.; Bazrgari, B. Persons with unilateral transfemoral amputation experience larger spinal loads during level-ground walking compared to able-bodied individuals. *Clin. Biomech.* **2016**, *32*, 157–163. [CrossRef] [PubMed]
14. Lamoth, C.J.; Meijer, O.G.; Daffertshofer, A.; Wuisman, P.I.; Beek, P.J. Effects of chronic low back pain on trunk coordination and back muscle activity during walking: Changes in motor control. *Eur. Spine J.* **2006**, *15*, 23–40. [CrossRef]
15. Vogt, L.; Pfeifer, K.; Banzer, W. Neuromuscular control of walking with chronic low-back pain. *Man. Ther.* **2003**, *8*, 21–28. [CrossRef]
16. Winter, D.; Yack, H. EMG profiles during normal human walking: Stride-to-stride and inter-subject variability. *Electroencephalogr. Clin. Neurophysiol.* **1987**, *67*, 402–411. [CrossRef]
17. van der Hulst, M.; Vollenbroek-Hutten, M.M.; Rietman, J.S.; Schaake, L.; Groothuis-Oudshoorn, K.G.; Hermens, H.J. Back muscle activation patterns in chronic low back pain during walking: A "guarding" hypothesis. *Clin. J. Pain* **2010**, *26*, 30–37. [CrossRef]
18. Nair, K.; Masi, A.T.; Andonian, B.J.; Barry, A.J.; Coates, B.A.; Dougherty, J.; Schaefer, E.; Henderson, J.; Kelly, J. Stiffness of resting lumbar myofascia in healthy young subjects quantified using a handheld myotonometer and concurrently with surface electromyography monitoring. *J. Bodyw. Mov. Ther.* **2016**, *20*, 388–396. [CrossRef] [PubMed]
19. Campbell, K.; Lakie, M. A cross-bridge mechanism can explain the thixotropic short-range elastic component of relaxed frog skeletal muscle. *J. Physiol.* **1998**, *510*, 941–962. [CrossRef]
20. Lakie, M.; Robson, L.G. Thixotropic Changes in Human Muscle Stiffness and The Effects of Fatigue. *Q. J. Exp. Physiol.* **1988**, *73*, 487–500. [CrossRef]
21. Koppenhaver, S.; Gaffney, E.; Oates, A.; Eberle, L.; Young, B.; Hebert, J.; Proulx, L.; Shinohara, M. Lumbar muscle stiffness is different in individuals with low back pain than asymptomatic controls and is associated with pain and disability, but not common physical examination findings. *Musculoskelet. Sci. Pract.* **2020**, *45*, 102078. [CrossRef]
22. Benjamin, M.; Toumi, H.; Ralphs, J.; Bydder, G.; Best, T.; Milz, S. Where tendons and ligaments meet bone: Attachment sites ('entheses') in relation to exercise and/or mechanical load. *J. Anat.* **2006**, *208*, 471–490. [CrossRef]
23. Andonian, B.J.; Masi, A.T.; Aldag, J.C.; Barry, A.J.; Coates, B.A.; Emrich, K.; Henderson, J.; Kelly, J.; Nair, K. Greater resting lumbar extensor myofascial stiffness in younger ankylosing spondylitis patients than age-comparable healthy volunteers quantified by myotonometry. *Arch. Phys. Med. Rehabil.* **2015**, *96*, 2041–2047. [CrossRef] [PubMed]
24. Hu, X.; Lei, D.; Li, L.; Leng, Y.; Yu, Q.; Wei, X.; Lo, W.L.A. Quantifying paraspinal muscle tone and stiffness in young adults with chronic low back pain: A reliability study. *Sci. Rep.* **2018**, *8*, 1–10. [CrossRef]
25. White, A.; Abbott, H.; Masi, A.T.; Henderson, J.; Nair, K. Biomechanical properties of low back myofascial tissue in younger adult ankylosing spondylitis patients and matched healthy control subjects. *Clin. Biomech.* **2018**, *57*, 67–73. [CrossRef]
26. Marusiak, J.; Jaskólska, A.; Koszewicz, M.; Budrewicz, S.; Jaskólski, A. Myometry revealed medication-induced decrease in resting skeletal muscle stiffness in Parkinson's disease patients. *Clin. Biomech.* **2012**, *27*, 632–635. [CrossRef]
27. Chuang, L.-l.; Wu, C.-y.; Lin, K.-c.; Lur, S.-y. Quantitative mechanical properties of the relaxed biceps and triceps brachii muscles in patients with subacute stroke: A reliability study of the myoton-3 myometer. *Stroke Res. Treat.* **2012**, *2012*, 617694. [CrossRef] [PubMed]
28. Bizzini, M.; Mannion, A.F. Reliability of a new, hand-held device for assessing skeletal muscle stiffness. *Clin. Biomech.* **2003**, *18*, 459–461. [CrossRef]
29. Nourbakhsh, M.R.; Arab, A.M. Relationship between mechanical factors and incidence of low back pain. *J. Orthop. Sports Phys. Ther.* **2002**, *32*, 447–460. [CrossRef] [PubMed]
30. Merskey, H.E. Classification of chronic pain: Descriptions of chronic pain syndromes and definitions of pain terms. *Pain* **1986**, *3*, 226.
31. Sakai, F.; Ebihara, S.; Akiyama, M.; Horikawa, M. Pericranial muscle hardness in tension-type headache: A non-invasive measurement method and its clinical application. *Brain* **1995**, *118*, 523–531. [CrossRef]
32. Myoton. *Hand Helding Myoton Pro User Manual*; Myoton Ltd.: Tallinn, Estonia, 2013.
33. Bruno, A.G.; Burkhart, K.; Allaire, B.; Anderson, D.E.; Bouxsein, M.L. Spinal loading patterns from biomechanical modeling explain the high incidence of vertebral fractures in the thoracolumbar region. *J. Bone Miner. Res.* **2017**, *32*, 1282–1290. [CrossRef] [PubMed]
34. Lee, H.S.; Shim, J.S.; Lee, S.T.; Kim, M.; Ryu, J.S. Facilitating effects of fast and slope walking on paraspinal muscles. *Ann. Rehabil. Med.* **2014**, *38*, 514. [CrossRef] [PubMed]
35. Lo, W.L.A.; Yu, Q.; Mao, Y.; Li, W.; Hu, C.; Li, L. Lumbar muscles biomechanical characteristics in young people with chronic spinal pain. *BMC Musculoskelet. Disord.* **2019**, *20*, 1–9. [CrossRef] [PubMed]
36. Jubany, J.; Danneels, L.; Angulo-Barroso, R. The influence of fatigue and chronic low back pain on muscle recruitment patterns following an unexpected external perturbation. *BMC Musculoskelet. Disord.* **2017**, *18*, 161. [CrossRef]
37. Alsancak, S.; Sener, G.; Erdemli, B.; Ogun, T. Three dimensional measurements of pelvic tilt in trans-tibial amputations: The effects of pelvic tilt on trunk muscles strength and characteristics of gait. *Prosthet. Orthot. Int.* **1998**, *22*, 17–24. [CrossRef]
38. Anderson, F.C.; Pandy, M.G. Individual muscle contributions to support in normal walking. *Gait Posture* **2003**, *17*, 159–169. [CrossRef]
39. Ceccato, J.-C.; De Sèze, M.; Azevedo, C.; Cazalets, J.-R. Comparison of trunk activity during gait initiation and walking in humans. *PLoS ONE* **2009**, *4*, e8193. [CrossRef]

40. Kim, D.H.; Jung, Y.J.; Song, Y.E.; Hwang, D.H.; Ko, C.-Y.; Kim, H.S. 1C5-1 Measurement of Characteristic Change using MyotonPRO in Low Back Muscles during a Long-term Driving; Pilot Study. *Jpn. J. Ergon.* **2015**, *51*, S450–S453. [CrossRef]
41. Kim, C.; Kim, M. Mechanical properties and physical fitness of trunk muscles using Myoton. *Korean J. Phys. Educ.* **2016**, *55*, 633–642.
42. Crawford, R.; Gizzi, L.; Dieterich, A.; Ni Mhuiris, Á.; Falla, D. Age-related changes in trunk muscle activity and spinal and lower limb kinematics during gait. *PLoS ONE* **2018**, *13*, e0206514. [CrossRef] [PubMed]
43. Smith, H.E.; Anderson, D.G.; Vaccaro, A.R.; Albert, T.J.; Hilibrand, A.S.; Harrop, J.S.; Ratliff, J.K. Anatomy, biomechanics, and classification of thoracolumbar injuries. In *Seminars in Spine Surgery*; WB Saunders: Philadelphia, PA, USA, 2010; Volume 22, pp. 2–7. [CrossRef]
44. Hagg, G. Static work loads and occupational myalgia-a new explanation model. *Electromyogr. Kinesiol.* **1991**, *949*, 141–144.

Article

Analysis of Age-Based Bone Mineral Density in the Korean Adult Population Using Dual-Energy X-ray Absorptiometry

Jung Chul Lee [1], Chong Hoon Lee [2], Dong Wha Chung [3], Hee Joo Lee [4] and Jae Yong Park [5],*

1. Department of Exercise prescription, Dongshin University, 67, Dongshindae-gil, Naju-si, Jeollanma-do 58245, Korea; channel365@dsu.ac.kr
2. Department of Sports Sciences, Seoul National University of Science and Technology, 232 Gongneung-ro, Nowon-gu, Seoul 01811, Korea; leejh36@seoultech.ac.kr
3. Department of Sports industry, Sangmyung University, 31, Sangmyungdae-Gil, Choenan-si, Chungcheongnam-do 31066, Korea; mainz990@smu.ac.kr
4. Department of Nursing Science, Sang-Myung University, Sangmyeongdae-gil, Dongnam-gu, Cheonan-si, Chungcheongnam-do 31066, Korea; foremost@smu.ac.kr
5. Institute of Sports Health Science, Sunmoon University, 70, Sunmoon-ro 221 beon-gil, Tangjeong-myeon, Asan-si, Chungcheongnam-do 31460, Korea
* Correspondence: 2006076@sunmoon.ac.kr; Tel.: +82-10-9056-1953

Received: 8 October 2020; Accepted: 22 November 2020; Published: 27 November 2020

Abstract: Dual-energy X-ray absorptiometry (DEXA) provides a reliable and accurate measurement of bone density and bone mineral composition. This research examined the composition and bone density (bone mineral composition and bone mineral density; BMD) of the whole body and selected body parts using DEXA. The participants were 240 healthy adult men and women who were divided into three groups based on age. The total BMD of women amounted to an average of 1.14 g/cm^2 for those aged 20–39 years, 1.14 g/cm^2 for those aged 40–59 years, and 0.98 g/cm^2 for those aged 60–73 years. For men, the average BMD was 1.25 g/cm^2 for those aged 20–39 years, 1.20 g/cm^2 for those aged 40–59 years, and 1.17 g/cm^2 for those aged 60–73 years. The decrease in age-specific BMD was shown to have a correlation with both age and body mass index, and it is determined that exercising on a regular basis can prevent a reduction in BMD by maintaining appropriate muscle mass.

Keywords: dual-energy X-ray absorptiometry; bone mineral density; bone mineral content; osteoporosis; body mass index; aging

1. Introduction

Dual-energy X-ray absorptiometry (DEXA) is the most widely used method to measure bone mineral density (BMD), chiefly because it uses X-rays, which are noninvasive and inexpensive [1–3]. This measurement tool calculates the density of bone mass by measuring the rate differences of radiation transmittance in the analyzed bone mass when the radiation from the tool penetrates the body [4,5]. By using a tube voltage of 80 Kv Cerium filter, DEXA utilizes photon energies of 40 keV and 80 keV [6]. Thus, it can be used to assess bone health conditions in any part of the body. It is widely used to measure and assess the regions of the body and is typically used to assess full-body BMD, such as the lumbar spine and proximal femur [7].

Bones undergo mineralization and remodeling during their life cycle [8,9]. An imbalance in the absorption and generation of osseous tissue generally occurs in both men and women as they age. This process causes mineral synthetic imbalances of different body parts, which leads to reduced average BMD. The rate of mineral synthetic imbalance has been reported to be 26.59% for women and 14.56% for men [10].

A reduction in BMD, which causes diseases such as osteoporosis, is responsible for pain in various body parts and contributes to disabilities associated with old age [11]. More specifically, a decrease in BMD due to aging exponentially amplifies the risks of bone fracture [12], which can lead to disabilities and death and, ultimately, to increased social costs [13]. Moreover, a decline in BMD increases the risk of additional secondary fracture [14]. Mortality due to a reduction in BMD has been reported to be higher in men than in women [15].

Although studies on the process of mineralization and bone reformation have been conducted, there is a paucity of data on therapies, such as hormone therapy, diet therapy, and therapeutic exercise, which have been deemed important for adults with decreased BMD. These interventions not only delay bone loss but also help in the maintenance and development of bones [16]. The importance of maintaining a high BMD is highly emphasized in the medical community.

DEXA is necessary for accurately assessing and identifying bone conditions. According to the International Society for Clinical Densitometry (ISCD), DEXA is recommended as the most appropriate BMD measurement method that can then be applied to the diagnostic criteria of the World Health Organization [17,18]. According to research on osteoporosis and fractures, DEXA measurement can predict and assess the risk of bone fracture. A BMD-estimated T-score of <−2.5 (defined as osteoporosis) has a close correlation with the development of bone fractures [19].

In light of these findings, this paper seeks to provide an important reference for the pathophysiology and treatment of bone diseases, including osteoporosis, by analyzing the BMDs of Koreans based on sex and age.

2. Materials and Methods

2.1. Participants

All 240 participants (120 men, 120 women) were healthy adults living in Seoul, Republic of Korea between 20 and 73 years of age. Prior to participating in the experiment, enrolled participants were informed of the objectives and procedures of the study, and they provided written consent to participate. Patients with diabetes mellitus, cardiovascular disorders, and/or hypertension were excluded. Participants were divided into three groups based on their age. Group A included adults aged 20–39 years, Group B included participants aged 40–59 years, and Group C included older adult participants aged 60–73 years. The physical characteristics of participants are presented in Table 1.

Table 1. Physical characteristics of participants according to age and sex.

Sex	Age (Years)	Height (cm)	Weight (kg)	BMI (kg/m^2)
Male	20–39 ($n = 40$)	174.0 ± 5.70	75.72 ± 13.70	25.77 ± 3.70
	40–59 ($n = 40$)	167.4 ± 4.40	69.87 ± 8.10	24.50 ± 3.07
	60–73 ($n = 40$)	166.4 ± 5.60	68.93 ± 9.40	24.86 ± 3.36
	Total ($n = 120$)	169.77 ± 6.32	71.98 ± 11.40	25.04 ± 3.40
Female	20–39 ($n = 40$)	158.6 ± 4.80	59.08 ± 10.0	23.48 ± 3.84
	40–59 ($n = 40$)	155.1 ± 5.10	58.76 ± 7.50	24.29 ± 2.77
	60–73 ($n = 40$)	152.6 ± 4.50	57.06 ± 6.60	24.29 ± 3.18
	Total ($n = 120$)	155.5 ± 8.18	58.37 ± 5.37	24.02 ± 3.29

Values are mean ± standard deviation; BMI: body mass index, calculated by weight/height^2; (n): number of participants.

2.2. Experimental Procedure

The experimental procedure is shown in Figure 1.

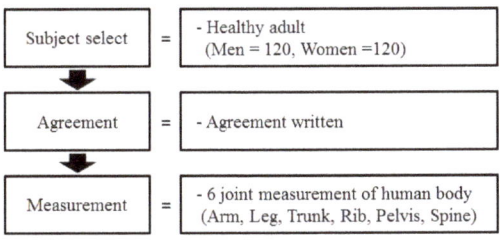

Figure 1. Experimental procedure.

2.3. DEXA Measurement

Participants underwent DEXA measurement in the morning on an empty stomach. DEXA was used to measure BMD and bone mineral content (BMC) of the whole body. During the measurement, participants were lightly dressed and were asked to lie still in a supine position on the scanning table. The presets for the applied DEXA (Lunna Radiation corp., Madison, WI, USA) were photon energy of 66 KeV and 40 KeV by conducting collimation at 1.68 mm intervals. For Scan type, DPX-L (GE-Lunar Corp., Madison, WI, USA) was used, and the software version for acquiring data was 3.1. The BMC and BMD of the left and right arms, legs, torso, and whole body were measured.

2.4. Data Analysis

SAS version 9.2 was used for statistical analysis. Mean and standard deviation for sex, age, height, weight, BMD, and BMC were calculated, and a two-way analysis of variance (ANOVA) was used to determine whether there were differences among the different age groups, and between men and women. Tukey's post-hoc adjustment was carried out for variables found to be statistically significant. The significance level (α) for testing hypotheses in this study was set at 0.05.

3. Results

3.1. Basic Statistics of BMD and BMC Factors Based on Sex and Age

The basic patient demographics of BMD and BMC based on sex and age are presented in Table 2 for men and Table 3 for women.

Table 2. The mean values weight, height, BMD, and BMC in various body segments of male participants.

Age \ Item	Group A: 20–39 Years	Group B: 40–59 Years	Group C: 60–79 Years
Weight (kg)	75.72 ± 13.7	69.87 ± 8.1	68.93 ± 9.4
Height (cm)	174.0 ± 5.7	167.4 ± 4.4	166.4 ± 5.6
BMD (arms)	0.99 ± 0.09	0.97 ± 0.11	0.93 ± 0.11
BMD (legs)	1.36 ± 0.10	1.29 ± 0.13	1.24 ± 0.12
BMD (trunk)	1.01 ± 0.08	0.95 ± 0.09	0.94 ± 0.12
BMD (ribs)	0.77 ± 0.06	0.72 ± 0.06	0.72 ± 0.09
BMD (pelvis)	1.26 ± 0.12	1.18 ± 0.15	1.11 ± 0.17
BMD (spine)	1.20 ± 0.13	1.15 ± 0.14	1.14 ± 0.18
BMD (total)	1.25 ± 0.00	1.20 ± 0.09	1.17 ± 0.11
BMC (arms)	396.5 ± 70.90	371.5 ± 62.33	353.3 ± 58.01
BMC (legs)	1192 ± 200.1	1038 ± 154.8	1004 ± 143.5
BMC (trunk)	990.2 ± 141.8	850.4 ± 149.7	819.6 ± 174.0
BMC (total)	3172 ± 421.2	2842 ± 389.2	2715 ± 372.8

All values are presented as mean ± standard deviation. BMD (g/cm^2): bone mineral density; BMC (g): bone mineral content.

Table 3. The mean values weight, height, BMD, and BMC in various body segments of female participants.

Age / Item	Group A: 20–39 Years	Group B: 40–59 Years	Group C: 60–79 Years
Weight (kg)	59.08 ± 10.0	58.76 ± 7.5	57.06 ± 6.6
Height (cm)	158.6 ± 4.8	155.1 ± 5.1	152. ± 64.5
BMD (arms)	0.81 ± 0.08	0.80 ± 0.15	0.69 ± 0.07
BMD (legs)	1.14 ± 0.10	1.14 ± 0.11	0.97 ± 0.10
BMD (trunk)	0.91 ± 0.09	0.90 ± 0.10	0.78 ± 0.08
BMD (ribs)	0.68 ± 0.06	0.68 ± 0.07	0.60 ± 0.05
BMD (pelvis)	1.11 ± 0.13	1.09 ± 0.13	0.92 ± 0.10
BMD (spine)	1.13 ± 0.15	1.12 ± 0.16	0.92 ± 0.13
BMD (total)	1.14 ± 0.08	1.14 ± 0.09	0.98 ± 0.08
BMC (arms)	222.6 ± 57.53	228.5 ± 52.11	190.1 ± 34.79
BMC (legs)	785.3 ± 158.6	772.5 ± 146.8	649.7 ± 96.81
BMC (trunk)	694.5 ± 176.0	694.3 ± 160.4	525.6 ± 114.7
BMC (total)	2261 ± 433.5	2266 ± 402.8	1830 ± 271.5

All values are presented as mean ± standard deviation. BMD (g/cm^2): bone mineral density; BMC (g): bone mineral content.

3.2. Differences in BMD Based on Sex and Age

The results of the two-way ANOVA for BMD of each sex according to age are presented in Table 4. In addition, the results of the post-hoc test are presented in Tables 5 and 6.

Table 4. The results of the two-way ANOVA for whole-body BMD of males and females according to age.

Source	DF	SS	MS	F Value	Pr > F
Model	5	1.61163354	0.32232671	40.09	0.0001
Error	234	1.88121320	0.00803937		
Sex	1	0.83994322	0.83994322	104.48	0.0001
Age	2	0.57732961	0.28866481	35.91	0.0001
Sex * Age	2	0.15328471	0.07664236	9.53	0.0001
Corrected Total	239	3.49284673			

Table 5. Tukey post-hoc test in male participants according to age.

Source	DF	SS	MS	F	Pr > F	Post-Hoc
Model	2	0.11420968	0.05710484	6.57	0.0020	
Error	111	0.96530018	0.00869640			
Age	2	0.11420968	0.05710484	6.57	0.0020	a b c
Corrected Total	113	1.07950986				

a = Group A (20–39 years); b = Group B (40–59 years); c = Group C (60–73 years).

Table 6. Tukey post-hoc analysis in female participants according to age.

Source	DF	SS	MS	F	Pr > F	Post-Hoc
Model	2	0.66760870	0.33380435	44.83	0.0001	
Error	123	0.91591302	0.00744645			
Age	2	0.66760870	0.33380435	44.83	0.0001	a b c
Corrected Total	125	1.58352171				

a = Group A (20–39 years); b = Group B (40–59 years); c = Group C (60–73 years).

According to a two-way ANOVA based on sex and age, there was a significant main effect of participant sex on whole-body BMD (F(1,234) = 104.48 ($p < 0.01$)). There was also a significant main effect of age on whole-body BMD (F(2,234) = 35.91 ($p < 0.01$)), and a significant interaction of sex by age (F(2,234) = 9.53 ($p < 0.01$)). Post-hoc analyses revealed a significant difference between the whole-body BMD of males and females, and certain distinctions were found between Groups A, B, and C.

A one-way ANOVA based on age showed a significant difference in whole-body BMD between the age groups among male participants (F(2,111) = 6.57 ($p < 0.01$)). There was a significant difference between Group A and Group C in the Tukey post-hoc.

The one-way ANOVA based on age showed a significant difference in whole-body BMD between the age groups among female participants (F(2,123) = 44.38 ($p < 0.001$)). There was a statistically significant difference between Groups A and B compared to Group C.

These results demonstrate that the decline in whole-body BMD with age is closely related to loss of muscle mass and a decrease in BMC.

3.3. Differences in BMC Based on Sex and Age

The results of the two-way ANOVA for the BMC of each sex according to age are presented in Table 7. In addition, the results of the posteriori test are presented in Tables 8 and 9.

Table 7. The results of the two-way ANOVA for whole-body BMC of males and females according to age.

Source	DF	SS	MS	F Value	Pr > F
Model	5	47,913,917.88	9,582,783.58	63.20	0.0001
Error	234	35,479,495.92	151,621.78		
Gender	1	36,614,251.09	36,614,251.09	241.48	0.0001
Age	2	7,409,161.57	3,704,580.78	24.43	0.0001
Gender * Age	2	1,479,315.02	739,657.51	4.88	0.0084
Corrected Total	239	83,393,413.80			

Table 8. Tukey post-hoc in male participants according to age.

Source	DF	SS	MS	F	Pr > F	Post-Hoc
Model	2	4,445,694.39	2,222,847.20	14.00	<0.0001	
Error	111	17,621,312.60	158,750.56			
Age	2	4,445,694.393	2,222,847.19	14.00	<0.0001	a b c
Corrected Total	113	22,067,006.99				

a = Group A (20–39 years); b = Group B (40–59 years); c = Group C (60–73 years).

Table 9. Tukey post-hoc in female participants according to age.

Source	DF	SS	MS	F	Pr > F	Post-Hoc
Model	2	4,836,043.54	2,418,021.77	16.65	0.0001	
Error	123	17,858,183.32	145,188.48			
Age	2	4,836,043.54	2,418,021.77	16.65	0.0001	a b c
Corrected Total	125	22,694,226.86				

a = Group A (20–39 years); b = Group B (40–59 years); c = Group C (60–73 years).

The two-way ANOVA based on sex and age showed a significant main effect of participant sex on whole body BMC (F(1,234) = 241.48 ($p < 0.01$)). There was also a significant main effect of age (F(2,234) = 24.43 ($p < 0.01$)) and a significant interaction of sex by age (F(2,234) = 4.88 ($p < 0.01$)).

The Tukey post-hoc tests demonstrated a significant difference in whole-body BMC between male and female participants, and differences based on age were found in each group. A one-way ANOVA based on age demonstrated a significant difference in whole-body BMC among male participants (F(2,111) = 14.00 ($p < 0.01$)). There was a statistically significant difference in whole-body BMC between Groups B and C compared to Group A in the Tukey post-hoc.

A one-way ANOVA based on age showed a significant difference in whole-body BMC based on age among female participants (F(2,123) = 16.65 ($p < 0.01$)). A Tukey post-hoc test demonstrated a statistically significant difference between Groups A and B compared to Group C.

Based on these results, the most influential factors for BMD were revealed to be sex and age. With age in particular, there was a decrease in BMD and BMC along with a decrease in height and weight. In addition, of the females, postmenopausal participants showed a significant decrease in BMC and BMD in the group over 60 years old. Therefore, it can be considered that changes in body composition due to aging drastically reduces whole-body BMD and BMC.

4. Discussion

The bones function to mechanically support the body and protect deep organs. They become the center of exercise and serve as a reservoir of various minerals. Bones continuously develop throughout the growth period, until the age of 30 to 40 years when the structural growth of the bone is completed. Therefore, BMD continues to increase throughout growth, resulting in peak bone mass and solidification at the end of structural development. The most common metabolic bone disease, osteoporosis, is a condition of reduced BMD. Osteoporosis is a serious metabolic disease accompanied by qualitative changes in bone microstructure and can lead to fractures of the spine, femur, and radius. Patients suffering from osteoporosis are at risk of bone fractures, even from less forceful impact to the bones [20]. Although osteoporosis is more common in women, previous studies have reported that osteoporotic fractures are also frequent in men [21,22]. Osteoporosis, therefore, should be recognized as a major disease that affects both women and men.

Based on this rationale, this study analyzed the relationship between BMC and age in adults to examine changes in bone density according to sex and age. The purpose of this research was to examine changes in the distribution of bone density in relation to menopause for various future medical purposes and practices related to osteoporosis.

DEXA is the most commonly used clinical tool for the diagnosis of osteoporosis. It is considered safe because it has relatively less radiation exposure and a short inspection time. In addition, it can directly measure total bone mass and has a rate of high diagnostic accuracy, sensitivity, and reproducibility.

The indicators of bone health are bone mass, BMC, and BMD, while BMD alone is used as a standard for diagnosing osteoporosis [23,24]. In this study, the mean BMD in male and female participants was inversely correlated with age. These findings were similar to the results of Ohmura's study [25], which effectively demonstrated that the BMDs of Japanese women in their 20s and 70s were inversely proportional to their age. Moreover, the differences in BMC and BMD between age groups demonstrated the total mineral contents of males aged 20–39 years were the highest when compared to older age groups, and females aged 20–59 years had similar results. In addition, BMC was significantly different between age groups among both male and female participants, with BMC decreasing with age.

Park et al. [26] reported age has the highest inverse correlation with BMD. Other factors associated with BMD included race, family history of osteoporosis, estrogen hormone, calcium intake, weight, and physique. In addition, age was reported as a major predictor of BMD and osteoporosis [27]. In this study, male participants aged 20–39 years had the highest total BMC. Male participants aged 40–59 years also had a relatively high BMC in comparison to male participants aged 60–79 years. Female participants aged 20–39 years and 40–59 years demonstrated a similar pattern of relatively high BMC compared to older female participants (aged 60–73 years). These results are similar to those of previous studies [25,27], which showed a correlation between age and weight as factors that influence bone density. Our results are also consistent with the findings of Ohmura et al. [25], which showed that Japanese women have low BMDs, and the difference is several times greater for women after menopause.

Decreases in BMD and in BMC with increasing age are thought to be due to a decrease in lean mass, and increased bone resorption of osteoclasts caused by the lack of estrogen secretion from the ovaries after menopause. In addition, as noted by Tremollieres and Ribot [27], race, family history of osteoporosis, calcium intake, weight, and physique may affect BMD and BMC.

Our study was inconsistent with previous studies [28,29], which demonstrated a slight increase in BMC after the age of 30 years and a rapid decrease after the age of 50 years, both before and after menopause. Ohmura et al. [25] also mentioned that premenopausal Japanese women had 5% lower BMD than premenopausal Caucasian women in America or Europe, and this difference multiplied after menopause. Unlike women, osteoporosis in men can be classified as primary (with uncertain pathogenic determinants) and secondary (with clear underlying cause). Men more often suffer from secondary osteoporosis caused by low body mass index, smoking, excessive alcohol consumption, and lack of exercise.

In bone growth and maintenance, calcium is an essential nutrient that is necessary to lower the bone replacement rate and reduce bone resorption [30]. Reduced calcium absorption rates in the bone can lead to reduced bone density and bone mineral quantity in both men and woman as they age. In addition to reduced secretion of phosphorous- and calcium-regulating hormones, changes in bone metabolism, decreased physical activity, and inadequate diet can reduce BMD and BCD in both men and women. For older women after menopause, the reason behind the reduction in BMD and BMC in this study is considered to be reduced estrogen, which increases osteoclastic bone resorption. This was demonstrated in the female participants of our study, as there was a significant difference in BMD and BMC between those under the age of 60 years and those over the age of 60 years. We confirmed that there was no difference in BMC and BMC according to age before menopause, and - there was a change corresponding to the time when estrogen deficiency became apparent, as menopause typically occurs before the age of 60 years old. In contrast, low body mass index, smoking, excess alcohol intake, and a lack of exercise are thought to cause BMD reduction in tandem with the influences of hormones in men [31]. In our study, however, there was a significant difference in BMD and BMC between younger male participants (20–39 years) and older male participants (60–79 years) and not between middle aged male participants and either of the two other groups. It is thought that hormone changes are relatively small in the males of the same age group as females. It seems, therefore, that some factors affecting BMD and BMC for women and men are different.

This study indicates that the BMD of adult Korean women is remarkably lower than that of Caucasian women, and BMD reduction accelerates after menopause. This phenomenon is considered to have a close relationship with reduction in muscle mass, especially that of legs. Therefore, we suggest that exercising on a regular basis is critical to maintain muscle mass and BMD before menopause. Specific exercise-related education and nutrition guides are required according to sex and age. Finally, we hope that the findings of this study will be helpful to predict the risk of osteoporosis in the future by evaluating the bone density of Koreans according to age group. We believe that this study can help medical practitioners make appropriate decisions to help patients cope with reductions in the ability to exercise caused by aging and reductions in BMD due to changes in dietary habits. We hope this study also encourages the creation of detailed health education guides.

This study should be interpreted considering the limitation that results cannot be extrapolated to people living in different environments.

5. Conclusions

In order to prevent osteoporosis in middle aged adults, it is necessary to routinely measure BMD and BMC using accurate equipment such as DEXA. Sufficient protein, calcium, and vitamin D intake as well as resistive exercises can prevent older adults from becoming underweight and prevent reductions in BMD and BMC. Moreover, for women near or approaching menopause, proper dietary controls and continuous exercise can protect against drastic declines in body fat, muscle mass, and BMD. This study has identified age- and sex-specific differences in BMD and BMC in city-dwelling Koreans. Further studies, however, are required for extrapolation of these findings to a larger population. Comparative studies for adults with different living conditions, such as residents in large cities and rural areas, and studies that compare and analyze the correlation between factors related to BMD and BMC are suggested.

Author Contributions: Conceptualization, J.C.L., C.H.L. and J.Y.P.; methodology, D.W.C., H.J.L. and J.Y.P.; software, J.C.L.; formal analysis, J.Y.P. and H.J.L.; investigation, J.C.L. and J.Y.P.; resources, J.C.L.; data curation, C.H.L., J.C.L.; writing—original draft preparation, D.W.L., J.Y.P.; writing—review and editing, J.C.L., H.J.L. and J.Y.P.; visualization, C.H.L. and J.Y.P.; supervision, J.C.L. and J.Y.P.; project administration, C.H.L., and D.W.C. All authors have read and agreed to the published version of the manuscript.

Funding: This research received no external funding.

Conflicts of Interest: The authors declare no conflict of interest.

References

1. Zhong, R.; Chen, Q.; Zhang, X.; Li, M.; Liang, J.; Lin, W. Bone Mineral Density Loss in People With Epilepsy Taking Valproate as a Monotherapy: A Systematic Review and Meta-Analysis. *Front. Neurol.* **2019**, *10*, 1171. [CrossRef] [PubMed]
2. Batur, P.; Rice, S.; Barrios, P.; Sikon, A. Osteoporosis Management. *J. Women Health* **2017**, *26*, 918–921. [CrossRef] [PubMed]
3. Gilsanz, V. Bone density in children: A review of the available techniques and indications. *Eur. J. Radiol.* **1998**, *26*, 177–182. [CrossRef]
4. Blake, G.M.; Fogelman, I. Bone densitometry and the diagnosis of osteoporosis. *Semin. Nucl. Med.* **2001**, *31*, 69–81. [CrossRef]
5. Jain, R.K.; Vokes, T. Dual-energy X-ray Absorptiometry. *J. Clin. Densitom.* **2017**, *20*, 291–303. [CrossRef]
6. Lorente Ramos, R.M.; Azpeitia Armán, J.; Arévalo Galeano, N.; Muñoz Hernández, A.; García Gómez, J.M.; Gredilla Molinero, J. Dual energy X-ray absorptimetry: Fundamentals, methodology, and clinical applications. *Radiologia* **2012**, *54*, 410–423. [CrossRef]
7. Lane, N.E. Epidemiology, etiology, and diagnosis of osteoporosis. *Am. J. Obstet. Gynecol.* **2006**, *194*, S3–S11. [CrossRef]
8. Glimcher, M.J. Mechanism of calcification: Role of collagen fibrils and collagen-phosphoprotein complexes in vitro and in vivo. *Anat. Rec.* **1989**, *224*, 139–153. [CrossRef]
9. Katsimbri, P. The biology of normal bone remodeling. *Eur. J. Cancer Care* **2017**, *26*. [CrossRef]
10. Looker, A.C.; Orwoll, E.S.; Johnston, C.C., Jr.; Lindsay, R.L.; Wahner, H.W.; Dunn, W.L.; Calvo, M.S.; Harris, T.B.; Heyse, S.P. Prevalence of low femoral bone density in older U.S. adults from NHANES III. *J. Bone Miner. Res.* **1997**, *12*, 1761–1768. [CrossRef]
11. Kim, H.S.; Jeong, E.S.; Yang, M.H.; Yang, S.O. Bone Mineral Density Assessment for Research Purpose Using Dual Energy X-ray Absorptiometry. *Osteoporos. Sarcopenia* **2018**, *4*, 79–85. [CrossRef] [PubMed]
12. Watts, N.B.; Manson, J.E. Osteoporosis and Fracture Risk Evaluation and Management: Shared Decision Making in Clinical Practice. *JAMA* **2017**, *317*, 253–254. [CrossRef] [PubMed]
13. Clarke, B.L.; Ebeling, P.R.; Jones, J.D.; Wahner, H.W.; O'Fallon, W.M.; Riggs, B.L.; Fitzpatrick, L.A. Predictors of Bone Mineral Density in Aging Healthy Men Varies by Skeletal Site. *Curr. Radiol. Rep.* **2002**, *70*, 137–145. [CrossRef] [PubMed]
14. Bliuc, D.; Alarkawi, D.; Nguyen, T.V.; Eisman, J.A.; Center, J.R. Risk of Subsequent Fractures and Mortality in Elderly Women and Men With Fragility Fractures With and Without Osteoporotic Bone Density: The Dubbo Osteoporosis Epidemiology Study. *J. Bone Miner. Res.* **2015**, *30*, 637–646. [CrossRef] [PubMed]
15. Van Der Klift, M.; Pols, H.A.; Geleijnse, J.M.; Van Der Kuip, D.A.; Hofman, A.; De Laet, C.E. Bone mineral density and mortality in elderly men and women: The Rotterdam Study. *Bone* **2002**, *30*, 643–648. [CrossRef]
16. Hong, A.R.; Kim, S.W. Effects of Resistance Exercise on Bone Health. *Endocrinol. Metab.* **2018**, *4*, 435–444. [CrossRef]
17. Kanis, J.A.; Glüer, C.C. An update on the diagnosis and assessment of osteoporosis with densitometry. Committee of Scientific Advisors, International Osteoporosis Foundation. *Osteoporos. Int.* **2000**, *11*, 192–202. [CrossRef]
18. Kanis, J.A. Assessment of Fracture Risk and Its Application to Screening for Postmenopausal Osteoporosis: Synopsis of a WHO Report. WHO Study Group. *Osteoporos. Int.* **1994**, *4*, 368–381. [CrossRef]

19. Stone, K.L.; Seeley, D.G.; Lui, L.Y.; Cauley, J.A.; Ensrud, K.; Browner, W.S.; Nevitt, M.C.; Cummings, S.R. BMD at multiple sites and risk of fracture of multiple types: Long-term results from the Study of Osteoporotic Fractures. *J. Bone Miner. Res.* **2003**, *18*, 1947–1954. [CrossRef]
20. Ross, A.C.; Manson, J.E.; Abrams, S.A.; Aloia, J.F.; Brannon, P.M.; Clinton, S.K.; Durazo-Arvizu, R.A.; Gallagher, J.C.; Gallo, R.L.; Jones, G.; et al. The 2011 report on dietary reference intakes for calcium and vitamin D from the Institute of Medicine: What clinicians need to know. *J. Clin. Endocrinol. Metab.* **2011**, *96*, 53–58. [CrossRef]
21. Schuitt, S.C.; Van der Klift, M.; Weel, A.E.; Laet, C.E.; Burger, H.; Seeman, E.; Hofman, A.; Itterlinden, A.G.; Van Leeuwen, J.P.; Pols, H.A. Fracture incidence and association with bone mineral density in elderly men and women: The Rotterdam Study. *Bone* **2004**, *34*, 195–202. [CrossRef] [PubMed]
22. Dhanwal, D.K.; Cooper, C.; Dennison, E.M. Geographic variation in osteoporotic hip fracture incidence: The growing importance of Asian influences in coming decades. *J. Osteoporos.* **2010**, *2*, 757102. [CrossRef] [PubMed]
23. Michaëlsson, K.; Wolk, A.; Langenskiöld, S.; Basu, S.; Warensjö Lemming, E.; Melhus, H.; Byberg, L. Milk intake and risk of mortality and fractures in women and men: Cohort studies. *BMJ* **2014**, *349*, 6015. [CrossRef] [PubMed]
24. Warriner, A.H.; Saag, K.G. Osteoporosis diagnosis and medical treatment. *Orthop. Clin. N. Am.* **2013**, *44*, 125–135. [CrossRef] [PubMed]
25. Ohmura, A.; Kushida, K.; Yamazaki, K.; Okamoto, S.; Katsuno, H.; Inoue, T. Bone density and body composition in Japanese women. *Calcif. Tissue Int.* **1997**, *61*, 117–122. [CrossRef] [PubMed]
26. Park, K.K.; Kim, S.J.; Moon, E.S. Association between bone mineral density and metabolic syndrome in postmenopausal Korean women. *Gynecol. Obstet. Investig.* **2010**, *69*, 145–152. [CrossRef]
27. Tremollieres, F.; Ribot, C. Bone mineral density and prediction of non-osteoporotic disease. *Maturitas* **2010**, *65*, 348–351. [CrossRef]
28. Kopiczko, A. Bone mineral density in old age: The influence of age at menarche, menopause status and habitual past and present physical activity. *Arch. Med. Sci.* **2020**, *16*, 657–665. [CrossRef]
29. Sanada, K.; Miyachi, M.; Tabata, I.; Miyatani, M.; Tanimoto, M.; Oh, T.W.; Yamamoto, K.; Usui, C.; Takahashi, E.; Kawano, H.; et al. Muscle mass and bone mineral indices: Does the normalized bone mineral content differ with age? *Eur. J. Clin. Nutr.* **2009**, *63*, 465–472. [CrossRef]
30. Son, G.S. Effect of soybean intake on bone mineral density and bone turnover markers in postmenopausal Women. *J. Korean Acad. Nurs.* **2006**, *36*, 933–941. [CrossRef]
31. Adler, R.A. Osteoporosis in Men: A Review. *Bone Res.* **2014**, *2*, 14001. [CrossRef] [PubMed]

Publisher's Note: MDPI stays neutral with regard to jurisdictional claims in published maps and institutional affiliations.

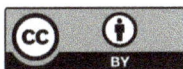

© 2020 by the authors. Licensee MDPI, Basel, Switzerland. This article is an open access article distributed under the terms and conditions of the Creative Commons Attribution (CC BY) license (http://creativecommons.org/licenses/by/4.0/).

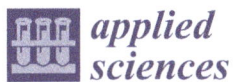

Article

Analysis of Random Dynamics of Cell Segmented by a Modified Active Contour Method

Ji Yeon Hyun [1], Seungeon Ha [1], Jongmin Baek [1], Junghun Han [1], Honggi An [1], Sung-Hun Woo [2], Yoon Suk Kim [2], Sang Woo Lee [1], Sejung Yang [1,*] and Sei Young Lee [1,*]

[1] Department of Biomedical Engineering, Yonsei University, Wonju, Kangwon 26427, Korea; jiyeun212@naver.com (J.Y.H.); tmddjs0307@naver.com (S.H.); jongmin311@naver.com (J.B.); cheque@yonsei.ac.kr (J.H.); kkwa999@yonsei.ac.kr (H.A.); yusuklee@yonsei.ac.kr (S.W.L.)
[2] Department of Biomedical Laboratory Science, Yonsei University, Wonju, Kangwon 26427, Korea; sunghun2120@gmail.com (S.-H.W.); yoonsukkim@yonsei.ac.kr (Y.S.K.)
* Correspondence: syang@yonsei.ac.kr (S.Y.); syl235@yonsei.ac.kr (S.Y.L.); Tel.: +82-33-760-2459 (S.Y.); +82-33-760-2888 (S.Y.L.)

Received: 3 September 2020; Accepted: 24 September 2020; Published: 28 September 2020

Abstract: To understand the dynamics of a living system, the analysis of particular and/or cellular dynamics has been performed based on shape-based center point detection. After collecting sequential time-lapse images of cellular dynamics, the trajectory of a moving object is determined from the set of center points of the cell analyzed from each image. The accuracy of trajectory is significant in understanding the stochastic nature of the dynamics of biological objects. In this study, to localize a cellular object in time-lapse images, three different localization methods, namely radial symmetry, circular Hough transform, and modified active contour, were considered. To analyze the accuracy of cellular dynamics, several statistical parameters such as mean square displacement and velocity autocorrelation function were employed, and localization error derived from these was reported for each localization method. In particular, through denoising using a Poisson noise filter, improved localization characteristics could be achieved. The modified active contour with denoising reduced localization error significantly, and thus allowed for accurate estimation of the statistical parameters of cellular dynamics.

Keywords: random dynamics; mean localization error; mean square displacement; radial symmetric; modified active contour

---

1. Introduction

Recently, it has become an essential theme of biology to understand the dynamics of living systems, such as cell migration [1,2], embryogenesis [3,4], and transport of organelles within a cell [5]. Characterization of living organisms can be performed not only by measuring their biochemical properties, but also by analyzing their dynamic properties including trajectories, velocities, and diffusion coefficients. For example, cellular migration is caused by the dynamics of cytoskeletal proteins such as actin and microfilaments within the cell, which indicate that cellular biochemical properties can be correlated to dynamic properties of the cell [1]. Sometimes, the dynamics of intracellular organelles can be explained by analysis of deformation of a migrating cell [5]. However, since cells do not have ultrasmooth surfaces, and there is no ultrasensitive method to capture cell images, there always exist localization errors when analyzing cellular movement. Therefore, a highly sensitive method must be developed to remove unnecessary signals such as noise through advanced filtering or an advanced device to capture a spatiotemporally high-resolution image [6–8]. The spatiotemporal resolution of a dynamic target object is determined by its photo-physical properties, the signal to noise ratio, and the speeds of the moving objects [9].

Advancement of imaging techniques enables imaging of moving cells and macromolecules. Furthermore, with a live cell imaging system, which provides a controlled environment for cells under a microscope, it is possible to run a long-term experiment with living cells. The long-term recording of cell migration or macromolecules requires processing of a large number of time-lapse images. Tracking algorithms for analyzing such images have two types of errors, determinate (accuracy or bias error) and indeterminate (precision or standard deviation) [9–11]. Determinate errors are responsible for inaccuracies inherently caused by the algorithm, whereas indeterminate errors, which are caused by individual fluctuating random measurements, result from the noise of the image [9,12].

Single-particle tracking algorithms have been developed to localize particles with subpixel displacement [10,11,13]. A microscopic image of a point object appears as a diffraction pattern in that intensity distribution following the point spread function (PSF), which is radially symmetric and shows Gaussian distribution [12,14]. Direct Gaussian fitting of the intensity distribution is a superior algorithm in terms of both accuracy and precision [9]. First, the most common Gaussian fitting method for the measured PSF intensity profile is the nonlinear least squares algorithm [15,16]. The main principle of this algorithm is to search for parameters that minimize weighted squared errors between the fit and the data. Least squares fitting is accurate but is a very costly algorithm [17,18]. Second, while the maximum likelihood method is more accurate [19], Gaussian fitting requires much computational cost due to the large number of iterations and superfluous parameters like amplitude and width of the function necessary to locate the particle center [18,20]. Third, the radial symmetry method localizes the center of the PSF through only one linear matrix calculation. The radial symmetry method has been shown to be as accurate as Gaussian fitting and more rapidly calculable [18].

Alternatively, segmentation of the target image is also applicable to localize the cellular image. Edges of objects that have different intensities from the background can be detected using this method. Many different thresholding algorithms have been developed and applied to analyze the shapes of target images from grey scale images [21,22]. The simplest segmentation is intensity thresholding [23,24]. Despite its simplicity, intensity thresholding is difficult to apply to cell images due to poor contrast or the halo effect. Diverse segmentation approaches, such as template matching [25,26], watershed transformations [27,28], and deformable models [29,30], have been developed. However, to detect complex cell boundaries, several specific methods such as the level set method [31,32] and active contour [30] can be employed. Recently, time-lapse living cell data have been analyzed with deformable models considering the evolving contour of a cell from that in the previous frame [31,33].

The dynamics of cells or biological particles suspended in a solution are usually analyzed as a random process [2,31,32]. Based on accurate analysis of particle/cell trajectory, basic random process characteristics can be found using mean square displacement (MSD), which provides information regarding diffusion characteristics. It is well known that normal diffusion shows a linear relationship between MSD and time, and the slope of the linear fit is known as the diffusion coefficient (D). If linearity is disrupted, the process is called abnormal diffusion. When MSD$\propto t^\alpha$ and $\alpha > 1$, the process is called superdiffusion. When MSD$\propto t^\alpha$ and $\alpha > 1$, it is called subdiffusion [34]. The velocity autocorrelation function (VACF) can be employed to distinguish other mechanisms for abnormal diffusion [32,35].

To understand the random dynamic characteristics of particles or cells suspended in a solution, accurate localization of the object in a microscopic image is fundamental and significant. Clinically, it is important to discriminate the cellular type in diagnosis and therapeutics, since the therapeutic strategy and prognosis are strongly dependent on the cellular type [36]. In addition to this, ultimately, we are interested in the application of cellular dynamics to the discrimination of cell condition. For example, metastasis is known to be mediated by the circulating tumor cell (CTC) in the blood of the patient. Thus, it is important to find the specific cell type in the blood sample through simple method such as just observing the cellular dynamics to minimize the cost and time to detect. The method applied in this study could provide the accurate cellular trajectory so that it can be applied to the discrimination of different cellular types through the different cellular random dynamics. Specifically, the image of a cell is different from that of a particle in terms of appearance and intensity profile. Generally, the shape of a cell is more irregular and deformable than those of a particle, and the intensity distribution is noisier. The asymmetric shape and disturbed distribution of intensity might cause significant localization errors, which negatively impact analysis of the random variables estimated based on trajectory. Hence, in this study, we compared three localization methods, namely the radial symmetry algorithm, circular Hough transform method, and modified active contour method with denoising, to determine the most accurate way to localize cellular images. We employed stochastic parameters, such as MSD and VACF, to estimate the accuracy.

2. Materials and Methods

2.1. Cell Culture

MCF-7 cells were cultured in Dulbecco's Modified Eagle Medium (DMEM, Lonza, Switzerland) supplemented with 10% (v/v) fetal bovine serum (FBS; Gibco, USA) and 1% (v/v) penicillin-streptomycin (Invitrogen, USA) and incubated at 37 °C and 5% CO_2. For the Brownian motion experiment, cells were cultured in 6-well plates and, after 24 h, were detached by treatment with 0.25% trypsin EDTA (Gibco) for 5 min. After trypsinization, DMEM with 10% FBS inactivated the trypsin, and the cells were washed with experimental buffer (8.6% [w/w] sucrose, 0.3% [w/w] glucose, and 1.0 mg/mL bovine serum albumin) and re-suspended. Cells were diluted with buffer to 8×10^4/mL to prevent interactions among them.

2.2. Measurement of Particle/Cell Random Motion

Diluted solutions containing 300 μL of particles or cells were dropped onto a sterile glass bottom chamber. On top of the dropped experimental solution, 1 mL of mineral oil was loaded to avoid vibrations from external effects and to prevent the solution from into the surroundings. Before capturing the Brownian motion, the cells suspended in the solution were stabilized for about 10 min, and the temperature was maintained at 22 °C to limit natural convection due to the temperature difference between the solution and the surrounding. The random motions of the cells were imaged at 40× magnification with a frame rate of 25 hz for 43.60 s, using a FASTCAM Mini UX 100 (Photron, Japan).

2.3. Particle/Cell Tracking and Random Dynamics Analysis

By cropping the image of 121 × 121 pixels, a single particle/cell trajectory was obtained for 43.6 s. To localize the center point of the particle/cell, three tracking algorithms were employed: the radial symmetric method [18], the circular Hough transformation method embedded in MATLAB 2017b [37], and the modified active contour method [38]. From the center point information obtained experimentally by the three localization methods, the two-dimensional MSD of the particle/cell was calculated as [34]

$$\langle x^2 \rangle = \frac{1}{N-\tau} \sum_{t=1}^{N-\tau} (x(t+\tau) - x(t))^2 = 4D\tau \quad \tau = 1, \cdots, N-1 \quad (1)$$

where r is the position vector of the cell at the ith time step, D is the diffusion coefficient, τ is the time lag, which is the time between two position vectors, from 1 to $N-1$, and N is the total number of time steps. The experimentally measured trajectory possessed intrinsic noise, possibly originating from image noise. The measured position $\widetilde{x}(t)$ can be modelled as follows:

$$\widetilde{x}(t) = x(t) + \varepsilon(t) \quad (2)$$

where $x(t)$ is the actual position, and $\varepsilon(t)$ is the localization error caused by the noise, with $\langle \varepsilon(t) \rangle = 0$ and $\langle \varepsilon^2(t) \rangle = \sigma^2$. When Equation (2) is squared and ensemble-averaged,

$$\langle \tilde{x}^2(t) \rangle = \langle x^2(t) \rangle + \sigma^2. \tag{3}$$

The experimentally determined MSD was fitted with Equation (3) using Origin Lab 9.0, and the localization errors were estimated for different particles/cells and different image localization methods, such as the radial symmetric method [18], circular Hough transform [36], and modified active contour.

The VACF, which represents the correlation of velocity vectors within one trajectory, was calculated for the velocity vectors obtained from the tracking methods as follows:

$$C_\delta(\tau) = \langle \vec{v}(t+\tau) \cdot \vec{v}(t) \rangle \tag{4}$$

where $\bar{v} = \frac{1}{\delta}(x(t+\delta) - x(t))$ is the cellular velocity, τ is the time between velocity vectors, and δ is the time between successive frames in the time-lapse images. Thus, multiple VACFs can be calculated according to δ value for a single-cell trajectory experiment.

2.4. Modified Active Contour

The active contour model is a method of detecting boundaries by expressing the properties of an image using the spline as an energy function with various forces governing the image and minimizing the energy function. As the function is minimized, it approaches the boundary line; thus, this method is widely used for detecting a boundary line of an image.

The energy of the active contour can be divided into internal energy, image energy, and external energy. The internal energy is that representing the characteristics related to the shape of the active contour and its fit to a smooth and gentle curve. Image energy is that of the image itself has and is the most important influence on internal movement of the active contour. Finally, external energy is related to external constraints, which allow the user to make subjective judgments and provides power to change the situation to move the active contour in the expected direction. The total energy of the active snake model is given by Equation (5) [30].

$$\begin{aligned} E_T &= \int_0^1 E_{int}(v(s)) + E_{image}(v(s)) + E_{con}(v(s)) ds, \\ v(s) &= (x(s), y(s)), \end{aligned} \tag{5}$$

where x and y are the coordinates of the two-dimensional curve, v is the spline parameter in the range 0~1, and s is a linear parameter $\in [0, 1]$.

During cell tracking, the parameters of the model obtained through analysis in the previous frame were used as the initial values for analysis of the current frame. Therefore, the setting of the initial mask has a crucial influence on boundary detection, and if an error occurs due to a change in a minor value, it is difficult to detect the desired boundary due to the large influence on the resultant image even if the error is small.

We present two methods to overcome the problems of the existing active contour model. The first is to automate the initial values of the active contour model. When the edge detection method is performed, the region where the change in brightness is large represents the boundary of the object, and the region where the brightness is not significant is the boundary surface. Therefore, if we detect only a region with large difference in brightness change value, the boundaries of the objects in the image can be extracted. The Sobel operation is one of the edge detection algorithms and uses a 3×3 size matrix [39]. In this method, the center of the matrix is set as a reference, and the center value of the image is compared to detect the change amount. The grayscale image is extracted by a 3×3 mask, and the result is computed horizontally and vertically to obtain the sum of the absolute values of the axes, finally recognizing the edges. Second, to improve the performance of boundary detection of the active contour, we adopt a method that ignores the difference in distance from the center of mass of the previous frame in the case of incorrect detection. Since the interval between frames is very short, there is no significant difference in the results of cell image tracking, even when ignoring the image in which the boundary detection is not performed.

3. Results & Discussion

3.1. Difference of Trajectory between cPMS Particles and MCF-7 Cells

Accurate measurement of the reference location of the targeted image is one of the most significant factors when analyzing random dynamics of nano/micro-sized objects. When the object is spherical and non-transparent, there are many traditional methods to find the center or reference point of the object. Unfortunately, our interest is not limited to a spherical hard sphere but is extended to cells or even proteins, which could have diverse irregular shapes and translucent features. Figure 1a,b illustrates representative two-dimensional intensity profiles of carboxylated polystyrene microspheres (cPMS, nominal dimeter 16.1 µm) and the MCF-7 breast cancer cell line, respectively. The diameters of cPMS and MCF-7 are estimated as 34.2 pixels and 32.8 pixels, corresponding to 15.39 µm and 14.76 µm, respectively. As shown in Figure 1a, at the center region of the particle, the intensity value reaches 255, which corresponds to the white center region of the particle image in the inset of Figure 1a, and the intensity sharply decreases like a Gaussian point spread function to below 50 as it extends to the edge of the particle. At the edge, a dark circle is formed. At the outside of the edge, a mildly bright circular band is shown, and the background noise around the particle is also observed in Figure 1a. On the other hand, as in Figure 1b, the intensity distribution of MCF-7 is quite different from that of cPMS. An irregular intensity distribution as well as the irregular shape of the cell are observed, even though an edge darker than the background intensity is also shown, like the intensity distribution of the particle edge. However, the intensity value is much higher than those of the cPMS edge, and the uniformity of the intensity along the cellular edge is much more irregular. At the outside of the cellular edge, a bright circular band and the background noise around the particle are also visible.

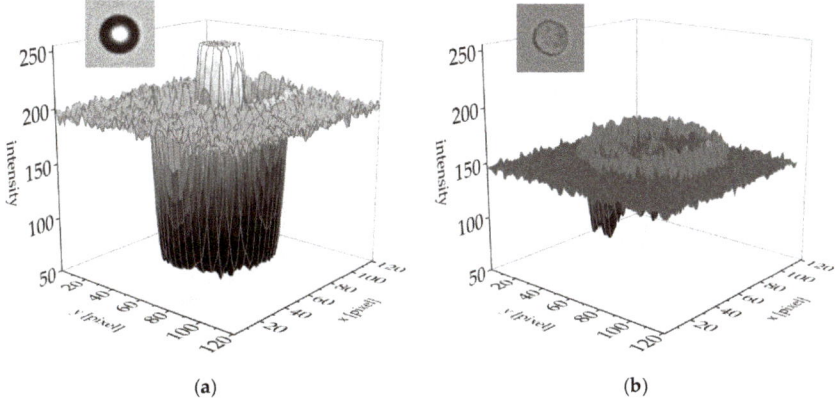

Figure 1. Intensity profiles of 2-dimensional bright field images of (**a**) carboxylated polystyrene microspheres and (**b**) the MCF-7 breast cancer cell line.

To understand the effect of intensity distribution and the uniformity of image, the comparison of random dynamics between cPMS and MCF-7 is performed. When particles or cells are suspended in a solution, they are continuously contacted by surrounding water molecules due to thermal energy. These interactions result in random motion of particles or cells, as shown in Figure 2a,b, which are the trajectories of cPMS and MCF-7, respectively, as analyzed by the radial symmetry localization method [18]. Both trajectories seem to be random, but there are definite differences between them. The MSD of cPMS in the log-log plot in Figure 2c is linear, while that of MCF-7 in Figure 2d shows nonlinear characteristics over a short time scale ($\tau \lesssim 1$ s). Comparing the trajectories of cPMS and MCF-7 shows that overall displacement of the particle is much smaller than that of the MCF-7 cell in the experimentally smallest time scale ($\Delta t = 0.04$ s), and the movement of MCF-7 appears to change its direction sharply.

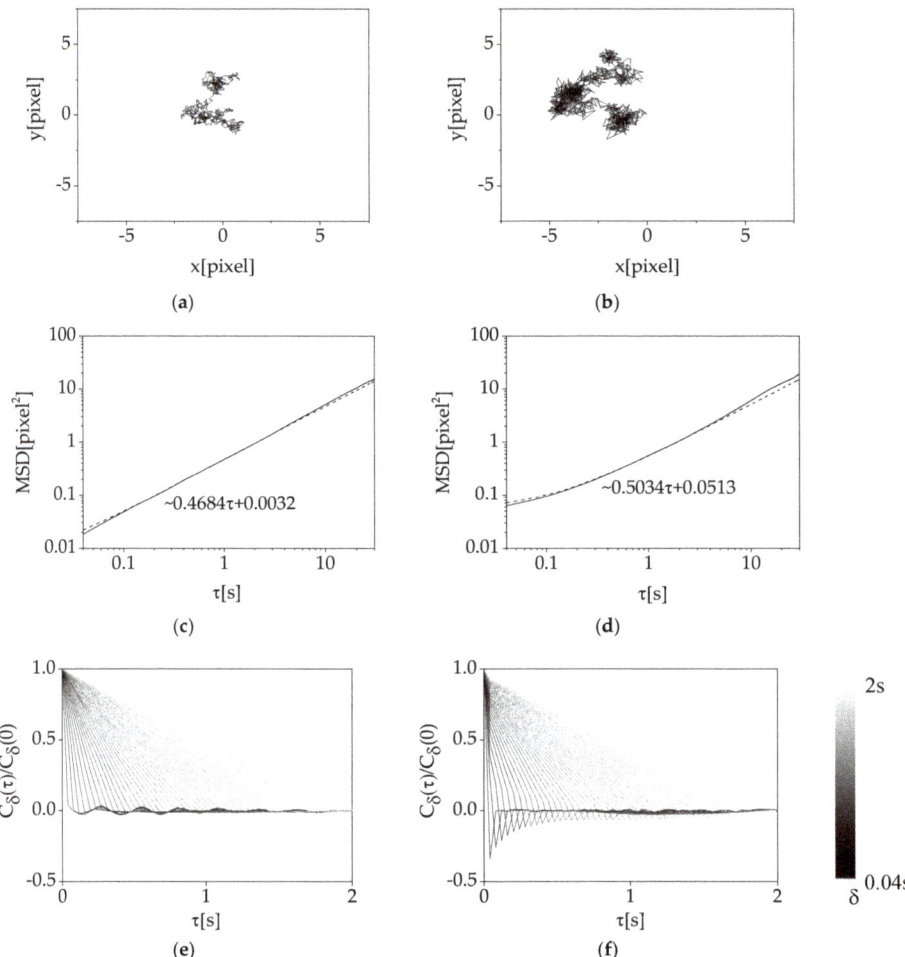

Figure 2. Representative trajectories of random motion of (**a**) cPMS and (**b**) MCF-7 cells calculated using the radial symmetry method. The ensemble-averaged MSDs of (**c**) cPMS and (**d**) MCF-7 cells calculated from the trajectories and the VACFs of (**e**) cPMS and (**f**) MCF-7 cells, δ from 0.04 to 2 s (black to white).

To characterize the differences in these two random processes, VACF-based analysis is performed, as shown in Figure 2e,f for cPMS and MCF-7, respectively. The VACFs are normalized to a value of $\tau = 0$. A previous report showed that the VACF can provide useful information to distinguish effects on the random process, such as localization errors, confinement, and moderate elasticity. The VACF of the trajectory with localization error has a sharp negative peak over a short time scale, and the peak decays as time δ increases. In the case of confined conditions, the VACF decays quickly to zero after it reaches to −0.5 at $\tau = \delta$ [40]. The VACF of the cPMS is different from that of the MCF-7. The VACF of cPMS does not show a peak value for any δ, which indicates that the particle follows random dynamics. On the other hand, the VACF of the MCF-7 cell shows a peak distribution according to δ, which corresponds to the peak distribution with localization error, that is, a sharp leak over the short time scale and peaks decay as δ increases.

Following the error analysis in single-particle tracking [41], the MSD can be fitted using Equation (3) so that the mean localization error, $\sigma = \sqrt{\langle \varepsilon^2(t) \rangle}$, can be estimated as a parameter of the degree of noise in position measurement. As shown in Figure 2c,d, $\sigma_{cPMS} \approx 0.0566$ and $\sigma_{MCF-7} \approx 0.2265$, which can be interpreted to signify that the analyzed trajectory of MCF-7 possesses approximately 5.4 times more localization error than that of cPMS. It also confirms that the VACF of cPMS follows random dynamics, whereas the VACF of MCF-7 shows a peculiar peak distribution depending on δ, possible evidence of localization error in the trajectory data. According to the results shown in Figure 2, localization of the cell requires a different approach to minimize localization error. Thus, in this study, a modified active contour method is introduced for analysis of cellular trajectory and random dynamics and is compared to other methods as follows.

3.2. Comparison of Image Analysis Methods

Before the discussion about random dynamics of particles and cells analyzed by the localization methods, we explain how each method detects the local point from the bright field microscopy image using the cPMS image. Figure 3a shows the intensity distribution of a cPMS image of 121 by 121 pixels, localized by three methods, namely radial symmetry [18], circular Hough transform [36], and modified active contour.

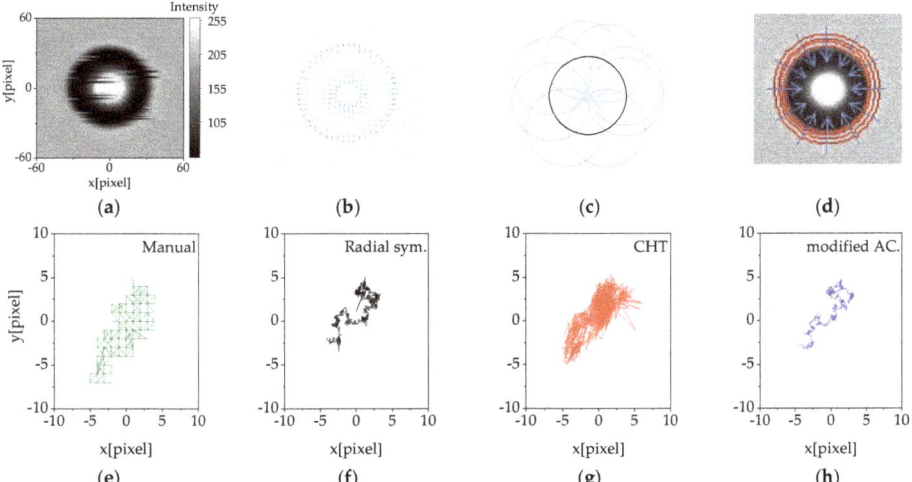

Figure 3. (**a**) The intensity distribution of a cPMS image. (**b**–**d**) The illustration of the 3 different localization methods; (**b**) radial symmetry, (**c**) circular Hough transformation and (**d**) modified active contour method. (**e**–**h**) The representative trajectory of MCF-7 cell using different localization method; (**e**) manual localization, (**f**) radial symmetry, (**g**) circular Hough transformation and (**h**) modified active contour method.

First, the radial symmetry method localizes the target image based on local intensity gradient. At the outset, it defines the midpoint of each grid in the entire image (x_k, y_k) [18]. At the defined midpoint, the intensity gradient across the grid is calculated. The whole intensity gradient of the cPMS image in Figure 3a is shown in Figure 3b. The intensity gradients have large magnitudes at the bright center region and at the boundary of the particle and point to the center point of the particle. The center point is that where the weighted sum of the distance to the lines of all midpoints is minimal.

In the weighted sum process, the weighting factor is proportional to the magnitude of the intensity gradient, so that the longer vectors toward the center in Figure 3b have a greater effect in determining the center point than do the smaller ones. Radial symmetry is very useful when the resolution of the image is low or the target image is small. On the other hand, when the size of an image is so large that the intensity variation of the target image could possibly affect the overall intensity distribution, it could be treated as noise. Moreover, if the size of the target image was relatively so small that the background represents a large portion of the image, background noise could influence the overall intensity distribution.

Second, the circular Hough transform (CHT) embedded in MATLAB 2018b is used to characterize the center point of the circular particle. First, the peripheral edge of an object in the whole image is detected through an edge gradient threshold automatically chosen using the graythresh function, which determines the threshold that minimizes intraclass variance of the selected black and white pixels following Otsu's method [42], embedded in MATLAB 2018b. On the determined edge in the image, the circular Hough transform considers and counts all circles on the expected circumference. Figure 3c shows possible candidates of the circle in the range of radii. The probable center point is the position of the maximum counting point. The circular Hough transform is simple in detecting circular objects with relatively strong edges. However, for a suspended cell, which is not perfectly circular and has an irregular shape, it is hard to automatically detect a strong edge.

Lastly, the modified active contour method is a segmentation technique with energy forces and constraints for discrimination of the pixels of interest from the image for further analysis. It does not depend on limited information because it considers the information obtained in the surrounding space as well as the brightness change in expressing the boundary part in the image, as shown in Figure 3d. This method considers the intensity of local edges obtained in the image to search for projected areas such as edges, lines, and subjective judgments in the image. In addition, it makes available a wider range of data by considering the internal relationship of the active contour. Since the conventional active contour method is sensitive to the initial boundary, we modified this method to overcome it. Thus, the proposed method is relatively robust in boundary conditions and performs cell tracking successfully.

To compare the effect on the trajectory of different localization methods, the representative MCF-7 cell trajectories of manual localization, radial symmetry, CHT and modified active contour are depicted in Figure 3e–h, respectively. When the manual localization is used, the position vector of cellular centroid is expressed only by integer number, since it comes from pixel of the image. Therefore, as shown in Figure 3e, the trajectory follows the integer point in the 2D plane. To accurately localize the position of cell, subpixel detection of particle/cell position is required. As shown in Figure 3f–h, it is possible to localize subpixel position using all of three different localization methods compared in this study. However, the resulting trajectory from three methods are quite different. It the next section, three different localization methods are compared through the analysis of random dynamics of MCF-7 cell.

3.3. Analysis of Cellular Random Motion by the Image Analysis Methods

By comparing the three methods, we concluded that the effect of localization error on particle position should be considered when the image of the cell is analyzed to localize the cellular position. Thus, to compare the effects of localization errors originating from the three image analysis methods, the trajectory of the MCF-7 cells and the MSD and VACF derived from that trajectory are depicted in Figure 4. Figure 4a–c are the trajectories of the MCF-7 cells (N = 36) analyzed by the radial symmetry method, circular Hough transform method, and modified active contour method, respectively. Comparing the three trajectories shows that, even though the trajectory computed by the radial symmetry method (Figure 4a) produces relatively decent trajectory results compared to that derived by the circular Hough transform method (Figure 4b), it still possesses a relatively large amount of localization error in comparison to the modified active contour method presented in Figure 4c.

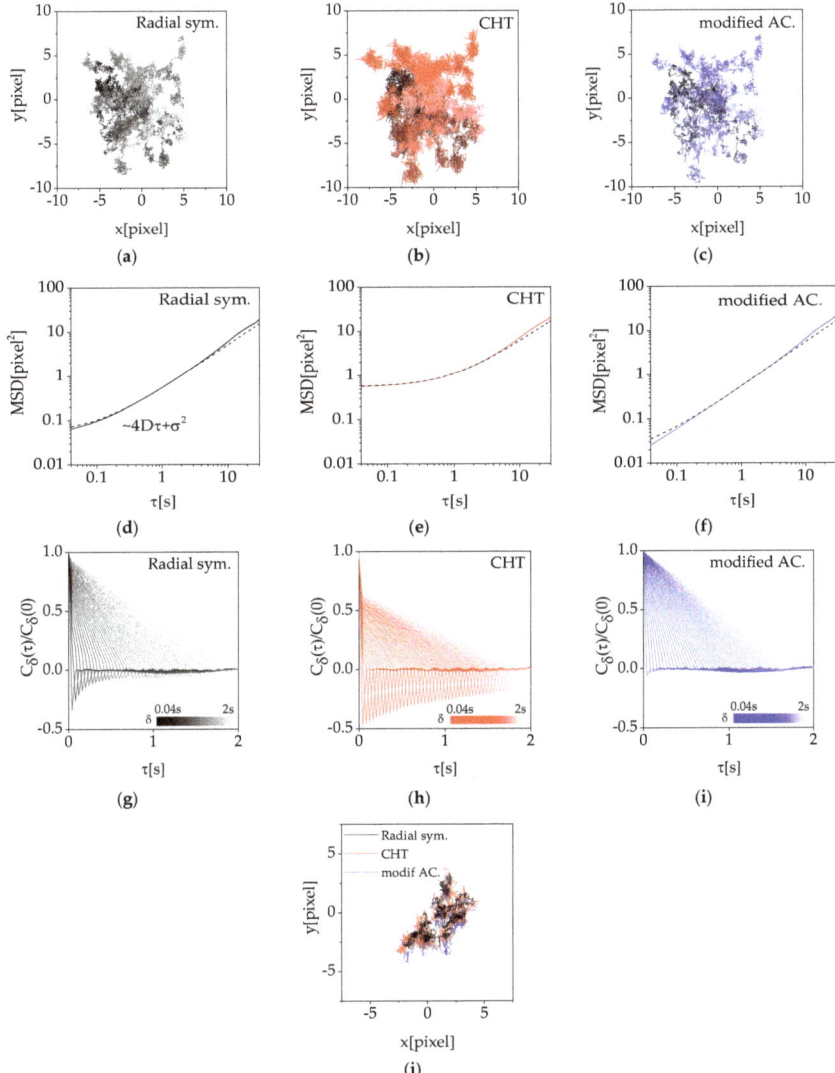

Figure 4. Random dynamics of MCF-7 cells analyzed by the tracking methods. The (**a**–**c**) trajectories, (**d**–**f**) MSDs, and (**g**–**i**) VACFs δ from 0.04 to 2 s calculated by the radial symmetry, circular Hough transform, and modified active contour methods (N = 36). (**j**) The comparison of the representative trajectory achieved from 3 different localization methods.

To quantify localization errors associated with the three image analysis methods, log-log MSD plots of MCF-7 cells acquired by the radial symmetric method, circular Hough transform method, and modified active contour method are presented in Figure 4d–f, respectively, and the VACFs are shown in Figure 4g–i. Over a short timescale, a nonlinear MSD region is observed, and the time scale of nonlinear MSD is lengthened in the order of the modified active contour method, radial symmetry method, and circular Hough transform method. This is attributed to the characteristics shown in Figure 4a–c such that the trajectory analyzed by the circular Hough transform method is noisier than the other two methods, and the modified active contour method exhibits the least noise. In Figure 4d–f, the fitting results with Equation (3) are expressed along with the experimental results produced by the three methods. From the fitting results, the mean localization error, σ, associated with the radial symmetric method, circular Hough transform method, and modified active contour method is estimated as 0.2265, 0.7467, and 0.1153, respectively. As expected from the trajectory results in Figure 4a–c, the circular Hough transform has the largest mean localization error, the modified active contour has the lowest, and the radial symmetric method is in the middle. Figure 4d–f, which present the VACF results acquired by the three methods up to $\tau \leq 2$ s, show the same characteristics of the methods considered. For the radial symmetric method, the sharp negative peak appears at the smallest δ and decreases quickly. In contrast, for the circular Hough transform method, the diminishing rate of the peak value of VACF is much slower than that in the radial symmetric method. The modified active contour shows a very small negative peak relative to the other two methods, which indicates that it is associated with less noise than the others. To compare the trajectory difference according to the localization methods, the representative trajectories are presented in Figure 4j.

3.4. Effects of Denoising

Using the radial symmetric method, image analysis is performed not only for the cells themselves, but also for the background. To exclude the effects of the background noise in image analysis, a denoising process using a Poisson noise filter is applied before localization, as shown in Figure 5. After denoising, background noise is rarely seen, and the edge of the cell looks clear. Based on the denoised image, the trajectory, MSD, and VACF of an MCF-7 cell are acquired for the three localization methods, as shown in Figure 6. The effect of denoising is clearly seen in the trajectory calculated by the radial symmetric method when Figure 6a is compared to Figure 4a. Even though the circular Hough transform method depicted in Figure 6b and the modified active contour method in Figure 6c show differences from the trajectories in Figure 4b,c, the difference is not as large as that observed in the radial symmetric method. This can be quantitatively confirmed by the MSD data in Figure 6d–f. The curves are fitted using Equation (3), and the diffusion coefficient D and the mean localization error σ are shown in Table 1. From the diffusion coefficient of three methods, cells randomly move with 4D of ~0.5. The mean localization error of the radial symmetry method, circular Hough transform method, and modified active contour are reduced to 0.1292, 0.7117, and 0.1963, respectively. Specifically, the mean localization error by radial symmetry is reduced by 0.0973, from 0.2265 to 0.1292, while the circular Hough transform method and modified active contour method show a reduction in localization error by 0.0350 and 0.0090, respectively. As mentioned, the radial symmetric method considers the whole image including the noisy background, and the effect of background noise becomes significant when analyzing the intensity gradient. In other words, if denoising is applied to these images, the level of localization error caused by the radial symmetric method ($\sigma = 0.1292$) can be reduced to the level of that caused by the modified active contour method without denoising ($\sigma = 0.1153$). To compare the trajectory difference according to the localization methods after denoising, the representative trajectories are presented in Figure 6j.

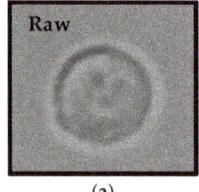

(a)

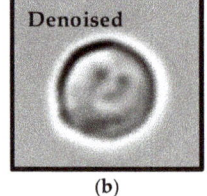

(b)

Figure 5. (a) A bright field image of MCF-7 cells and (b) the image after denoising.

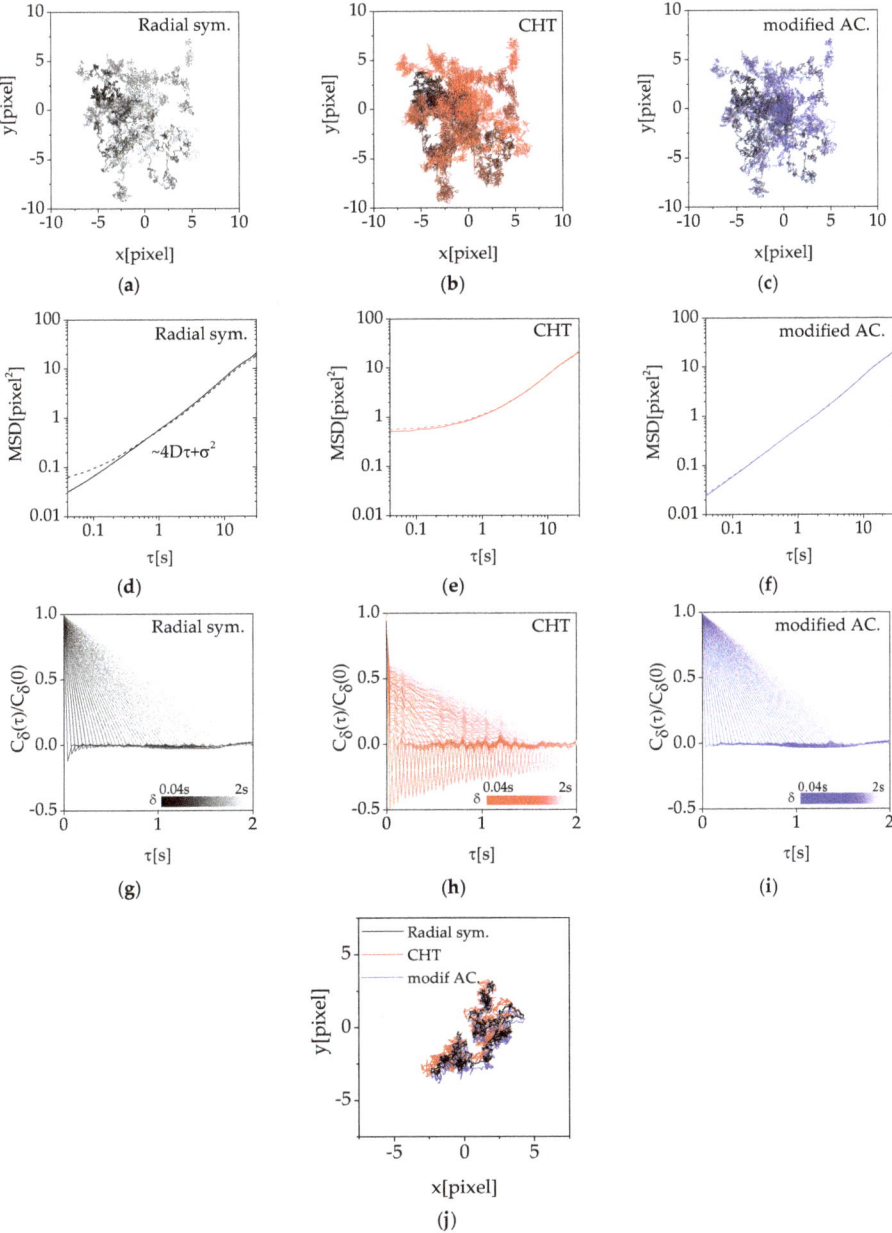

Figure 6. Random dynamics of MCF-7 cells analyzed by the tracking methods after denoising. The (**a**–**c**) trajectories, (**d**–**f**) (dashed line) MSD for raw image and (solid line) MSD for denoised image, and (**g**–**i**) VACFs (δ from 0.04 to 2 s) calculated by the radial symmetry, circular Hough transform, and modified active contour methods (N = 36) (**j**) The comparison of the representative trajectory achieved from 3 different localization methods.

Table 1. The diffusion coefficient D and the square of mean localization error σ^2 for the 3 different tracking method.

Method	Radial sym.		CHT		Modified AC	
	Raw	Denoised	Raw	Denoised	Raw	Denoised
4D	0.503	0.555	0.554	0.568	0.545	0.550
σ^2	0.051	0.017	0.558	0.507	0.013	0.011

4. Conclusions

The random dynamics of a cPMS particle and MCF-7 cell recorded at a frame rate of 25 hz were measured, and sub-pixel resolution analyses were performed using three localization methods, the radial symmetric method, circular Hough transform method, and modified active contour method. To understand the effects of different image analysis methods in localizing the position of a cell in an image for random dynamics analysis, the trajectory, MSD, and VACF of the measured objects were compared, and we found that the modified active contour method presented the smallest localization error compared to the other two methods considered. In addition, the effect of denoising on the stochastic dynamics of the MCF-7 cell was discussed for different image analysis methods.

An iterative fitting-based localization method has been used in single-particle tracking, where the considered particle size is on the order of a nanometer so that the image can be approximately modeled as a point spread function such as a Gaussian function. The radial symmetry method, however, determines a direction of center from every pixel by calculating the gradient of the point spread function at each pixel instead of using Gaussian fitting. When it is applied to the image of a nanosized object or of an object that is radially symmetric and has a clear gradient about the centroid, the radial symmetry method is appropriate for tracking. As shown in Figure 2 for cPMS, the radial symmetry method found the center of the cPMS and reported the MSD and VACF with little localization error, even though the size of the particle was on the micron scale. When studying cellular dynamics or migration, the size of the target object is on the micron scale; in our study, it was approximately 14.32 µm. Additionally, unlike a particle image, cellular images contain many irregular components such as non-circular shapes and small signal to noise ratios. Due to such weak radial symmetric properties, the radial symmetric method is not suitable for detecting the center point of a cellular image and has an enhanced likelihood of generating localization errors for algorithms detecting an object based on a circular shape. The localization error from the circular Hough transform method was the largest among the methods considered, as shown in Figure 4. The circular Hough transform method finds the center point, assuming that the object is circular. The non-circular shape of the cell and unclear edges of cell images can be major sources of localization errors. In addition to non-circularity, there are many dynamic noise sources in the interior of the cell. The morphology of the cell is inhomogeneous due to diverse cellular components such as the nucleus, ER, and mitochondria. As time elapses, these cellular components move freely within the cellular membrane. As discussed, both the radial symmetry method and the circular Hough transform method can be influenced by noise inside and/or outside of a cell; in particular, the radial symmetry method can be significantly influenced by background noise. Therefore, it could be useful to consider only the boundary of the cell for cellular localization in a dynamic cellular image. The modified active contour method employed in this study considers the boundary of the cell and calculates the center based on this boundary, decreasing the possibility of localization errors.

After the denoising process was applied to the bright field image, the boundaries of the cells became clear, and the cell outline detection was more effective than in the images without denoising. This preprocessing could reduce localization error through analysis of MSD and VACF, as shown in Figure 6. Thus, we conclude that it is helpful to employ a denoising process on a bright field image and/or to analyze the position using the modified active contour method to minimize the effects of localization error in cellular dynamics measurements.

Author Contributions: Conceptualization, S.Y.L.; methodology, J.Y.H., S.H., J.B., J.H., H.A., S.-H.W.; software, J.Y.H., S.H., J.B., J.H., H.A.; validation, J.Y.H. and S.Y.L.; formal analysis, J.Y.H. and S.Y.L.; investigation, J.Y.H. and S.Y.L.; resources, S.Y. and S.Y.L.; data curation, J.Y.H. and S.Y.L.; writing—original draft preparation, J.Y.H., S.Y. and S.Y.L.; writing—review and editing, S.W.L., Y.S.K., S.Y. and S.Y.L.; visualization, J.Y.H.; supervision, S.Y.L.; project administration, S.Y.L.; funding acquisition, S.Y.L. All authors have read and agreed to the published version of the manuscript.

Funding: This research was supported by the Basic Science Research Program through the National Research Foundation of Korea (NRF) funded by the Ministry of Education (NRF-2016R1D1A1A02937019), Republic of Korea.

Conflicts of Interest: The authors declare no conflict of interest.

References

1. Gupton, S.L.; Anderson, K.L.; Kole, T.P.; Fischer, R.S.; Ponti, A.; Hitchcock-DeGregori, S.E.; Danuser, G.; Fowler, V.M.; Wirtz, D.; Hanein, D.; et al. Cell migration without a lamellipodium: Translation of actin dynamics into cell movement mediated by tropomyosin. *J. Cell Biol.* **2005**, *168*, 619–631. [CrossRef] [PubMed]
2. Wu, P.-H.; Giri, A.; Sun, S.X.; Wirtz, D. Three-dimensional cell migration does not follow a random walk. *Proc. Natl. Acad. Sci. USA* **2014**, *111*, 3949–3954. [CrossRef] [PubMed]
3. Hyman, A.A.; White, J.G. Determination of cell division axes in the early embryogenesis of Caenorhabditis elegans. *J. Cell Biol.* **1987**, *105*, 2123–2135. [CrossRef] [PubMed]
4. Murray, J.I.; Bao, Z.; Boyle, T.J.; Waterston, R.H. The lineaging of fluorescently-labeled Caenorhabditis elegans embryos with StarryNite and AceTree. *Nat. Protoc.* **2006**, *1*, 1468–1476. [CrossRef] [PubMed]
5. Koslover, E.F.; Chan, C.K.; Theriot, J.A. Cytoplasmic flow and mixing due to deformation of motile cells. *Biophys. J.* **2017**, *113*, 2077–2087. [CrossRef] [PubMed]
6. Celebrano, M.; Kukura, P.; Renn, A.; Sandoghdar, V. Single-molecule imaging by optical absorption. *Nat. Photonics* **2011**, *5*, 95–98. [CrossRef]
7. Kukura, P.; Celebrano, M.; Renn, A.; Sandoghdar, V. Single-molecule sensitivity in optical absorption at room temperature. *J. Phys. Chem. Lett.* **2010**, *1*, 3323–3327. [CrossRef]
8. Wieser, S.; Schütz, G.J. Tracking single molecules in the live cell plasma membrane—Do's and Don't's. *Methods* **2008**, *46*, 131–140. [CrossRef]
9. Cheezum, M.K.; Walker, W.F.; Guilford, W.H. Quantitative comparison of algorithms for tracking single fluorescent particles. *Biophys. J.* **2001**, *81*, 2378–2388. [CrossRef]
10. Rogers, S.S.; Waigh, T.A.; Zhao, X.; Lu, J.R. Precise particle tracking against a complicated background: Polynomial fitting with Gaussian weight. *Phys. Biol.* **2007**, *4*, 220–227. [CrossRef]
11. Thompson, R.E.; Larson, D.R.; Webb, W.W. Precise nanometer localization analysis for individual fluorescent probes. *Biophys. J.* **2002**, *82*, 2775–2783. [CrossRef]
12. Manzo, C.; Garcia-Parajo, M.F. A review of progress in single particle tracking: From methods to biophysical insights. *Rep. Prog. Phys.* **2015**, *78*, 124601. [CrossRef] [PubMed]
13. Crocker, J.C.; Grier, D.G. Methods of digital video microscopy for colloidal studies. *J. Colloid Interface Sci.* **1996**, *179*, 298–310. [CrossRef]
14. Liu, Z.; Lavis, L.D.; Betzig, E. Imaging live-cell dynamics and structure at the single-molecule level. *Mol. Cell* **2015**, *58*, 644–659. [CrossRef] [PubMed]
15. Press, W.H.; Flannery, B.P.; Teukolsky, S.A.; Vetterling, W.T. *Numerical Recipes*; Cambridge University Press: Cambridge, UK, 1989.
16. Shen, H.; Tauzin, L.J.; Baiyasi, R.; Wang, W.; Moringo, N.; Shuang, B.; Landes, C.F. Single particle tracking: From theory to biophysical applications. *Chem. Rev.* **2017**, *117*, 7331–7376. [CrossRef]
17. Berglund, A.J.; McMahon, M.D.; McClelland, J.J.; Liddle, J.A. Fast, bias-free algorithm for tracking single particles with variable size and shape. *Opt. Express* **2008**, *16*, 14064–14075. [CrossRef]
18. Parthasarathy, R. Rapid, accurate particle tracking by calculation of radial symmetry centers. *Nat. Methods* **2012**, *9*, 724–726. [CrossRef]
19. Smith, C.S.; Joseph, N.; Rieger, B.; Lidke, K.A. Fast, single-molecule localization that achieves theoretically minimum uncertainty. *Nat. Methods* **2010**, *7*, 373–375. [CrossRef]
20. Mashanov, G.; Molloy, J. Automatic detection of single fluorophores in live cells. *Biophys. J.* **2007**, *92*, 2199–2211. [CrossRef]

21. Lee, S.U.; Chung, S.Y.; Park, R.H. A comparative performance study of several global thresholding techniques for segmentation. *Comput. Vis. Graph. Image Process.* **1990**, *52*, 171–190. [CrossRef]
22. Sezgin, M.; Sankur, B. Survey over image thresholding techniques and quantitative performance evaluation. *J. Electron. Imaging* **2004**, *13*, 146–166.
23. Demou, Z.N.; McIntire, L.V. Fully automated three-dimensional tracking of cancer cells in collagen gels: Determination of motility phenotypes at the cellular level. *Cancer Res.* **2002**, *62*, 5301–5307. [PubMed]
24. Thurston, G.; Jaggi, B.; Palcic, B. Measurement of cell motility and morphology with an automated microscope system. *Cytometry* **1988**, *9*, 411–417. [CrossRef] [PubMed]
25. Kachouie, N.N.; Fieguth, P.; Ramunas, J.; Jervis, E. Probabilistic model-based cell tracking. *Int. J. Biomed. Imaging* **2006**, *2006*, 012186. [CrossRef]
26. Young, D.; Glasbey, C.; Gray, A.; Martin, N. Towards automatic cell identification in DIC microscopy. *J. Microsc.* **1998**, *192*, 186–193. [CrossRef]
27. Nandy, K.; Gudla, P.R.; Amundsen, R.; Meaburn, K.J.; Misteli, T.; Lockett, S.J. Automatic segmentation and supervised learning-based selection of nuclei in cancer tissue images. *Cytometry Part A* **2012**, *81*, 743–754. [CrossRef]
28. Wählby, C.; Sintorn, I.M.; Erlandsson, F.; Borgefors, G.; Bengtsson, E. Combining intensity, edge and shape information for 2D and 3D segmentation of cell nuclei in tissue sections. *J. Microsc.* **2004**, *215*, 67–76. [CrossRef]
29. Delgado-Gonzalo, R.; Uhlmann, V.; Schmitter, D.; Unser, M. Snakes on a Plane: A perfect snap for bioimage analysis. *IEEE Signal Process. Mag.* **2015**, *32*, 41–48. [CrossRef]
30. Kass, M.; Witkin, A.; Terzopoulos, D. Snakes: Active contour models. *Int. J. Comput. Vis.* **1988**, *1*, 321–331. [CrossRef]
31. Dzyubachyk, O.; Van Cappellen, W.A.; Essers, J.; Niessen, W.J.; Meijering, E. Advanced level-set-based cell tracking in time-lapse fluorescence microscopy. *IEEE Trans. Med. Imaging* **2010**, *29*, 852–867. [CrossRef]
32. Sethian, J.A. *Level Set Methods and Fast Marching Methods: Evolving Interfaces in Computational Geometry, Fluid Mechanics, Computer Vision, and Materials Science*; Cambridge University Press: Cambridge, UK, 1999; Volume 3.
33. Yang, F.; Mackey, M.A.; Ianzini, F.; Gallardo, G.; Sonka, M. Cell segmentation, tracking, and mitosis detection using temporal context. In Proceedings of the International Conference on Medical Image Computing and Computer-Assisted Intervention, Palm Springs, CA, USA, 26–29 October 2005; pp. 302–309.
34. Reif, F. *Fundamentals of Statistical and Thermal Physics*; Waveland Press: Long Grove, IL, USA, 2009.
35. Saxton, M.J.; Jacobson, K. Single-particle tracking: Applications to membrane dynamics. *Annu. Rev. Biophys. Biomol. Struct.* **1997**, *26*, 373–399. [CrossRef]
36. Hyun, J.; Kim, S.; Kim, D.; Choi, S.; Key, J.; Kim, Y.; Lee, S.; Lee, S. Comparison of the abnormal diffusion characteristics of tumor cells. *Microfluid. Nanofluid.* **2019**, *23*, 119. [CrossRef]
37. Yuen, H.; Princen, J.; Illingworth, J.; Kittler, J. Comparative study of Hough transform methods for circle finding. *Image Vis. Comput.* **1990**, *8*, 71–77. [CrossRef]
38. Xu, J.; Chutatape, O.; Chew, P. Automated optic disk boundary detection by modified active contour model. *IEEE Trans. Biomed. Eng.* **2007**, *54*, 473–482. [CrossRef] [PubMed]
39. Kanopoulos, N.; Vasanthavada, N.; Baker, R.L. Design of an image edge detection filter using the Sobel operator. *IEEE J. Solid State Circuits* **1988**, *23*, 358–367. [CrossRef]
40. Weber, S.C.; Thompson, M.A.; Moerner, W.; Spakowitz, A.J.; Theriot, J.A. Analytical tools to distinguish the effects of localization error, confinement, and medium elasticity on the velocity autocorrelation function. *Biophys. J.* **2012**, *102*, 2443–2450. [CrossRef]
41. Savin, T.; Doyle, P.S. Static and dynamic errors in particle tracking microrheology. *Biophys. J.* **2005**, *88*, 623–638. [CrossRef]
42. Otsu, N. A threshold selection method from gray-level histograms. *IEEE Trans. Syst. Man Cybern.* **1979**, *9*, 62–66. [CrossRef]

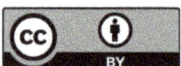

© 2020 by the authors. Licensee MDPI, Basel, Switzerland. This article is an open access article distributed under the terms and conditions of the Creative Commons Attribution (CC BY) license (http://creativecommons.org/licenses/by/4.0/).

Article

Silver Nanowire Micro-Ring Formation Using Immiscible Emulsion Droplets for Surface-Enhanced Raman Spectroscopy

Hyungdong Lee [1], Woojun Ye [1], Jaehyun Lee [1], Hyunggun Kim [2,*] and Doyoung Byun [1,*]

1. Department of Mechanical Engineering, Sungkyunkwan University, Suwon 16419, Korea; hyngdng.lee@gmail.com (H.L.); kittyluv007@gmail.com (W.Y.); pitts08@skku.edu (J.L.)
2. Department of Biomechatronic Engineering, Sungkyunkwan University, Suwon 16419, Korea
* Correspondence: hkim.bme@skku.edu (H.K.); dybyun@skku.edu (D.B.); Tel.: +82-31-290-7821 (H.K.); +82-31-299-4846 (D.B.)

Received: 21 October 2020; Accepted: 10 November 2020; Published: 12 November 2020

Abstract: Precise and rapid detection of biomolecules is a fast-growing research theme in the field of biomedical engineering. Based on the surface-enhanced Raman scattering, micro/nano-scale structures composed of noble metals (e.g., gold and silver) play a critical role in plasmonics. However, it is still limited to structuring nanomaterials in a specific manner. Here, we investigated a novel surface-enhanced Raman spectroscopy (SERS) application using one-dimensional nanomaterials and micro-encapsulation methods. With the immiscible nature of fluids, the nanomaterials were properly captured inside a number of droplets for encapsulation, deforming to micro-ring nanostructures. To yield uniform sizes of the silver micro-ring structures, a microchannel system was designed to characterize particle sizes via microscopic approaches. We were able to obtain printable silver nanowire micro-ring ink, and investigated the SERS substrate effect of the silver micro-ring structure. This fabrication method can be used in many other SERS-based biomedical engineering applications in the near future.

Keywords: micro-encapsulation; nanowire; immiscible solution; printing; surface-enhanced Raman spectroscopy

1. Introduction

In the past several decades, the surface plasmonics of self-assembled metallic nanostructures has been utilized for various biomedical applications such as biosensors, plasmonic filters, diagnostic devices, and photothermal-induced cancer therapy [1,2]. To precisely and rapidly detect biomolecules, micro/nano-scale structures composed of noble metals, e.g., gold (Au) and silver (Ag), play a critical role in the field of plasmonics. Surface-enhanced Raman spectroscopy (SERS) demonstrates that metal nanostructures can control the surface optical properties [3]. An ideal SERS substrate should have high uniformity and field enhancement. Such substrates can be prepared on a wafer scale, and fluctuations of SERS signals on such highly uniform, high-performance plasmonic metasurfaces can be demonstrated in label-free microscopy [4]. However, it is still difficult to structure nanomaterials due to the limitations of controlling the single nanoparticle without well-confined conditions such as atomic force microscopic (AFM) manipulation [5]. Furthermore, the fabrication cost of SERS substrates needs to be reduced via proper manufacturing techniques [6].

Among the conventional self-assembly methods for nanomaterials, the micro-encapsulation method in immiscible solution has been considered a promising technique due to its simplicity and cost-effectiveness [7,8]. For example, many researchers have tried to implement micro-encapsulation to enclose solid or fluid materials inside a microscale membrane made of two-dimensional (2D) soluble layers, which would allow for the control of dosing frequency and prevent degradation of the pharmaceutical materials. Thanks to the benefits of micro-encapsulation, this approach to exploit the SERS effect has also been investigated [9–11]. Although these studies proposed multifunctional micro-encapsulation platforms for pharmaceutical analysis or biosensor development, there still remains an unexplored area in investigating and manipulating one-dimensional (1D) metal nanowire-based encapsulation for the SERS effect. From the perspective of material properties, 1D nanomaterials have great mechanical flexibility and high thermal or electrical conductivity [12,13]. If SERS application can be adequately explored using these nanomaterials and micro-encapsulation methods, a newly proposed approach is expected, which could be helpful in future biomedical engineering applications [14,15].

In the present study, a formation method for micro-ring materials using micro-encapsulation in immiscible solution was introduced. In order to fabricate the ring structure, metallic nanowires and emulsion liquid droplets were used. In addition, a pinched flow fractionation (PFF) microchannel was experimentally investigated to uniformly and continuously separate the Ag nanowire micro-ring structure in different sizes. Printable ink containing Ag nanowire micro-ring structures was produced through a classification process. Lastly, a printing pattern for the ring-based ink was proposed and the ring patterns were characterized.

2. Materials and Methods

2.1. Materials and Method For Emulsion Droplet Formation

Ag nanowires with a length of 25 µm and a width of 30 nm dispersed in deionized (DI) water (0.1 wt%) were purchased (N&B Corporation, Ansan, Korea). N,N-Dimethylformamide (DMF), 1,2-Dichlorobenzene (DCB), $NH_3 \cdot H_2O$, and tetraethyl orthosilicate (TEOS) were purchased from Sigma-Aldrich (Seoul, Korea). For the DMF-based Ag nanowires, a centrifuge (1248, Labogene, Seoul, Korea) was used to separate Ag nanowire solution from water at 2000 rpm for 15 min. After removing water, the separated Ag nanowires were dispersed in DMF with 0.04 wt%. To formulate a water-in-oil emulsion, 200 µL of nanowire solution and 15 µL of $NH_3 \cdot H_2O$ were mixed. Afterward, 5 mL of DCB were added to the mixture at a proper ratio followed by adding 15 µL of TEOS. Before heating the solution, a sonicator (Sonics VCX-500, Sonics & Materials Inc, Newtown, CT, USA) was utilized for a short time (<1 min) to prevent the droplets from recombining. The mixture was heated at 60 °C for 30 min to form the silica shells.

2.2. Preparation of the Pinched Flow Fractionation Microchannel

Microchannel design was taken from the multi-outlet microchannel developed in a previous study [10]. A microchannel was designed with a depth of 50 µm, inlet width of 60 µm, pinched channel width of 30 µm, and outlet width of 100 µm. A microchannel mold on a silicon wafer was constructed by deep reactive ion etching (DRIE). For microchannel fabrication, silane coating on the mold substrate was conducted in a vacuum chamber for 2 h. Trichloro (1 h, 1 h, 2 h, 2 h-perfluorooctyl) silane (Sigma Aldrich, Seoul, Korea) was used for silane coating, and a sufficient amount of polydimethylsiloxane (PDMS) was poured on the mold substrate. The PDMS was placed in the vacuum chamber until most of the captured bubbles in the PDMS disappeared, and then baked at 120 °C for 2 h on a hotplate. The baked PDMS channel was detached from the substrate, punched through the inlet and outlet, and connected with a Teflon tube. To attach the PDMS channels to slide glasses, oxygen plasma coating was applied to each attachment surface. Lastly, the PMDS channel attached on the slide glass was heated at 80 °C for 30 min.

2.3. Printing Process Using the Ag Nanowire Micro-Ring Ink

An electrohydrodynamic jet printing device (Enjet Inc, Suwon, Korea) was used to print the sorted Ag nanowire micro-ring ink solution. The experiment was conducted under the following conditions:

flow rate of 0.75 μL/m, working height of 500 μm, voltage of 1.5 kV, substrate temperature of 50 °C, and printing velocity of 50 mm/s.

2.4. Characterization of the Ag Nanowire Micro-Rings and the Printing Pattern

The Ag nanowire micro-ring structure and printed pattern images were characterized by optical microscopy (Eclipse Series, Nikon Instruments Inc., Melville, NY, USA) with a polarizing filter and a field emission scanning electron microscope (JEM-2100F, JEOL, Peabody, MA, USA). The optical properties were determined by dispersive Raman spectroscopy (SENTERRA Raman, Bruker, Billerica, MA, USA). The Raman spectra of the Ag nanowire micro-ring patterned substrate and bare Si wafer at a 532 nm wavelength under the same experimental conditions were measured and compared.

3. Results and Discussion

3.1. Optimization of the Ag Nanowire Micro-Ring Structure Formation

In order to make the Ag nanowire micro-ring structure, we employed an immiscible emulsion droplet formation method. Figure 1 shows that emulsion droplets could be continuously generated by tip sonication-induced vibration in DMF and DCB solution. During the process, Ag nanowires were captured in micro-scale bubbles (i.e., encapsulation) due to high surface tension force compared to the yield strength of Ag nanowires. We have previously shown that micro-rings are formed inside droplets by the force balance between the compressive force of the droplet and the restoring force of the high aspect ratio nanowire material [16]. Based on this mechanism, we investigated whether the micro-ring composed of Ag nanowire could be constructed in immiscible solution (Figure 2). The Ag nanowire micro-ring structure with a diameter in the sub-micron scale was successfully deposited on the substrate (Figure 2a,b). However, random generation of the emulsion droplets led to several entangled Ag nanowires in a single droplet. Figure 2c,d demonstrate that the entangled Ag nanowire micro-rings had a larger diameter (4–5 μm) compared to the single Ag nanowire micro-rings (<4 μm). This result led us to the next stage to sort the fabricated single and bundled Ag nanowire micro-rings with respect to droplet size using the PFF microchannel.

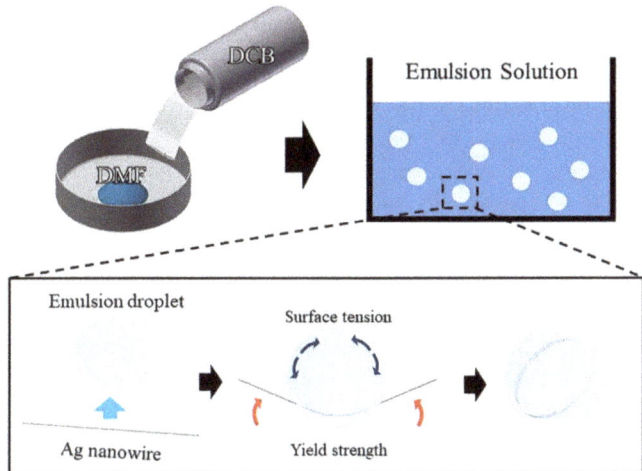

Figure 1. A schematic of the coiling nanowire inside a water-in-oil emulsion droplet.

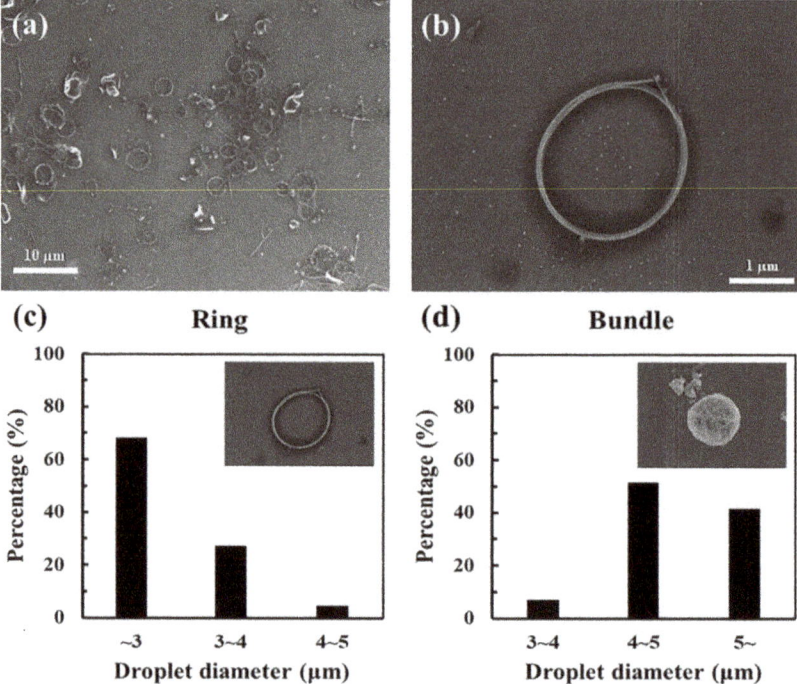

Figure 2. (**a**,**b**) SEM images of coiled silver nanowires, (**c**) droplet diameters of a single Ag nanowire, and (**d**) droplet diameters of entangled Ag nanowires.

3.2. Separation of the Droplets Using the Microchannel

Prior to sorting the Ag nanowire micro-ring structures, hollow glass particles with a diameter of 10 μm were utilized to test whether the microchannel would be suitable to efficiently sort the Ag nanowire micro-rings (Figure 3). DCB was used as a solvent for the glass particles to disperse as in the micro-ring formation process. DCB with and without glass particles was released at different flow rates (A:B = 1:1, 1:4, and 1:10) simultaneously at each inlet. In this feasibility test, almost all the glass particles were collected through outlet 1 (downstream) when the flow rate ratio was fixed to 1:10 (Figure 3d). It has been reported that moving the particle close to the wall can initiate a dispersing effect, resulting in sorting the particles by size distribution [10]. This indicates that the ratio of two different flow rates can determine the separation of particles in various sizes using a pinched channel.

Following this feasibility test with hollow glass particles, the same experimental setting was implemented to apply to the immiscible emulsion with the Ag nanowire micro-rings (Figure 4). Figure 4b demonstrates that approximately 50% of the Ag nanowire micro-ring structures with 2–3 μm diameters could be collected at outlet 1. Further detailed evaluation of the size distribution revealed that the Ag nanowire micro-rings with a relatively smaller size (<2.5 μm) could be collected in outlet 1 compared to outlet 2 (Figure 4c). Using this separation process with the micro-ring particles, we were able to collect Ag nanowire micro-ring structures of a similar size dispersed in the organic solvent. Next, we applied this Ag nanowire micro-ring material to printing ink, and investigated a printing pattern with the Ag nanowire micro-ring structures to enhance the surface plasmonic scattering for biological applications.

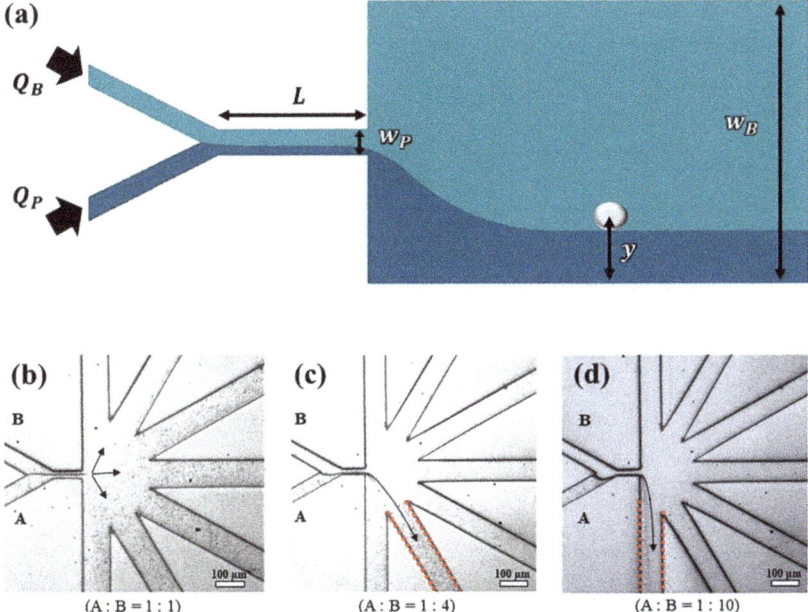

Figure 3. (**a**) A schematic of the pinched flow fractionation microchannel with a particle. Trajectory of 10 μm of hollow glass particles in different flow rate ratios of (**b**) 1:1, (**c**) 1:4, and (**d**) 1:10 (μL/min).

3.3. Printing Pattern and Its Application

Experiments were carried out to make patterns through the electrohydrodynamic (EHD) jet printing process with the micro-ring dispersion ink (Figure 5a). First, we tried to print a line pattern containing the micro-rings through the dispensing method by heating the substrate to induce an evaporation rate of the toluene solvent. Figure 5b demonstrates the detailed pattern with the micro-ring array along the printing direction. Due to the coffee ring effect originating from the capillary flow induced by the differential evaporation rates across the drop [17], the micro-rings were concentrated at the edge of the pattern.

SERS substrates can be offered as one of the biological applications with these Ag nanowire micro-rings. The substrates are used to determine the minimum quantity of biomolecules and allow us to detect biological species in biofluids. Therefore, this technique can enhance the Raman scattering by molecules adsorbed onto metallic structures. We measured the Raman spectrum of the Ag nanowire micro-ring patterned substrate and bare Si wafer at 532 nm wavelength under the same measurement conditions, and clearly observed enhanced total surface background intensity values (Figure 5c). The shape and size of the metallic nanostructures affect the enhancement strength due to the factors influencing the ratio of absorption and scattering [18]. Moreover, self-assembled metallic nanoparticles such as Ag and Au nanostructures can actively enhance the Raman scattering. These data suggest that our Ag nanowire micro-ring structure could be utilized in SERS substrate as the Ag nanowire micro-rings have nanoscale widths (<25 nm), thus offering great printability on surfaces.

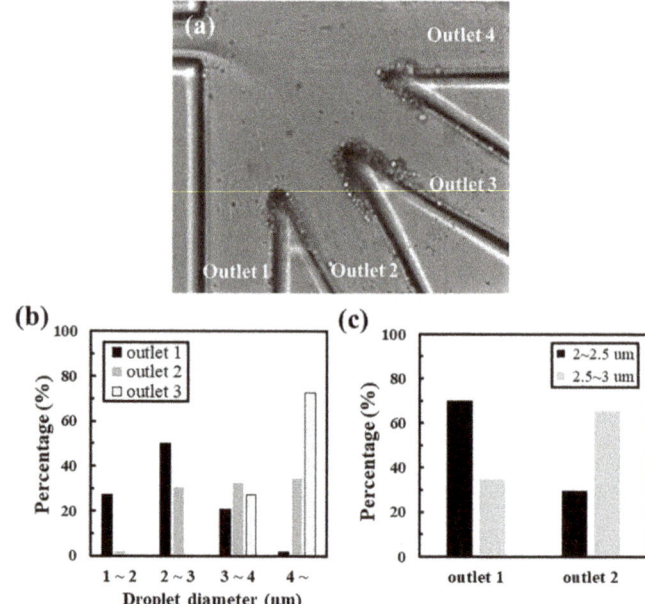

Figure 4. (**a**) A microscopic image of the sorting process in the pinched flow fractionation (PFF) microchannel, (**b**) Ag nanowire rings in dispersed solution from outlet 1, and (**c**) droplet diameters of the sorted droplets in outlets 1 and 2.

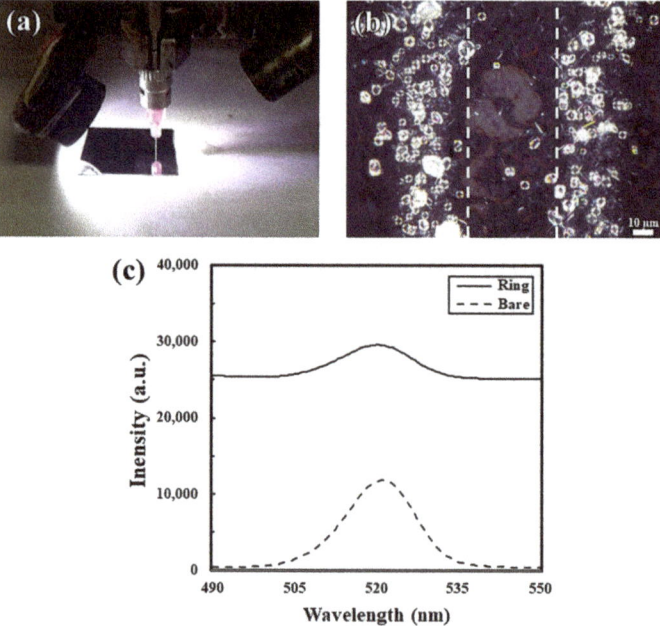

Figure 5. (**a**) Patterning with the micro-ring solution using electrohydrodynamic (EHD) jet printing, (**b**) a microscopic image of the micro-ring distribution, and (**c**) diagram of the Raman spectra for the Ag nanowire micro-ring structure and bare wafer.

4. Conclusions

In this study, we proposed a potential material for printing ink using ring-shaped microscale structures. A large amount of ring-shaped material was formed using Ag nanowires, immiscible emulsion solution, and silica shells. In order to utilize the micro-ring solution as printing ink, two alternatives were implemented. First, the solution was dispersed again using a sonicator to prevent the droplets surrounding the nanowire from recombination before the silica shell was formed. The size of the droplets with rings and those with bundles formed during the synthesis were determined, and the droplets were classified by size using the PFF microchannel to increase the micro-ring ratio in the solution. The Ag nanowire micro-ring solution was patterned using EHD jet printing. The optical characteristics of the micro-ring pattern fabricated by EHD jet printing were analyzed using a dispersive Raman spectrometer. This novel method to fabricate Ag nanowire micro-rings can be used in many other SERS-based biomedical engineering applications in the near future.

Author Contributions: Conceptualization, H.K., D.B.; methodology, H.L., W.Y., J.L.; formal analysis, H.L., W.Y.; investigation, H.L., W.Y., H.K., D.B.; resources, D.B.; writing—original draft preparation, H.L., W.Y.; writing—review and editing, H.K., D.B.; visualization, W.Y., J.L.; funding acquisition, D.B. All authors have read and agreed to the published version of the manuscript.

Funding: This research was funded by the Basic Science Research Program through the National Research Foundation of Korea (NRF), funded by the Ministry of Science, ICT & Future Planning (NRF-2017R1E1A1A01075353).

Conflicts of Interest: The authors declare no conflict of interest.

References

1. Toriyama, S.; Mizeikis, V.; Ono, A. Fabrication of silver nano-rings using photo-reduction induced by femtosecond pulses. *Appl. Phys. Express* **2019**, *12*, 015004. [CrossRef]
2. Kahraman, M.; Mullen, E.R.; Korkmaz, A.; Wachsmann-Hogiu, S. Fundamentals and applications of sers-based bioanalytical sensing. *Nanophotonics* **2017**, *6*, 831–852. [CrossRef]
3. Lane, L.A.; Qian, X.; Nie, S. Sers nanoparticles in medicine: From label-free detection to spectroscopic tagging. *Chem. Rev.* **2015**, *115*, 10489–10529. [CrossRef] [PubMed]
4. Ayas, S.; Cinar, G.; Ozkan, A.D.; Soran, Z.; Ekiz, O.; Kocaay, D.; Tomak, A.; Toren, P.; Kaya, Y.; Tunc, I.; et al. Label-free nanometer-resolution imaging of biological architectures through surface enhanced raman scattering. *Sci. Rep.* **2013**, *3*, 2624. [CrossRef] [PubMed]
5. Kim, S.; Shafiei, F.; Ratchford, D.; Li, X. Controlled afm manipulation of small nanoparticles and assembly of hybrid nanostructures. *Nanotechnology* **2011**, *22*, 115301. [CrossRef] [PubMed]
6. Bernatova, S.; Donato, M.G.; Jezek, J.; Pilat, Z.; Samek, O.; Magazzu, A.; Marago, O.M.; Zemanek, P.; Gucciardi, P.G. Wavelength-dependent optical force aggregation of gold nanorods for sers in a microfluidic chip. *J. Phys. Chem. C* **2019**, *123*, 5608–5615. [CrossRef]
7. Teng, X.R.; Shchukin, D.G.; Mohwald, H. Encapsulation of water-immiscible solvents in polyglutamate/polyelectrolyte nanocontainers. *Adv. Funct. Mater.* **2007**, *17*, 1273–1278. [CrossRef]
8. Sakai, S.; Hashimoto, I.; Ogushi, Y.; Kawakami, K. Peroxidase-catalyzed cell encapsulation in subsieve-size capsules of alginate with phenol moieties in water-immiscible fluid dissolving H_2O_2. *Biomacromolecules* **2007**, *8*, 2622–2626. [CrossRef] [PubMed]
9. Stetciura, I.Y.; Markin, A.V.; Bratashov, D.N.; Sukhorukov, G.B.; Gorin, D.A. Nanoencapsulated and microencapsulated sers platforms for biomedical analysis. *Curr. Opin. Pharmacol.* **2014**, *18*, 149–158. [CrossRef] [PubMed]
10. Yamada, M.; Nakashima, M.; Seki, M. Pinched flow fractionation: Continuous size separation of particles utilizing a laminar flow profile in a pinched microchannel. *Anal. Chem.* **2004**, *76*, 5465–5471. [CrossRef] [PubMed]
11. Markina, N.E.; Markin, A.V.; Zakharevich, A.M.; Goryacheva, I.Y. Calcium carbonate microparticles with embedded silver and magnetite nanoparticles as new sers-active sorbent for solid phase extraction. *Microchim. Acta* **2017**, *184*, 3937–3944. [CrossRef]

12. Lin, J.; Cretu, O.; Zhou, W.; Suenaga, K.; Prasai, D.; Bolotin, K.I.; Cuong, N.T.; Otani, M.; Okada, S.; Lupini, A.R.; et al. Flexible metallic nanowires with self-adaptive contacts to semiconducting transition-metal dichalcogenide monolayers. *Nat. Nanotechnol.* **2014**, *9*, 436–442. [CrossRef] [PubMed]
13. Sannicolo, T.; Lagrange, M.; Cabos, A.; Celle, C.; Simonato, J.P.; Bellet, D. Metallic nanowire-based transparent electrodes for next generation flexible devices: A review. *Small* **2016**, *12*, 6052–6075. [CrossRef] [PubMed]
14. Vo-Dinh, T.; Liu, Y.; Fales, A.M.; Ngo, H.; Wang, H.N.; Register, J.K.; Yuan, H.; Norton, S.J.; Griffin, G.D. Sers nanosensors and nanoreporters: Golden opportunities in biomedical applications. *Wiley Interdiscip. Rev. Nanomed. Nanobiotechnol.* **2015**, *7*, 17–33. [CrossRef] [PubMed]
15. Zong, C.; Xu, M.; Xu, L.J.; Wei, T.; Ma, X.; Zheng, X.S.; Hu, R.; Ren, B. Surface-enhanced raman spectroscopy for bioanalysis: Reliability and challenges. *Chem. Rev.* **2018**, *118*, 4946–4980. [CrossRef] [PubMed]
16. Seong, B.; Park, H.S.; Chae, I.; Lee, H.; Wang, X.; Jang, H.S.; Jung, J.; Lee, C.; Lin, L.; Byun, D. Self-assembly of silver nanowire ring structures driven by the compressive force of a liquid droplet. *Langmuir* **2017**, *33*, 3367–3372. [CrossRef] [PubMed]
17. Deegan, R.D.; Bakajin, O.; Dupont, T.F.; Huber, G.; Nagel, S.R.; Witten, T.A. Capillary flow as the cause of ring stains from dried liquid drops. *Nature* **1997**, *389*, 827–829. [CrossRef]
18. Lu, H.F.; Zhang, H.X.; Yu, X.; Zeng, S.W.; Yong, K.T.; Ho, H.P. Seed-mediated plasmon-driven regrowth of silver nanodecahedrons (nds). *Plasmonics* **2012**, *7*, 167–173. [CrossRef]

Publisher's Note: MDPI stays neutral with regard to jurisdictional claims in published maps and institutional affiliations.

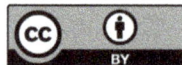

© 2020 by the authors. Licensee MDPI, Basel, Switzerland. This article is an open access article distributed under the terms and conditions of the Creative Commons Attribution (CC BY) license (http://creativecommons.org/licenses/by/4.0/).

 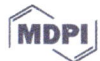

Article

A Novel Patient-to-Image Surface Registration Technique for ENT- and Neuro-Navigation Systems: Proper Point Set in Patient Space

Ahnryul Choi [1,2], Seungheon Chae [2], Tae-Hyong Kim [2], Hyunwoo Jung [2], Sang-Sik Lee [1], Ki-Young Lee [1] and Joung-Hwan Mun [2,*]

1. Department of Biomedical Engineering, College of Medical Convergence, Catholic Kwandong University, Gangneung-si 25601, Korea; achoi@cku.ac.kr (A.C.); lsskyj@cku.ac.kr (S.-S.L.); kylee@cku.ac.kr (K.-Y.L.)
2. Department of Bio-Mechatronic Engineering, College of Biotechnology and Bioengineering, Sungkyunkwan University, Suwon-si 16419, Korea; chd8806a@skku.edu (S.C.); sanctified@skku.edu (T.-H.K.); alex1130@skku.edu (H.J.)
* Correspondence: jmun@skku.edu; Tel.: +82-31-290-7827

Abstract: Patient-to-medical image registration is a crucial factor that affects the accuracy of image-guided ENT- and neurosurgery systems. In this study, a novel registration protocol that extracts the point cloud in the patient space using the contact approach was proposed. To extract the optimal point cloud in patient space, we propose a multi-step registration protocol consisting of augmentation of the point cloud and creation of an optimal point cloud in patient space that satisfies the minimum distance from the point cloud in the medical image space. A hemisphere mathematical model and plastic facial phantom were used to validate the proposed registration protocol. An optical and electromagnetic tracking system, of the type that is commonly used in clinical practice, was used to acquire the point cloud in the patient space and evaluate the accuracy of the proposed registration protocol. The SRE and TRE of the proposed protocol were improved by about 30% and 50%, respectively, compared to those of a conventional registration protocol. In addition, TRE was reduced to about 28% and 21% in the optical and electromagnetic methods, respectively, thus showing improved accuracy. The new algorithm proposed in this study is expected to be applied to surgical navigation systems in the near future, which could increase the success rate of otolaryngological and neurological surgery.

Keywords: patient-to-image registration; image-guided ENT- and neurosurgery system; surface registration; piecewise cubic Hermite interpolation

1. Introduction

An image-guided surgery system visualizes the three-dimensional position of a surgical tool using preoperative medical images and provides the location of lesions and surrounding areas in real time [1,2]. The imaging information of this type of system allows surgeons to perform minimally invasive surgery and plan a path to the lesion in advance, thereby improving the quality of the surgery and reducing the operating time [3]. Therefore, this technology is widely used for different types of neurosurgery, such as tumor biopsy and resection, craniotomy, and deep brain stimulation [4], as well as in head and neck surgery, including sinusitis surgery [5]. Spatial registration, one of the core elements of image-guided ENT- and neurosurgery systems, is the process of aligning the coordinates of a medical image taken before surgery with the spatial coordinates of the patient acquired during surgery in the same space [6]. If the registration between the two spaces is not accurate, a gap arises between the position of the actual surgical tool and that of the virtual surgical tool displayed on the image. Therefore, the registration technology is a crucial factor that affects the accuracy of an image-guided ENT- and neurosurgery system [3,4,7].

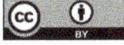

Patient-to-medical image registration methods can be divided into point registration and surface registration methods [8]. A surface registration method finds the transformation matrix based on a point cloud in the patient space and the medical image space, and does not require attachment of specific fiducial markers [9,10]. Therefore, this type of registration method is free from problems such as skin swelling due to attachment of fiducial markers [11], and additional medical imaging is unnecessary, thereby eliminating cost and hassle [2]. In surface registration, also called marker-less registration, many corresponding points in each space are matched up through a sequential process of coarse and precise registration [12]. Coarse registration, which is rough and relatively inaccurate, is performed using the initial anatomical landmarks of each space, then precise registration is performed by applying an iterative closest point (ICP) algorithm. ICP is an optimization method that iteratively finds the medical image coordinates that satisfy the minimum distance from the point cloud in the patient space, and a transformation matrix is acquired when the sum of the Euclidean distances between corresponding points is minimal [13,14]. Unfortunately, despite the various advantages of surface registration, its accuracy continues to be controversial. Several studies reported that the accuracy of the technique is similar to that of point registration [15], but many other studies reported significantly lower accuracy [2,16]. Therefore, despite the various advantages of the surface registration technique, concerns about its accuracy remain.

The acquisition and processing of the point sets of each space are essential to improving the accuracy of a surface registration method that is based on the point sets in the patient and medical image space [12]. While medical images such as CT often show excellent resolution and accuracy [3,17], most previous studies focused on the extraction of a point cloud in patient space; these studies showed that accuracy can be affected by such factors as equipment performance or clinical proficiency [2,9,12,18]. The approaches to extraction of the point cloud in patient space can be divided into contact-type approaches that extract points by tracing probes on the surface of the face and non-contact approaches that collect points using additional scanner devices [6]. In the latter, a scanner device can be used to avoid contact with the surface of the face, thereby reducing the error due to deformation of soft skin when obtaining the point cloud. Furthermore, this method has the advantage of being able to obtain more point sets, which increases the accuracy of registration. Recent studies reported on methods to reduce target registration error (TRE), which utilize mobile 3D scanners to collect point clouds across the whole head [4,7]. However, scanners with guaranteed precision are generally very expensive [3]. In addition, since the device differs from that used for commercial image-guided surgery systems, an additional coordinate transformation process must be performed, which may result in accumulation of errors [19].

Therefore, the commercial image-guided surgery systems that are currently in use extract point clouds in patient space through contact with the surface of the face. Accordingly, in neurosurgery or head and neck surgery, clinicians perform surface registration by placing a probe on the patient's face as a convenient method of extracting the point cloud; several clinical case reports of the surgical effects of this method have been conducted [5,20–22]. However, in all of these studies, only the original patient space coordinates obtained through facial surface tracing were used, and no attempts have been made to improve the point cloud in order to reduce the surface registration error. Therefore, the main purpose of this study is to propose a novel registration protocol that extracts the point cloud in patient space using the contact approach to increase the accuracy of surface registration of an image-guided surgery system. The proposed registration protocol consists of a two-step process: augmentation of the point clouds and creation of a proper point cloud. The secondary purpose of this study is to validate the proposed registration protocol using a hemisphere mathematical model and a plastic facial phantom.

2. Proposed Registration Strategy

The surface registration method used for image-guided surgery systems refers to a process of matching point clouds between preoperative medical image space and intraoperative patient space. The 3D structure is first reconstructed based on pre-operative tomographic medical images such as CT, and the point cloud on the facial surface is then extracted. In addition, the point cloud of the facial surface is acquired using a probe or scanner during surgery. Points in different spaces are used to perform coarse registration using three or four representative fiducial markers. The final process is a precise registration process that aims to minimize the distance between the corresponding points. In this study, a novel protocol is used to create a point cloud in patient space between the initial coarse registration stage and the precise registration stage. The detailed process is illustrated in Figure 1.

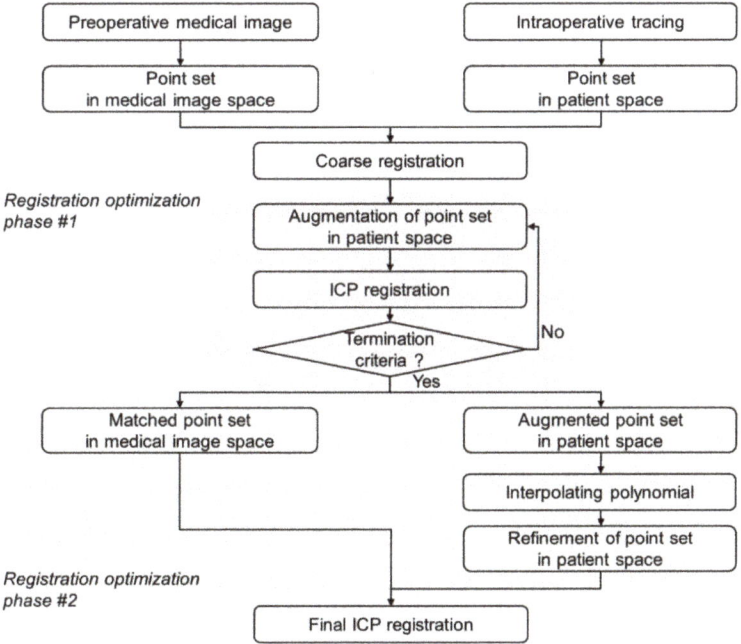

Figure 1. Workflow of the proposed registration strategy.

2.1. Registration Optimization Phase 1: Augmentation of the Number of Points in Patient Space

In general, medical images include a large number of points due to their high resolution. However, the point cloud in patient space is determined by the duration of the facial tracing and the available camera samples of the surgical probe. Due to practical limitations, it is difficult to obtain a large number of points in real surgical situations. Therefore, starting with the point cloud obtained by tracing, the point cloud is augmented using an interpolation technique and the surface registration performance is evaluated according to the precise registration process (Figure 1). Here, the point cloud is increased by 5% compared to the previous step. Furthermore, the precision registration method utilizes the ICP method, which is the most widely utilized method (see Section 2.3 for details). The surface registration error (SRE) is evaluated according to augmentation of the point cloud, and the termination criteria are set when the absolute value of the difference in SRE between two consecutive ICPs in the current and previous steps is within 0.1%.

2.2. Registration Optimization Phase 2: Proper Point Set in Patient Space

In the second step, the proper point cloud is extracted to match the medical image-based spatial point cloud using the augmented point cloud in patient space (Figure 2). An interpolation polynomial is extracted based on the point cloud, and a virtual point cloud that satisfies the minimum distance to each point in the corresponding medical image space in the previous step (registration optimization phase #1) is extracted. In this study, the piecewise cubic Hermite interpolation method is used, which maintains a polynomial form consisting of coordinate points with less overshoot and undershoot [23]. The process of converting the interval of $[x_k, x_{k+1}]$ to intervals of $[0,1]$ and obtaining the coefficients a_0, a_1, a_2, a_3 of the arbitrary cubic polynomial $p(u)$ is shown below [24].

$$P(u) = a_0 + a_1 u + a_2 u^2 + a_3 u^3 \qquad (1)$$

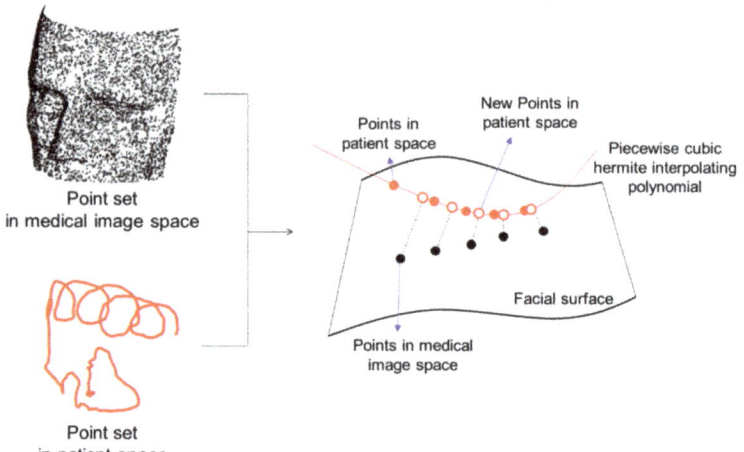

Figure 2. Refinement of the point set in patient space using a piecewise cubic Hermite interpolating polynomial.

The above cubic polynomial consists of four interpolation conditions, corresponding to two function values and two differential values at both endpoints, as follows.

$$P(0) = P_0, \ P(1) = P_1, \ P'(0) = \nabla P_0, \ P'(1) = \nabla P_0 \qquad (2)$$

Polynomials that meet the above conditions can be expressed in the form of a matrix, as follows.

$$P(u) = [u^3 \ u^2 \ u \ 1] \begin{bmatrix} 2 & -2 & 1 & 1 \\ -3 & 3 & -2 & -1 \\ 0 & 0 & 1 & 0 \\ 1 & 0 & 0 & 0 \end{bmatrix} \begin{bmatrix} P_0 \\ P_1 \\ \nabla P_0 \\ \nabla p_1 \end{bmatrix} \qquad (3)$$

2.3. Final ICP Refinement

The extracted medical images and patient spatial point clouds are finally matched by applying the ICP algorithm [15]. The ICP algorithm calculates and matches rotational and translation matrices such that the mean difference between two spatial points is minimized, and is defined by the following formula:

$$\mathbf{f}(R,t) = \mathrm{argmin}_f \sum_{i=1}^{N} \| (Rs_i + t) - c_i \|^2 \qquad (4)$$

Here, *R* and *t*, respectively, refer to the rotational and translation matrices that can minimize the positional error of the two-point cloud. s_i and c_i denote the point cloud in patient space and medical image space, respectively. Optimization processing is done as follows. The distance from one point in the reference space to all points in the transform space is calculated, and the closest point is set as the corresponding point. Corresponding points are extracted by repeating the above process for all points in the reference space, and rotation and translation transformation matrices between the two point sets of the corresponding relationship are calculated. Coordinate transformation is performed through the transformation matrix, and the final transformation matrix is iteratively calculated until the criteria are satisfied. The algorithm iterates until it reaches one of two convergence criteria: either the absolute value of the difference in SRE between two consecutive iterations is below 0.001 or the number of maximum iterations is reached (set as 30 iterations) [25].

3. Validation Study Based on Hemisphere Model

3.1. Hemisphere Modeling

To evaluate the performance of the proposed surface registration algorithm, a hypothetical hemisphere model [26] was created using MATLAB R2018b (MathWorks, Inc., Natick, MA, USA). The surface points of the hemisphere were constructed so that the distribution of points was uniform (Figure 3A). In order to uniformly distribute the points on the surface of the hemisphere, the outer area of a hemisphere with a radius (*r*) of 1 was divided by the number of points *N*. A square was obtained, with area *A* and side length *d*.

$$A = \frac{4\pi r^2}{N} \tag{5}$$

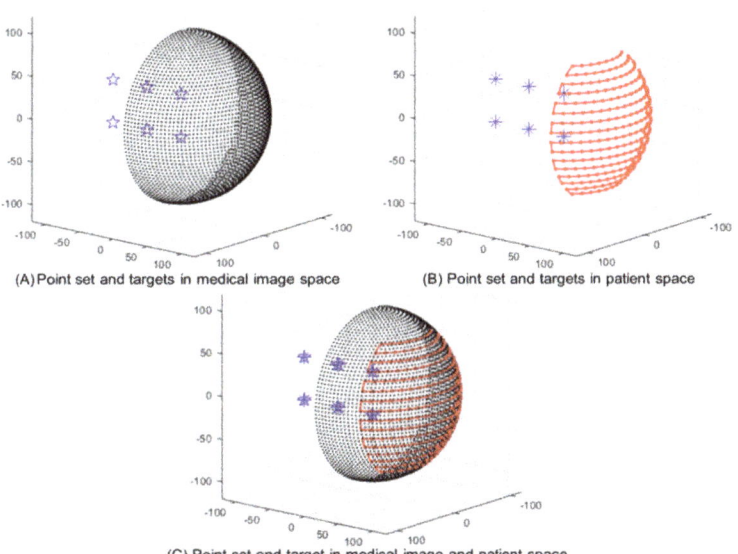

Figure 3. Hemisphere model (**A**–**C**).

The unit angle M_θ was calculated by dividing a semicircle with the arc π belonging to the hemisphere by the length (*d*) of one side of the square (*A*) and rounding up the result.

$$M_\theta = round\left(\frac{\pi}{d}\right) \tag{6}$$

The length π of the semicircle with a radius (r) of 1 was divided by the unit angle M_θ to calculate the gap d_θ between circles with a constant latitude, and the width of the square A was divided by d_θ to calculate the gap (d_φ) between points with constant hardness.

$$d_\theta = \frac{\pi}{M_\theta} \quad \text{and} \quad d_\varphi = \frac{A}{d_\theta} \tag{7}$$

The set of points was placed at constant intervals (d_φ) in circles with constant latitudes and d_φ values, using the previously calculated values of d_θ and d_φ. The radius of the hemisphere was set to 100 mm considering the size of the human face, and it was modeled for eight cases, ranging from 1527 points to 12,100 points, to evaluate the effectiveness of the number of medical image point clouds. The point cloud in the patient space represented the patient's face traced in a left-to-right motion (Figure 3B). The point sets were constructed in the same form as the hemisphere model, and the number of point clusters was limited to 200.

The six target positions (3 rows × 2 columns) were located inside the hemisphere model to evaluate the TRE. The interval between targets was set at 50 mm. The coordinates of each target were [0,0,25], [0,−50,25], [0,−100,25], [0,0,−25], [0,−50,−25], and [0,−100,−25].

3.2. Performance Evaluation of the Proposed Registration Strategy

The performance of registration was evaluated by SRE and TRE. The SRE was obtained by calculating the average distance between the point cloud in the medical image space ($i = 1\ldots n$) and the point cloud that was augmented and registered with the proposed strategy ($i = 1\ldots n$). TRE was obtained by calculating the distance between the target location in the medical image space and the target location in the transformed patient space by applying the transformation matrix obtained through the ICP algorithm [27].

$$SRE = \frac{\sum_{i=1}^{n} \| CT\ point_i - Patient\ point_i \|}{n} \tag{8}$$

$$TRE = \| Target_{CT}P - Target_{Camera}P \| \tag{9}$$

Here, $CT\ point_i$ denotes the ith point of the medical image and $Patient\ point_i$ denotes the ith point of the patient after the transformation is applied. In addition, $Target_{CT}P$ denotes the location of the target measured in the medical image space, and $Target_{Camera}P$ denotes the points that were generated after applying the transformation matrix of the target measured in the patient space.

3.3. Results of the Proposed Registration Strategy Using the Hemisphere Model

To evaluate the proposed registration method, the initial condition (coarse registration effect) was set to coincide with the origin of the hemisphere model composed of the point sets in the medical image and patient space. The rotation matrix was calculated using the ICP optimization process due to the mismatch between the points in each space. The SRE and TRE values were calculated by transforming the points in patient space (Figures 4 and 5). Compared to the initial condition, the SRE was reduced by approximately 1.3% and 33% for the conventional and proposed method, respectively. As the number of points in the medical image increases, the overall trend of SRE decreases. Overall, the error when the proposed algorithm is applied is reduced by an average of about 0.4 (0.2) mm compared to the error when the conventional registration method is used. When the registration results of the proposed method are visualized, the number of points in patient space increases, but the overall error value decreases (Figure 4).

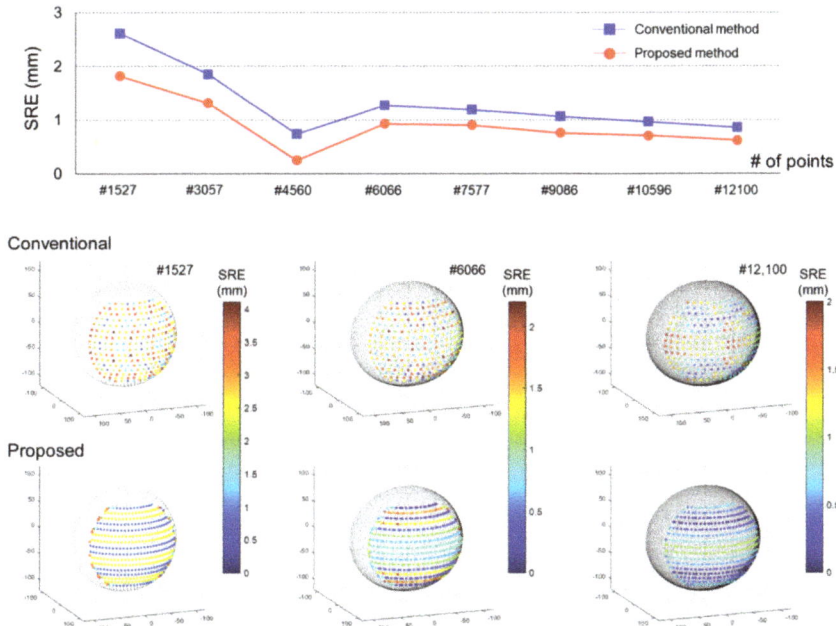

Figure 4. Comparison of surface registration error (SRE) between the conventional and proposed registration strategies using the hemisphere model.

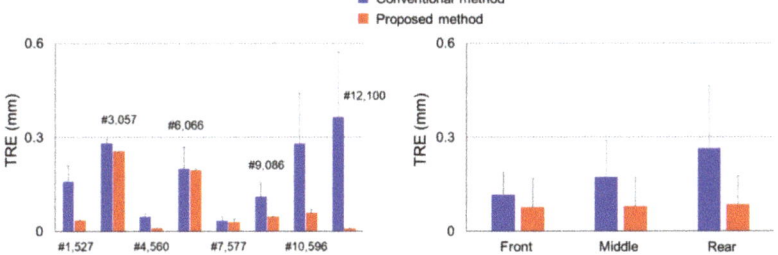

Figure 5. Comparison of target registration error (TRE) between the conventional and proposed registration strategies using the hemisphere model.

TRE using the conventional registration protocol and the proposed registration protocol is demonstrated in Figure 5. Depending on the number of points in the medical image space (8 cases), the TRE varies by about 0.6 mm for the conventional method, and the registration using the proposed protocol was found to be 0.2 (0.1) mm smaller on average. In addition, as the target was located at an inferior position, the conventional registration method showed a larger TRE. However, there was almost no difference in TRE (0.075–0.083 mm) according to the target location.

4. Application to Plastic Facial Phantom

4.1. Design of the Plastic Facial Phantom

To evaluate the applicability of the proposed registration strategy, a plastic facial phantom was created. The basic structure of the phantom consisted of the upper part of a mannequin (the upper part of the chest, the neck, and the head; Figure 6B) and a frame to show the location of the lesion to be inserted inside the mannequin (Figure 6C). The lesion location was printed using an industrial 3D printer (ZPrinter 650, 3Dsystems, Rock Hill, SC, USA) and consisted of three rows in the center on the coronal plane. To evaluate the TRE, 5 lesion targets were placed from the surface of the face towards the back of the head at 20 mm intervals, and a frame with a total of 15 lesion targets (5 targets × 3 rows) was fabricated.

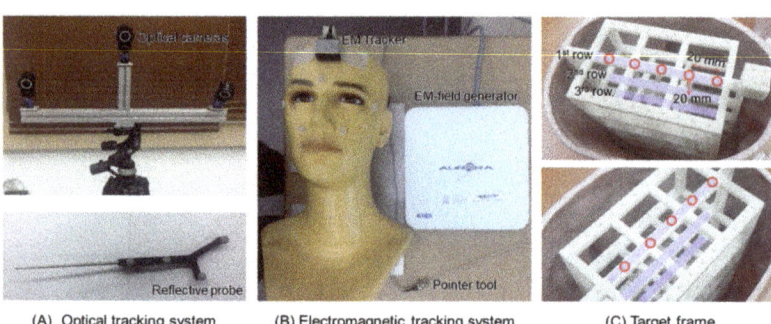

Figure 6. Apparatus and experimental setup (**A–C**).

4.2. Apparatus and Experimental Protocol

CT was performed using medical imaging equipment (Brivo CT 385, General Electronics Medical Systems, Milwaukee, WI, USA) to acquire the location information of the phantom surface. Cross-sectional CT images were taken at 0.5 mm intervals (resolution, 512 × 512 pixels). In addition, an optical tracking device and an electromagnetic tracking device, which are commonly used in clinical practice, were used to acquire the points in the patient space. For the optical devices, three optical cameras (Optitrack Flex 3, Natural points, Corvallis, OR, USA), like those that are generally used for motion capture systems [28,29], and a passive surgical probe (Northern Digital Inc., Waterloo, ON, Canada) were used (Figure 6A). The 3D coordinates of four infrared markers attached to passive probes were obtained using the optical system. The optical system consisted of the three optical cameras, the data acquisition S/W, and the surgical probe. An Aurora electromagnetic tracking system (Northern Digital Inc., Waterloo, ON, Canada) was used to acquire the point cloud of the facial surface (Figure 6B). The system consisted of an electromagnetic field generator, a tracker attached to the surface of the forehead, and a pointer tool to extract the point cloud of the facial surface.

The Medical Imaging Interaction Toolkit (MITK) library was used to acquire 2D tomographic images and the 3D shape of the facial phantom from CT DICOM files. The 3D point sets of the facial surface were extracted using the marching cube technique, and the acquisition range of the 3D points was limited in range from the lip area to the top of the forehead. Patient space coordinates were obtained by tracing the surface of the face using the optical and electromagnetic equipment. The tracing time did not exceed 20 s in order to accurately reflect real clinical situations.

4.3. Experimental Results of the Proposed Registration Strategy

For initial registration (coarse registration) of the point cloud acquired from the medical image and patient space, four coordinate points on the facial surface that could easily be identified were roughly selected. The locations of the four feature points in this study were the tip of the nose, the tips of both eyes, and the glabellar. Subsequently, the transformation matrix (rotation and translation) of the two spaces was extracted using the singular value decomposition method to perform the initial registration. Figure 7 illustrates a typical case of initial registration and shows the difference with ICP precision registration. The difference in the position of the point cloud between the initial registration and the ICP registration in all experimental cases using the plastic facial phantom was found to be about 2 mm on average. Successful initial registration was performed, leading to ICP refinement optimization without local minima.

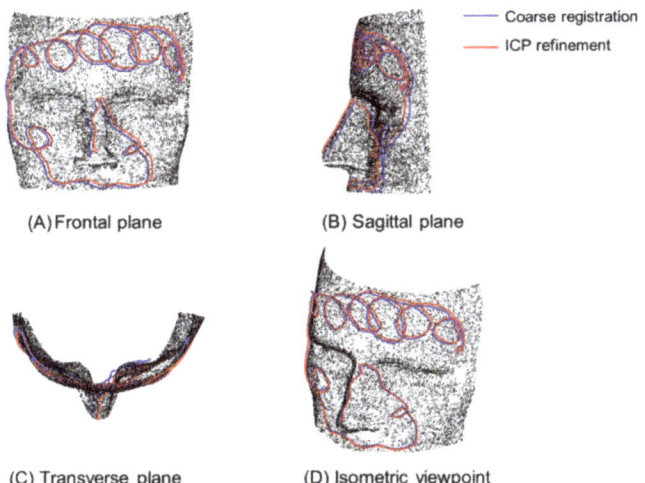

Figure 7. Coarse registration (representative trial) (**A–D**).

Figure 8 shows a comparison of the results of the conventional and proposed registration methods using experimental data from the plastic facial phantom. For the optical tracking system, the average SRE value using the conventional method was 1.36 mm, while the proposed registration method showed a reduced average SRE value of 1.07 mm and an increase in accuracy of about 21% ($p < 0.01$). Additionally, the SRE value in the proposed registration method decreased by about 15% compared to the conventional registration method, and the difference was significant ($p < 0.01$).

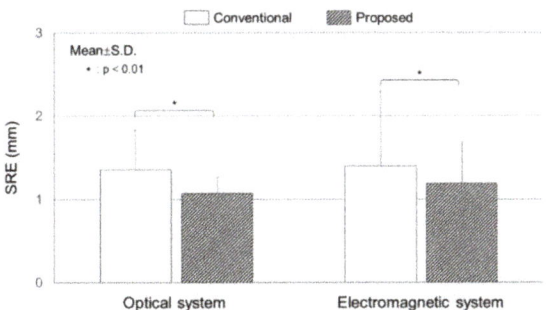

Figure 8. Comparison of SRE between the conventional and proposed registration strategies using the plastic facial phantom.

Figure 9 visually illustrates the difference in SRE between the conventional and proposed registration methods for representative experimental data from 20 replications. The colormap shown on the right side of the figure indicates that the SRE increases as the color goes from blue to red (i.e., blue represents zero). Both the optical and electromagnetic tracking systems produced a wide distribution of blue across the facial surface using the proposed registration method compared to the conventional method, and a significant reduction in errors (red). In the rest of the experiments, both the optical and electromagnetic systems produced similar results (color distributions).

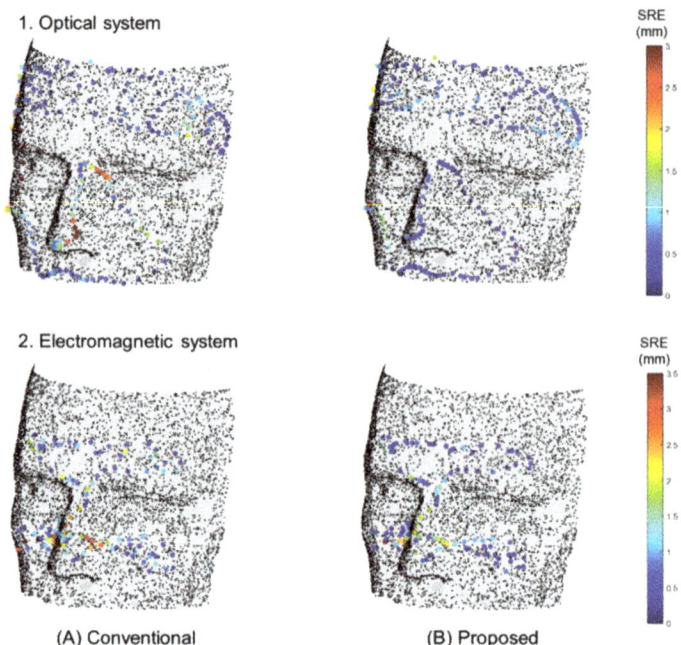

Figure 9. Visualized comparison of SRE between the conventional and proposed registration strategies (representative trials) (**A**,**B**).

Table 1 shows a comparison between the registration methodologies (conventional method vs. proposed method) and the TRE value according to the location of the diseased area. Compared to the existing method, the proposed registration method in this study showed reduced TRE values regardless of the location of the target.

Table 1. Comparison of TRE between the conventional and proposed registration strategies and between target locations in the optical and electromagnetic systems.

	Optical System		Electromagnetic System	
	Conventional	Proposed	Conventional	Proposed
Front	3.10 (0.8)	1.79 (0.6)	4.23 (0.8)	3.37 (1.0)
Middle	3.55 (0.7)	2.65 (0.3)	4.44 (0.9)	3.58 (1.1)
Rear	4.16 (0.6)	3.32 (0.5)	4.90 (1.0)	3.78 (1.0)

5. Discussion

Various attempts have been made to improve the surface matching performance of surgical navigation systems. Recently, in an attempt to reduce the TRE, point clouds in patient space have been extracted using a non-contact method via scanners and other devices [2,7,9,12]. Cao et al. (2008) extracted patient space coordinates using a commercial laser range scanner. The facial surface and the cortical surface of the brain were measured using different cradles, and the size of the scanner device was large and cumbersome, which limited task performance. Recently, Fan et al. (2014, 2017) attempted to easily extract point clouds in patient space using a mobile scanner (Go!SCAN scanner, Sense 3D scanner). The authors were able to extract a point cloud by scanning up to the back of the actual head, resulting in improved matching accuracy. However, since scanners with guaranteed precision are generally expensive and are not integrated with commercial navigation systems [3], their use necessitates an additional coordinate transformation, and there is an increased possibility that cumulative errors will occur in this process. Therefore, the objective of this study is to propose a new protocol that can reduce the registration error by utilizing the face surface tracing method that is currently in widespread clinical use.

In the registration result of the hemisphere model, the SRE tended to decrease as the number of points increased, and the accuracy of the proposed registration protocol was excellent for all cases (Figures 4 and 5). Previous studies have attempted to increase the accuracy of registration by increasing the number of points acquired in the patient space, and the highest accuracy was achieved at 300,000 points [18]. Similar studies also showed that when the number of points increases (up to 40,000), the registration error (about 2 mm) decreases rapidly [7]. This is because the larger the number of points, the higher the positional accuracy of the corresponding points in different spaces. The more points that are located within the same area, the smaller the distance between the points in the corresponding space, thus reducing SRE [10]. However, since the acquisition of many points requires a lot of time and processing steps [7], an appropriate number of points must be determined. The first strategy proposed in this work is based on the results of the existing studies mentioned above. It aims to improve accuracy by performing the matching process in a stepwise manner and establishing appropriate thresholds of differences from previous-stage errors.

The optimal point cloud extraction strategy in patient space that is proposed in this study showed improved performance compared to the conventional registration method in all cases (hemisphere and plastic facial phantom) (Figures 4, 5, 8 and 9 and Table 1). The proposed registration protocol reduces SRE by generating patient space points that correspond as closely as possible to the medical image data cluster through the first point augmentation strategy. In this process, the target position error is decreased by reducing the residual rotation and translation error. Then, a new point cloud is generated in patient space by interpolation of the second strategy, in addition to the medical image and the point cloud in the patient space that has been mapped. In this process, the points in patient space that significantly affect residual rotation and translation error are eliminated and a new point cloud in patient space that best corresponds to the one in medical image space is created. Therefore, we believe that additional reductions in SRE and TRE are possible. As discussed by Yoo et al. (2020b), the registration accuracy can be improved in some cases by acquiring new point sets in patient space through least squares projection. We believe that the registration performance was improved in the present study for similar reasons. In addition, we expect that further improvements in registration accuracy can be achieved by combining the proper point set in patient space proposed in this study.

The limitations of this study are as follows. First, since only a few lesion locations were used for TRE analysis, the accuracy of registration for the locations of various actual lesions could not be conclusively evaluated. In this study, TRE was evaluated using only six lesion locations in the hemisphere model and 15 target lesion locations in the plastic facial phantom. However, it was possible to confirm the superiority of the registration accuracy of the proposed algorithm despite the limited set of lesion locations, and we found that the error rate was reduced by 20% even when the locations of the target lesions were very deep as compared to the existing algorithm. In the future, CT images of actual human faces must be used to evaluate the error rate, given an accurate reflection of human anatomical structure. Second, as the skin tissue of the plastic facial phantom is hard, it was not possible to study the soft tissue of actual human skin and utilize the new technique in actual clinical practice. When obtaining a point cloud in patient space, there are inherent errors in the data due to the flexibility of actual human skin during probe tracing. Future research is required to verify the new registration algorithm, including further experiments on phantoms with skin-like soft tissue and, ultimately, actual clinical validation experiments.

In conclusion, in this study, a new surface registration protocol was proposed to improve the accuracy of a surgical navigation system. To extract the optimal point cloud in patient space before registration, we propose a multi-step registration protocol consisting of augmentation of the point cloud and creation of an optimal point cloud in patient space that satisfies the minimum distance from the point cloud in medical image space. Compared with the conventional method of surface registration, the new protocol showed improvements in SRE and TRE of about 30% and 50%, respectively. In addition, a plastic facial phantom was designed, which was used to verify the accuracy and usefulness of the proposed registration method. The point cloud on the facial surface was obtained in the patient space using optical and electromagnetic systems. As a result of registration, TRE was reduced to about 28% and 21% in the optical and electromagnetic systems, respectively, thus showing improved accuracy. The proposed algorithm is expected to be applied to surgical navigation systems in the near future, which could increase the success rate of otolaryngological and neurological surgery.

Author Contributions: Conceptualization, A.C. and J.-H.M.; methodology, A.C.; validation, S.-S.L. and K.-Y.L.; data curation, S.C. and H.J.; writing—original draft preparation, A.C.; revision, T.-H.K. All authors have read and agreed to the published version of the manuscript.

Funding: This research was supported by the Ministry of Trade, Industry & Energy (MOTIE), Korea Institute for Advancement of Technology (KIAT) through the Encouragement Program for the Industries of the Economic Cooperation Region (P0002272).

Institutional Review Board Statement: Not applicable.

Informed Consent Statement: Not applicable.

Data Availability Statement: Not applicable.

Acknowledgments: Not applicable.

Conflicts of Interest: The authors declare no conflict of interest.

References

1. Min, Z.; Zhu, D.; Ren, H.; Meng, M.Q.H. Feature-guided nonrigid 3-D point set registration framework for image-guided liver surgery: From isotropic positional noise to anisotropic positional noise. *IEEE Trans. Autom. Sci. Eng.* **2021**, *18*, 471–483. [CrossRef]
2. Fan, Y.; Jiang, D.; Wang, M.; Song, Z. A new markerless patient-to-image registration method using a portable 3D scanner. *Med. Phys.* **2014**, *10*, 101910. [CrossRef]
3. Wang, M.N.; Song, Z.J. Properties of the target registration error for surface matching in neuronavigation. *Comput. Aided Surg.* **2011**, *16*, 161–169. [CrossRef] [PubMed]
4. Fan, Y.; Yao, X.; Xu, X. A robust automated surface-matching registration method for neuronavigation. *Med. Phys.* **2020**, *47*, 2755–2767. [CrossRef]
5. Wick, E.H.; Mark, E.; Whipple, M.H.H.; Kris, S.M. Computer-aided rhinoplasty using a novel "navigated" nasal osteotomy technique: A pilot study. *Ann. Otol. Rhinol. Laryngol.* **2021**. [CrossRef]
6. Liu, Y.; Song, Z.; Wang, M. A new robust markerless method for automatic image-to-patient registration in image-guided neurosurgery system. *Comput. Assist. Surg.* **2017**, *22*, 319–325. [CrossRef]
7. Dong, Y.; Zhang, C.; Ji, D.; Wang, M.; Song, Z. Regional-surface-based registration for image-guided neurosurgery: Effects of scan modes on registration accuracy. *Int. J. Comput. Assist. Radiol. Surg.* **2019**, *14*, 1303–1315. [CrossRef] [PubMed]
8. Manning, W.; Zhijian, S. Distribution templates of the fiducial points in image-guided neurosurgery. *Oper. Neurosurg.* **2010**, *66*, ons-143–ons-151. [CrossRef]
9. Cao, A.; Thompson, R.C.; Dumpuri, P.; Dawant, B.M.; Galloway, R.L.; Ding, S.; Miga, M.I. Laser range scanning for image-guided neurosurgery: Investigation of image-to-physical space registrations. *Med. Phys.* **2008**, *35*, 1593–1605. [CrossRef]
10. Yoo, H.; Choi, A.; Kim, H.; Mun, J. A novel surface registration for image-guided neurosurgery: Effects of intervals of points in patient space on registration accuracy. *J. Med. Imaging Health Inform.* **2020**, *10*, 1466–1472. [CrossRef]
11. Eggers, G.; Mühling, J.; Marmulla, R. Image-to-patient registration techniques in head surgery. *Int. J. Oral. Maxillofac. Surg.* **2006**, *35*, 1081–1095. [CrossRef]
12. Fan, Y.; Xu, X.; Wang, M. A surface-based spatial registration method based on sense three-dimensional scanner. *J. Craniofac. Surg.* **2017**, *28*, 157–160. [CrossRef] [PubMed]
13. Min, Z.; Wang, J.; Pan, J.; Meng, M.Q.H. Generalized 3-D point set registration with hybrid mixture models for computer-assisted orthopedic surgery: From isotropic to anisotropic positional error. *IEEE Trans. Autom. Sci. Eng.* **2020**. [CrossRef]
14. Besl, P.J.; McKay, N.D. Method for registration of 3-D shapes. *Int. Soc. Opt. Photonics* **1992**, *1611*, 586–606. [CrossRef]
15. Paraskevopoulos, D.; Unterberg, A.; Metzner, R.; Dreyhaupt, J.; Eggers, G.; Wirtz, C.R. Comparative study of application accuracy of two frameless neuronavigation systems: Experimental error assessment quantifying registration methods and clinically influencing factors. *Neurosurg. Rev.* **2010**, *34*, 217–228. [CrossRef]

16. Mascott, C.R.; Sol, J.C.; Bousquet, P.; Lagarrigue, J.; Lazorthes, Y.; Lauwers-Cances, V. Quantification of true in vivo (application) accuracy in cranial image-guided surgery: Influence of mode of patient registration. *Neurosurgery* **2006**, *59*, 146–156. [CrossRef]
17. Yoo, H.; Choi, A.; Kim, H.; Mun, J. Acquisition of point cloud in CT image space to improve accuracy of surface registration: Application to neurosurgical navigation system. *J. Mech. Sci. Technol.* **2020**, *34*, 2667–2677. [CrossRef]
18. Marmulla, R.; Lüth, T.; Mühling, J.; Hassfeld, S. Automated laser registration in image-guided surgery: Evaluation of the correlation between laser scan resolution and navigation accuracy. *Int. J. Oral. Maxillofac. Surg.* **2004**, *33*, 642–648. [CrossRef]
19. Jiang, L.; Zhang, S.; Yang, J.; Zhuang, X.; Zhang, L.; Gu, L. A robust automated markerless registration framework for neurosurgery navigation. *Int. J. Med. Robot.* **2015**, *11*, 436–447. [CrossRef]
20. Velusamy, A.; Anand, A.; Hameed, N. Navigation assisted frontal sinus osteoplastic flap surgeries—A case series. *Indian J. Otolaryngol. Head Neck Surg.* **2021**. [CrossRef]
21. Keeble, H.; Lavrador, J.P.; Pereira, N.; Lente, K.; Brogna, C.; Gullan, R.; Bhangoo, R.; Vergani, F.; Ashkan, K. Electromagnetic navigation systems and intraoperative neuromonitoring: Reliability and feasibility study. *Oper. Neurosurg.* **2021**, *20*, 373–382. [CrossRef] [PubMed]
22. Liu, Y.; Yu, H.; Zhen, H. Navigation-assisted, endonasal, endoscopic optic nerve decompression for the treatment of nontraumatic optic neuropathy. *Craniomaxillofac. Surg.* **2019**, *47*, 328–333. [CrossRef]
23. Hintzen, N.T.; Piet, G.J.; Brunel, T. Improved estimation of trawling tracks using cubic Hermite spline interpolation of position registration data. *Fish. Res.* **2010**, *101*, 108–115. [CrossRef]
24. Kulkarni, P.G.; Sahasrabudhe, A.D. A dynamic model of ball bearing for simulating localized defects on outer race using cubic hermite spline. *J. Mech. Sci. Technol.* **2014**, *28*, 3433–3442. [CrossRef]
25. Lee, J.D.; Huang, C.H.; Wang, S.T. Fast-MICP for frameless image-guide surgery. *Med. Phys.* **2010**, *37*, 4551–4559. [CrossRef] [PubMed]
26. Deserno, M. *How to Generate Equidistributed Points on the Surface of a Sphere*; Max-Planck-Institut fur Polymerforschung: Mainz, Germany, 2004.
27. Min, Z.; Zhu, D.; Liu, J.; Ren, H.; Meng, M.Q.H. Aligning 3D curve with surface using tangent and normal vectors for computer-assisted orthopedic surgery. *IEEE Trans. Med. Robot. Bionics* **2021**, *3*, 372–383. [CrossRef]
28. Kim, H.; Moon, J.; Ha, H.; Lee, J.; Yu, J.; Chae, S.; Mun, J.H.; Choi, A. Can a deep learning model estimate low back torque during a golf swing? *Int. J. Biotech. Sports Eng.* **2021**, *2*, 59–65.
29. Choi, A.; Kang, T.G.; Mun, J.H. Biomechanical evaluation of dynamic balance control ability during golf swing. *J. Med. Biol. Eng.* **2016**, *36*, 430–439. [CrossRef]

Article

Detection of Movement Intention for Operating Methods of Serious Games

Jung-Hyun Park [1], Ho-Sang Moon [2], Hyunggun Kim [3,*] and Sung-Taek Chung [1,*]

1. Department of Computer Engineering, Korea Polytechnic University, Siheung 15073, Korea; andi95@kpu.ac.kr
2. Department of Advanced Technology Fusion, Korea Polytechnic University, Siheung 15073, Korea; hosang0815@kpu.ac.kr
3. Department of Biomechatronic Engineering, Sungkyunkwan University, Suwon 16419, Korea
* Correspondence: hkim.bme@skku.edu (H.K.); unitaek@kpu.ac.kr (S.-T.C.); Tel.: +82-(31)-290-7821 (H.K.); +82-(10)-2770-2100 (S.-T.C.)

Abstract: In many post-stroke cases, patients show dysfunctions in movement, cognition, sense, and language, depending on the damaged area of the brain. Active and repetitive physical rehabilitation centered on the stroke-affected side is essential for effective and rapid neurological recovery of upper extremity dysfunction due to hemiplegia. A symmetric upper extremity trainer is utilized to assist the patient body, depending upon the degree of hemiplegia. In this study, we developed a novel balance handle as a symmetric upper extremity trainer capable of extension, flexion, pronation, and supination of the upper extremity. We collected the surface electromyogram (sEMG) signal data while the subjects were playing a serious game and recorded the electroencephalogram (EEG) signal data while the subjects were performing basic movements with the balance handle, to analyze the effectiveness of the device as an assistive tool for rehabilitation. The triceps brachii were activated during the extension movements, whereas the biceps brachii and deltoid muscles were activated during the flexion movements. With the balance handle, the peak event-related desynchronization (ERD) values were relatively lower while showing higher peak event-related synchronization (ERS) values compared to other types of operating methods, such as hand gripping and gamepad operation. Movement intention of tilting the balance handle for the α and β waves was clearly distinguished from the other tasks. These data demonstrated the potential of various applications using the developed proof-of-concept upper extremity trainer to bring out an excellent rehabilitative effect not only through muscle growth but also via identification of large movement intentions inducing brain activation exercise.

Keywords: bilateral movement training; event-related desynchronization; hemiplegia; serious game; symmetric upper extremity trainer

Citation: Park, J.-H.; Moon, H.-S.; Kim, H.; Chung, S.-T. Detection of Movement Intention for Operating Methods of Serious Games. *Appl. Sci.* **2021**, *11*, 883. https://doi.org/10.3390/app11020883

Received: 7 December 2020
Accepted: 15 January 2021
Published: 19 January 2021

Publisher's Note: MDPI stays neutral with regard to jurisdictional claims in published maps and institutional affiliations.

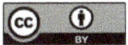

Copyright: © 2021 by the authors. Licensee MDPI, Basel, Switzerland. This article is an open access article distributed under the terms and conditions of the Creative Commons Attribution (CC BY) license (https://creativecommons.org/licenses/by/4.0/).

1. Introduction

1.1. Background

A commendable outcome, in recent years, of the enormous advancement in medical science is the continuous decrease in mortality rate of stroke [1]. However, in many post-stroke cases, patients show dysfunctions in movement, cognition, sense, and language, depending on the damaged area of the brain [2]. In particular, hemiplegia that occurs on the opposite side of the damaged brain reduces locomotor function of the affected extremity and causes an unstable balance sense, which in turn reduces the activities of daily living (ADL), such as walking, eating, and dressing [3,4]. Symptoms of movement disorders due to hemiplegia are normally more notable in the upper extremity than the lower one [5]. Upper extremity functions are closely related to the activities of exploring and manipulating the surrounding environment; therefore, the upper extremity is particularly important for the ADL and workability. Thus, active and repetitive physical rehabilitation centered on the stroke-affected side is essential for effective and rapid neurological recovery of upper extremity dysfunction due to hemiplegia [6].

The methods to improve the stroke-affected movement functions of the upper extremity include constraint-induced movement therapy, rehabilitation robotics, mirror therapy, and bilateral movement training [7–9]. Specifically, the bilateral movement training utilizes substitution, in which the neural network of the healthy side compensates for the functions of the neural network of the stroke-affected side by simultaneously activating the neural networks of both the healthy and pathologic sides [10]. In general, a symmetric upper extremity trainer is utilized to assist the patient body, depending upon the degree of hemiplegia. Recent studies have attempted to associate the rehabilitation equipment used to improve or treat physical abilities with serious games, applying game elements such as fun and challenge. Such programs are considered to increase the patients' intention to rehabilitate and effectively recovers the physical abilities by reducing the rejection or boredom of treatment that patients may have [11]. Moreover, it can help users actively perform steady repetitive exercises, which are the most important in rehabilitation, by offering them a sense of reality beyond the limited user interface of the serious games, consisting of a keyboard, mouse, and specific buttons and sticks [12,13].

In this study, a novel balance handle was manufactured as a symmetric upper extremity trainer to enable bilateral rehabilitation movements, such as extension, flexion, pronation, and supination of the upper extremity. The balance handle was connected to a serious game, and a surface electromyogram (sEMG) was measured for the triceps brachii, biceps brachii, and deltoid to assess the muscular activation while the users played the game. The sEMG signal has the advantage of quantitatively evaluating physical function and tracking the results of the rehabilitation treatment by measuring and analyzing the motor signals expressed in the central nervous system (CNS) in muscle nerves. Additionally, an electroencephalogram (EEG) was used to evaluate brain activation while the subjects performed the rehabilitation movement process with the symmetric upper extremity trainer. Reorganization of the damaged CNS was confirmed by evaluating the activation of the motor cortex from the EEG signals [14]. In order to analyze the activation of the motor cortex quantitatively, the signals measured by the symmetrical upper extremity trainer were compared with other types of operating methods for serious games, such as hand gripping and gamepad.

The EEG signals associated with the movement function helps analyze all the time points of body movement pertaining to an idle rhythm, a state in which a set of neurons in the motor cortex simultaneously displays a periodic signal. Movement intention can then be predicted by analyzing the signal that appears before actual movement occurs [15]. When movement intention of the body is found in the idle rhythm state, an event-related desynchronization (ERD) phenomenon, in which the power decreases at a specific frequency band by the excitatory postsynaptic potential (EPSP), occurs. Following the motion, an event-related synchronization (ERS) phenomenon, in which the power increases again at a specific frequency band by the inhibitory postsynaptic potential (IPSP), occurs. The movement intention can be analyzed using ERD and ERS and employed as a good indicator to quantitatively measure the willingness and movement of patients participating in training, as it demonstrates a statistical difference between rest and movement as well as between different types of movement [16]. The movement intention was calculated through the ERD/ERS analysis that can show the CNS activities based on the spontaneous shifting of the measured EEG signals. The difference between the groups according to the operating methods was compared by verifying the normality and performing the two-way analysis of variance (ANOVA).

1.2. Related Work

Recent studies compared the effects of upper extremity trainers as well as attempted to quantitatively measure movements or increase the effectiveness of rehabilitation. A variety of customized trainers were developed to rehabilitate specific areas of the upper extremities.

Movements of an end-effector robot capable of horizontal plane movement of the unilateral forearm were quantitatively evaluated by moving a hand on a desk [17]. Assist-as-needed training was conducted using an end-effector upper limb rehabilitation robot that helps patients keep their arm close to a specific trajectory [18]. Information technology (IT), including virtual reality (VR) and mobile applications, was integrated for accessible and structured rehabilitation. VR has great strength in interaction and was employed as a therapeutic treatment tool for rehabilitation of the upper extremities of stroke patients [19]. A mobile application was also developed as a useful tool for subject-specific rehabilitation of the upper extremity following stroke [20].

The balance handle developed in this study can assist movement with respect to the various axes, including extension, flexion, pronation, and supination of the upper extremity, by allowing movements on the coronal and sagittal planes unlike traditional trainers applying along a single axis. Improved effectiveness of rehabilitation is expected by symmetrically performing bilateral movements of both upper extremities at the same time compared to performing unilateral movements. Furthermore, this balance handle can be utilized to quantitively measure movement data with respect to various tilting angles and collect real time feedback data via Bluetooth connection.

2. Materials and Methods

2.1. Manufacture of the Balance Handle

We developed a novel balance handle as a symmetrical upper extremity trainer for extension, flexion, pronation, and supination of the upper extremity. The balance handle comprised a balance ball, arm holders, and handles (Figure 1).

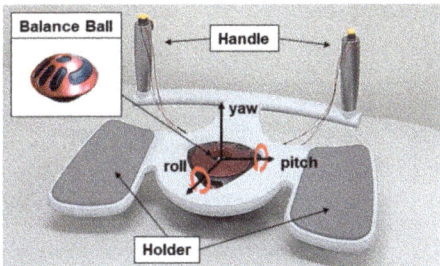

Figure 1. The components of the balance handle.

The spherical balance ball positioned at the center between the arm holders was designed to calculate its slope through an inertial measurement unit (IMU) sensor and send the data through a Bluetooth module that did not interfere with the user movement. A user with weak upper extremity muscle can comfortably place both upper extremity forearms on the holders, hold the handle, and move it freely towards the longitudinal and lateral axes. Furthermore, the user can push the buttons on the edges of both handles to add more input data if needed. We used an AM530 sensor (Laxtha, Daejeon, Korea) to measure the sEMG signals and a cap-type EMOTIV EPOC Flex (Emotiv, San Francisco, CA, USA) to measure the EEG signals through up to 32 channels to examine the muscular (sEMG data) and brain (EEG data) activation of the subjects while using the balance handle.

2.2. Measurement of the Muscular Activation Using the Balance Handle

Users activated the major upper extremity muscles by moving the balance handle forward, backward, leftward, or rightward. Figure 2 displays the serious game developed to induce these movements. Figure 2a shows the jet ski moving up and down as the user tilted the balance handle forward and backward through extension and flexion of the upper extremity. Figure 2b demonstrates the jet ski moving leftward and rightward as the user tilts the balance handle to the left and to the right through pronation and supination of both upper extremity forearms. The user gained score points, the competitive element of the serious game, by acquiring the displayed fuel and increase the content execution time. The score was deducted if the user failed to avoid an obstacle. The highest score among the participants was displayed on the screen to encourage competition.

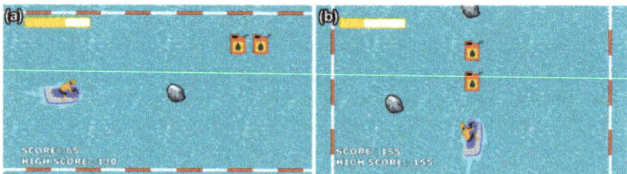

Figure 2. Serious game contents for surface electromyogram (sEMG) measurement: (**a**) forward–backward inclination; (**b**) left–right inclination.

2.3. Movement Intention Test

Ten adults (eight males and two females) in their twenties (average age 25.0 ± 1.7 years old) with no experience of a damaged upper extremity participated in the experimental tests to perform three operations: hand gripping, gamepad operation, and operation of the symmetric upper extremity trainer similar to the Oddball Paradigm, to compare the movement intention according to the operation methods for the serious game content (Figure 3).

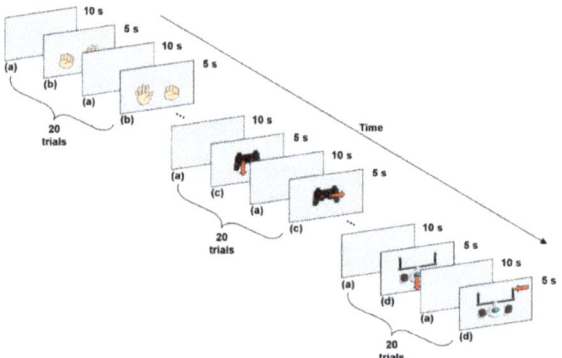

Figure 3. Sequence of the experimental task: (**a**) inter-stimulus interval; (**b**) grip task; (**c**) gamepad task; and (**d**) balance handle task.

All the tasks were divided into preparation, stimulation, and rest stages, to reduce their mutual influences before and after each task. A performance of 5 s was classified as a single trial, and each operation was repeated 20 times to minimize any error during the test process. Figure 3a demonstrates the rest stage after the stimulation stage between the repeated tasks as a blank page in the preparation stage. The rest stage gives a measure of the reference in the idle rhythm state before presenting a visual stimulus. The purpose of the data measured at the preparation stage for 5 s was to measure the changes in the data related to movement, and the relative amplitude was then calculated from these data. The EEG signals of the reaction to the visual stimulus on the screen were recorded during the stimulation stage. The rest stage was the idle moment before performing the next task; therefore, no data during the rest stage were used in the analysis.

The grip task was to perform extension and flexion of the finger used in an intuitive operation, such as using a keyboard or touching the screen, while the upper extremity remained fixed. The contents were composed to indicate one of the hands to grip; this for the user to perform the same task shown on the screen without bending the wrist

(Figure 3b). A product from Joytron, consisting of nine general buttons, two analog sticks, one cross button, and two trigger buttons, was utilized to conduct the gamepad task. The screen displayed red arrows to instruct the user to move to the right or to the left with the analog stick or to press the specified general button (Figure 3c). Lastly, for the task involving the trainer interfaced with the serious game, the screen showed red arrows to instruct the users to tilt the symmetrical upper extremity trainer (i.e., the balance handle) forward, backward, leftward, or rightward, or press the button on the handle (Figure 3d). The system was configured so that the task instruction was displayed in a random order to prevent the test subjects from predicting and acting on the stimulus in each task, and the number of repetitions was set to be the same in all the directions for straightforward comparison.

2.4. Measurement of the EMG and EEG Signals

With the balance handle, the subjects performed extension and flexion of their upper extremity and pronation and supination movements of their joints, including shoulder, elbows, and forearms, according to the device tilting movement. In order to collect and analyze the sEMG signal data, an AM530 active surface EMG sensor (Laxtha, Daejeon, Korea) was attached to the deltoid, biceps, and triceps while the reference electrodes were attached to the elbow joint where there was no change in muscle activity (Figure 4). The sEMG signal data were collected at a 1-kHz sampling frequency via serial communication.

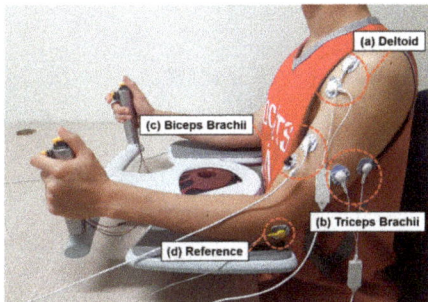

Figure 4. Positions of the electrodes attached to collect sEMG signals.

The EEG signal data were collected for analysis of brain activation at a sampling frequency of 1024 Hz and filtered through a band pass filter (BPF) ranging from 0.16 to 43 Hz and a notch filter at 50 and 60 Hz, such that the EEG signal data in the frequency band were selectively collected and the noises induced by the power were removed. Following the 10–20 international system of EEG electrode placement, 32 signal electrodes (hollow white) and 2 ground electrodes (solid black) were configured with two channels (C3 and C4) used to analyze the movement intention, displayed in red in Figure 5.

The C3 and C4 channels were positioned on the sensorimotor cortex encompassing the motor cortex and somatosensory cortex in the central part of the cerebrum. Activation of the sensorimotor cortex is closely associated with human body movement, which can be directly correlated with the analysis of movement intention [21]. Moreover, the ERD and ERS related to movement occur prominently in the opposite hemisphere of the moving body part, and therefore the EEG data collected in the opposite hemisphere of the moving hand were utilized for analyses of the hand gripping and gamepad operation. For the task of using the balance handle with both hands, arithmetic averages of the collected data from each hemisphere were analyzed.

2.5. Signal Processing and Data Analysis

The root mean square (RMS) values of the sEMG signal data measured from the upper extremities were calculated to quantify muscle energy. A 50-ms window was used to capture the rapid dynamic contraction of the joint movement of the upper extremity. In order to compare the muscle activation trends between the main upper extremity muscles according to basic movement, down-sampling was performed at 10-ms intervals, followed by smoothing through a moving average filter at 300 ms (Figure 6).

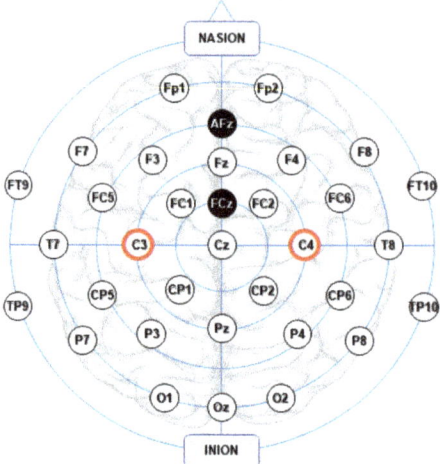

Figure 5. The 10–20 international system of EEG electrode placement.

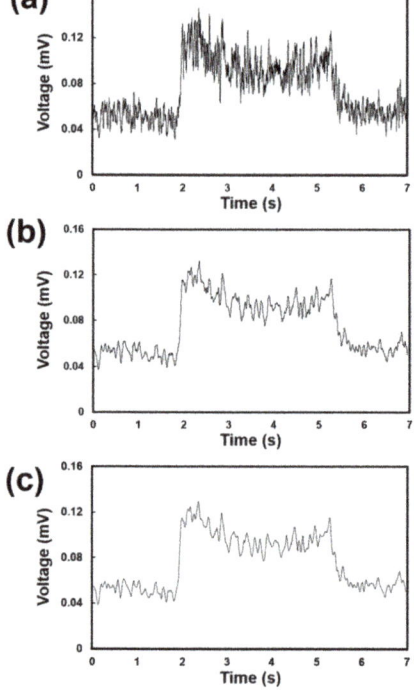

Figure 6. Signal processing procedures for sEMG data: (**a**) raw sEMG; (**b**) RMS for the raw data; and (**c**) down-sampling and moving averaging.

On the other hand, as the time series data of the EEG signals were vulnerable to noises from the surrounding environment, a signal-processing protocol, containing a suitable filter and quantification processes, was designed to calculate the ERD/ERS data (Figure 7).

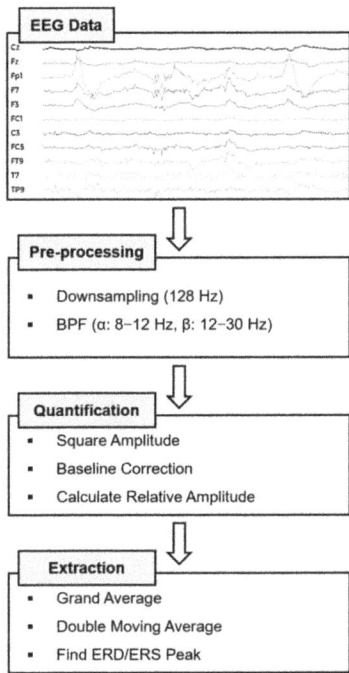

Figure 7. Flowchart of the signal processing for the event-related desynchronization (ERD)/event-related synchronization (ERS) calculation.

The EEG data collected at a frequency of 1024 Hz were down-sampled to 128 Hz, and since the length of the input signal was sufficiently long, the FIR (finite impulse response) filters for the α (8–12 Hz) and β (12–30 Hz) waves were employed to obtain the time series data for a specific frequency band and remove the high-frequency noises at the same time. The relative amplitude (RA) values for the idle rhythm state and the upper extremity movement due to the stimulus were calculated for quantification using Equations (1)–(3). Equation (1) signifies the rectification process that converts a negative EEG signal into a positive amplitude to assure that the sum of the amplitudes would not be zero. Equations (2) and (3) refer to extraction of the RA. In Equation (2), the pre-stimulus baseline is calculated to examine the relative impact of the stimulus. The RA is then calculated by subtracting the reference value from the time series data at each point in Equation (3). Here, N refers to the total number of executions, y to the BPF process data of the jth sample of the ith trial, $Act(j)$ to the average of the squared jth sample, and R to the reference, indicating the average of the section of 1 to 2 s prior to the stimulus.

$$Act_{(j)} = \frac{1}{N} \sum_{i=1}^{N} y_{ij} \qquad (1)$$

$$R = \frac{1}{k+1} \sum_{j=r_0}^{r_0+k} Act_{(j)} \qquad (2)$$

$$RA_{(j)}(\%) = \left(\frac{Act_{(j)} - R}{R}\right) \times 100 \tag{3}$$

Due to the difficulty in identifying the RA pattern only with a single trial, the average of the multi-trial data was employed to eliminate the extreme outliers in the data and minimize noise. Moreover, the double moving average was used to more clearly represent the data patterns. As the ERD peak was detected before a stimulus was given, the minimum value was selected among the data collected 1 to 2 s before a stimulus occurred. The ERS peak was selected as the maximum value at 1 s after occurrence on the stimulus. The minimum ERD and the maximum ERS values are the key states of the CNS that express participation in the activity of responses to movement or stimulus, indicating an induced response of changes in EEG oscillation [22]. Averaging the induced response allowed us to minimize the noise data and increase the signal-to-noise ratio (SNR). As the change in the stimulus became more notable in the idle state, the amplitudes were compared with each other to determine the cognitive characteristics.

The normality of each data group was verified to compare the movement intention according to the operating method, and the two-way ANOVA was performed with a statistical significance level of 0.05. This method allowed us to solve the increase in type-I error due to the multi-test problem when repeatedly using t-tests in multiple group comparisons, and also to validate the difference between groups with two or more independent variables. Therefore, we distinguished the tasks as a group of independent variables and set the α and β waves as independent variables and the ERD/ERS peak values as a dependent variable. The resulting F statistic was the difference between groups for intra-group differences, and the larger the F-value, the more pronounced the difference between the groups.

3. Results

3.1. sEMG during Operation of the Balance Handle

The sEMG signal data were recorded while the subjects operated the balance handle. In Figure 8a, "A" shows the inclination angles of the balance handle while the subjects performed the serious game by tilting the balance handle forward and backward. The sEMG signals measured while doing the extension and flexion movements from the triceps, biceps, and deltoid muscles are displayed in "B", "C", and "D", respectively. During extension movement by tilting the balance handle forward, the greatest muscle activation was found in the triceps muscle ("B"). During flexion movement by tilting the balance handle backward, the largest muscle activation was observed in the biceps ("C"). In Figure 8b, "A" demonstrates the inclination angles of the balance handle while the subjects performed the serious game by tilting the balance handle leftward and rightward. The muscle activation in the right deltoid muscle during tilting the balance handle to the left was displayed in "B", and the muscle activation in the left deltoid during tilting the balance handle to the right was displayed in "C". As the muscle activation while using the balance handle demonstrated a similar tendency as other conventional upper extremity trainers, it was successfully validated that our balance handle was appropriate for interfacing with a serious game to conduct rehabilitation exercise programs [23].

3.2. EEG for the Movement Intention Test

Figure 9 shows representative RA patterns of the three types of operational methods (hand gripping, gamepad operation, and balance handle operation). It was clearly observed that the ERD phenomenon of the α and β waves temporarily decreased immediately after the "start", which represented the occurrence time of the stimulus in the "stimuli" section. ERD generally refers to a temporary change in negative potential due to an instantaneous increase in the excitatory signals of the cortical neurons during the preparation for body movement; therefore, an analysis of ERD allows to determine the movement intention [24]. On the other hand, ERS occurring after an action is performed is accompanied with an increase in the α and β waves due to the positive potential changes following deactivation of the nervous system due to inhibitory signals. This refers to conversion into an idle state and, in the EEG tests, it was confirmed that ERS occurred after ERD in the "stimuli" section. Although the times of ERD/ERS in the RA patterns of the three operational methods were found to be similar, the magnitude of the amplitude with the balance handle was the largest, and the smallest magnitude of the amplitude was found with the gamepad.

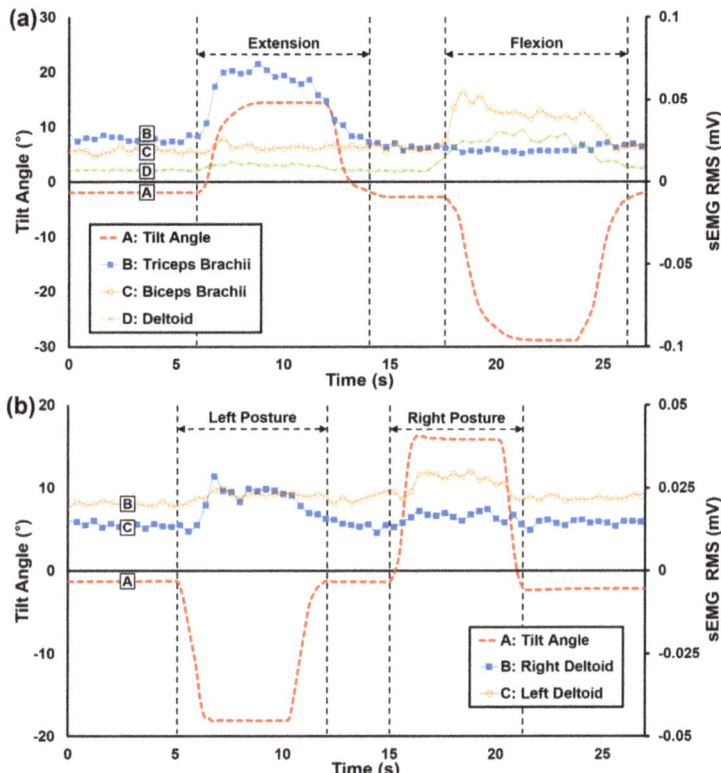

Figure 8. The sEMG signal data corresponding to the tilting angles of the balance handle: (**a**) extension and flexion; (**b**) pronation and supination.

Figure 10 demonstrates the box and whisker plots of the α and β waves of each task to quantitatively compare the magnitude of the amplitudes. As tilting the balance handle using the upper extremity was a physically different movement from pressing the buttons, tilting and button pressing were classified into Handle_I and Handle_B, respectively. The box represents the range of the first and third quartiles, the horizontal line in the box defines the second quartile, the x mark refers to the median, and the whisker indicates the range of the minimum and maximum values. The ERD/ERS peak distributions of the α and β waves were similar. The ERD peak indicated the lowest average value (α: −105.7%; and β: −81.1%) in the Handle_I task, whereas the ERS peak indicated the higher peak value of the Handle_I task (α: −188.9%; and β: 141.9%) and the Handle_B task (α: 171.3%; and β: 146.1%). A comparison of the average ERD values showed that tilting the balance handle resulted in the highest movement intention. Although pressing the button on the balance handle was physically not much different from hand gripping or pressing the button on the gamepad, a low ERD peak and a high ERS peak values were observed, expressing relatively high movement intention. However, several outliers were found in the Handle_B task due to the relatively low reproducibility of the ERS, resulting in large deviation. These outlier data are consistent with previous studies that reported that ERS might not be necessarily associated with signal generation or muscle activation in the motor cortex and rather reflected the short-term state to inhibit the motor cortex network [25]. Therefore, we intended to analyze the variance to verify the statistical significance of the ERD and ERS peak values for each task.

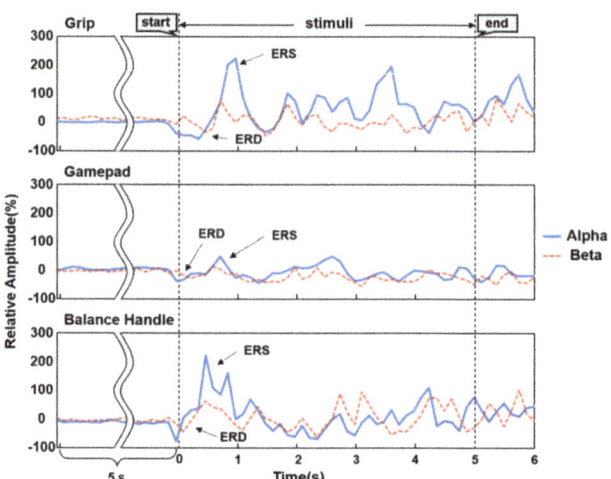

Figure 9. RA measurements with the hand gripping, gamepad operation, and balance handle operation.

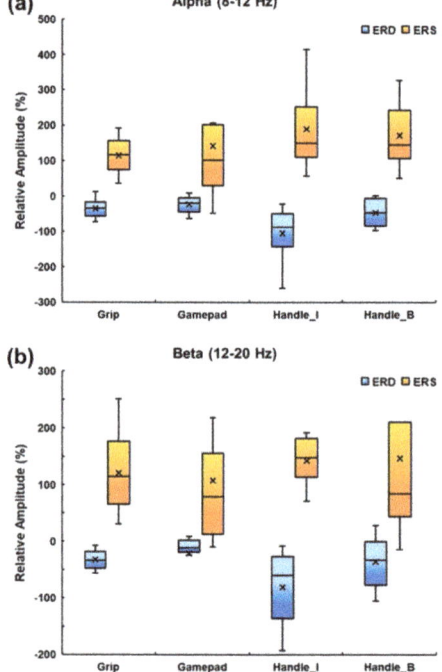

Figure 10. Box and whisker plots of the ERD/ERS peak values: (**a**) α wave (8–12 Hz); (**b**) β wave (12–20 Hz).

Table 1 shows the outcomes of the normality test. The Shapiro–Wilk method, suitable for less than 2000 samples, was used in the normality test. A normal distribution was considered if the *p*-value was larger than 0.05. The *p*-values for both the α and β waves of ERD were larger than 0.05, confirming that these data had a normal distribution. However, for the α wave ERS in the hand gripping and gamepad operation tasks, and for the β wave ERS in the balance handle button task, the normality was not verified, presumably attributing to the outliers found in the process of extracting the ERS peak values.

Table 1. Normality tests for the ERD and ERS peak values (* $p < 0.05$).

Peak	Rhythm	Task	Shapiro–Wilk Significance
ERD	α 8–12 Hz	Grip	0.111
		Gamepad	0.328
		Handle_I	0.278
		Handle_B	0.746
	β 12–30 Hz	Grip	0.198
		Gamepad	0.605
		Handle_I	0.052
		Handle_B	0.802
ERS	α 8–12 Hz	Grip	0.006 *
		Gamepad	0.023 *
		Handle_I	0.271
		Handle_B	0.589
	β 12–30 Hz	Grip	0.080
		Gamepad	0.090
		Handle_I	0.956
		Handle_B	0.005 *

Table 2 demonstrates the comparative data from the two-way ANOVA at a significance level 0.05 to identify the difference between the tasks with the operational methods and the post-hoc analysis using the Bonferroni method.

Table 2. Two-way ANOVA and post-hoc analysis (data shown as the mean ± SD, * $p < 0.05$).

	Rhythm	Task	Relative Amplitude (%)	F-Value	*p*-Value	Post-hoc
ERD	α 8–12 Hz	Grip (a)	−35.2 ± 26.4	6.914	<0.00 *	a, b, d > c (Bonferroni)
		Gamepad (b)	−23.1 ± 23.5			
		Handle_I (c)	−105.7 ± 72.0			
		Handle_B (d)	−46.8 ± 36.3			
	β 12–30 Hz	Grip (a)	−33.0 ± 16.4	3.567	<0.02 *	b > c (Bonferroni)
		Gamepad (b)	−21.4 ± 44.1			
		Handle_I (c)	−81.1 ± 60.9			
		Handle_B (d)	−36.3 ± 42.2			
ERS	α 8–12 Hz	Grip (a)	114.0 ± 48.2	0.782	0.512	
		Gamepad (b)	141.7 ± 175.4			
		Handle_I (c)	188.9 ± 122.7			
		Handle_B (d)	171.3 ± 86.5			
	β 12–30 Hz	Grip (a)	120.4 ± 67.1	0.247	0.863	
		Gamepad (b)	107.1 ± 117.9			
		Handle_I (c)	141.9 ± 40.5			
		Handle_B (d)	146.1 ± 186.1			

The α wave ERD revealed that the Handle_I task was more significant than the other three tasks ($F(3,6) = 6.914$, $p < 0.05$), and the F-value indicating the difference between the groups was clearly larger than the other groups. The β wave ERD showed that the Handle_I task significantly decreased for the gamepad operation task ($F(3,6) = 3.567$, $p < 0.05$). On the other hand, the ERS of the α and β waves demonstrated a large difference within the group but a small difference between the groups, and outliers were found in some data, indicating that these data were not suitable for comparison. Therefore, movement intention of tilting the balance handle for the α and β waves was clearly distinguished from the other tasks through ERD comparison; however, as the normality test of the ERS was not passed, there was no process characteristics found while recovering to the idle rhythm state after movement.

4. Discussion

Most of the post-stroke patients with hemiplegia have dysfunction of the upper extremity. The usage of an assistive trainer capable of bilateral exercise to help these patients exercise is an effective rehabilitation strategy [26]. Moreover, studies using serious games to reduce the rejection and boredom of patients toward treatment and induce voluntary participation have been actively ongoing in recent years [27]. In the present study, we developed a novel balance handle as a symmetric upper extremity trainer capable of extension, flexion, pronation, and supination of the upper extremity. We collected the sEMG signal data while the subjects were playing a serious game and recorded the EEG signal data while the subjects were performing basic movements with the balance handle, to analyze the effectiveness of the device as an assistive tool for rehabilitation. In particular, the effectiveness test using the EEG signals was conducted to compare the movement intention with the balance handle to the movement intention in other types of operational methods (hand gripping and gamepad operation) via analysis of the ERD and ERS values. Normality tests were also conducted, and two-way ANOVA and post-hoc analyses were performed for comparative studies.

The triceps brachii were activated during the extension movements, whereas the biceps brachii and deltoid muscles were activated during the flexion movements. The deltoid muscles on the opposite side were activated during the tilting of the balance handle to the left or to the right. This ensured that the extensor and flexor muscle activities, essential for increasing the hand and foot functions while moving the balance handle, were properly executed, demonstrating similar sEMG characteristics to other upper extremity trainers [28]. With the balance handle, the ERD peak values were relatively lower while showing higher ERS peak values compared to other types of operating methods. It was noteworthy that the task of pressing the balance handle button revealed a decrease in the ERD peak compared to the task of hand gripping and gamepad operation, which did not show much difference in exercise volume. The lower the ERD peak was, the higher the movement intention was; therefore, it can be inferred that a higher level of movement intention was expressed in the task of utilizing the balance handle [29]. However, for the ERS peak, the higher values reflected more short-term states of inhibiting movement, which corresponds to a previous study that the ERS phenomenon was not necessarily associated with muscle activation in motor cortical networks [30]. As there were some outliers found and data normality was not achieved, detailed classification of the frequency bands needs to be further conducted to reduce individual differences related to motor functions.

Most of the previous studies have demonstrated the prediction of movement intention for only a single type of upper extremity movement or either left or right side of the body movement using ERD analysis [31,32]. By contrast, the present study derived movement intention while users operated the balance handle, and showed a considerable difference compared to the other types of operational methods. These data demonstrated the potential for various applications using the upper extremity trainer to bring out an excellent rehabilitative effect, not only through muscle growth but also via identification of large movement intentions inducing brain activation. To develop specific applications to robot rehabilitation or nerve control using brain–computer interface (BCI) technologies, further studies are required to achieve consistent outcomes in securing and comparing the movement intention patterns; for example, by improving the signal processing methods.

Author Contributions: Conceptualization, S.-T.C.; methodology, J.-H.P.; formal analysis, J.-H.P. and H.-S.M.; investigation, J.-H.P., H.-S.M., H.K. and S.-T.C.; resources, S.-T.C.; writing—original draft preparation, J.-H.P. and H.-S.M.; writing—review and editing, H.K. and S.-T.C.; visualization, H.-S.M.; funding acquisition, S.-T.C. All authors have read and agreed to the published version of the manuscript.

Funding: This work was supported by "Emerging Technology Integrated Design Education program (P0012725)" program, a R&D project initiated by the Ministry of Trade, Industry and Energy, Republic of Korea, and by the ITRC (Information Technology Research Center) support program (IITP-2020-2018-0-01426) supervised by the IITP (Institute for Information & Communications Technology Planning & Evaluation) funded by the Ministry of Science and ICT, Republic of Korea.

Institutional Review Board Statement: All experiments were performed in accordance with the relevant guidelines of Korea Polytechnic University.

Informed Consent Statement: All participants provided informed written consent.

Data Availability Statement: The datasets generated during this study are available from the corresponding author on reasonable request.

Conflicts of Interest: The authors declare no conflict of interest.

References

1. Donkor, E.S. Stroke in the 21st century: A snapshot of the burden, epidemiology, and quality of life. *Stroke Res. Treat.* **2018**, *2018*, 3238165. [PubMed]
2. Franceschini, M.; Goffredo, M.; Pournajaf, S.; Paravati, S.; Agosti, M.; De Pisi, F.; Galafate, D.; Posteraro, F. Predictors of activities of daily living outcomes after upper limb robot-assisted therapy in subacute stroke patients. *PLoS ONE* **2018**, *13*, e0193235. [CrossRef] [PubMed]
3. Rafsten, L.; Danielsson, A.; Sunnerhagen, K.S. Anxiety after stroke: A systematic review and meta-analysis. *J. Rehabil. Med.* **2018**, *50*, 769–778. [CrossRef] [PubMed]
4. Lee, M.J.; Lee, J.H.; Koo, H.M.; Lee, S.M. Effectiveness of bilateral arm training for improving extremity function and activities of daily living performance in hemiplegic patients. *J. Stroke. Cerebrovasc. Dis.* **2017**, *26*, 1020–1025. [CrossRef] [PubMed]
5. Stinear, C.M.; Byblow, W.D.; Ackerley, S.J.; Barber, P.A.; Smith, M.C. Predicting recovery potential for individual stroke patients increases rehabilitation efficiency. *Stroke* **2017**, *48*, 1011–1019. [CrossRef]
6. Li, S. Spasticity, motor recovery, and neural plasticity after stroke. *Front. Neurol.* **2017**, *8*, 120. [CrossRef]
7. Figlewski, K.; Blicher, J.U.; Mortensen, J.; Severinsen, K.E.; Nielsen, J.F.; Andersen, H. Transcranial direct current stimulation potentiates improvements in functional ability in patients with chronic stroke receiving constraint-induced movement therapy. *Stroke* **2017**, *48*, 229–232. [CrossRef]
8. Bertani, R.; Melegari, C.; Maria, C.; Bramanti, A.; Bramanti, P.; Calabrò, R.S. Effects of robot-assisted upper limb rehabilitation in stroke patients: A systematic review with meta-analysis. *Neurol. Sci.* **2017**, *38*, 1561–1569. [CrossRef]
9. Hsieh, Y.W.; Lin, Y.H.; Zhu, J.D.; Wu, C.Y.; Lin, Y.P.; Chen, C.C. Treatment effects of upper limb action observation therapy and mirror therapy on rehabilitation outcomes after subacute stroke: A pilot study. *Behav. Neurol.* **2020**, *2020*, 6250524. [CrossRef]
10. Sheng, B.; Zhang, Y.; Meng, W.; Deng, C.; Xie, S. Bilateral robots for upper-limb stroke rehabilitation: State of the art and future prospects. *Med. Eng. Phys.* **2016**, *38*, 587–606. [CrossRef]
11. Sánchez-Herrera-Baeza, P.; Cano-de-la-Cuerda, R.; Oña-Simbaña, E.D.; Palacios-Ceña, D.; Pérez-Corrales, J.; Cuenca-Zaldivar, J.N.; Gueita-Rodriguez, J.; Balaguer-Bernaldo de Quirós, C.; Jardón-Huete, A.; Cuesta-Gomez, A. The impact of a novel immersive virtual reality technology associated with serious games in parkinson's disease patients on upper limb rehabilitation: A mixed methods intervention study. *Sensors* **2020**, *20*, 2168. [CrossRef] [PubMed]
12. Gutiérrez, Á.; Sepúlveda-Muñoz, D.; Gil-Agudo, Á.; de los Reyes Guzmán, A. Serious game platform with haptic feedback and EMG monitoring for upper limb rehabilitation and smoothness quantification on spinal cord injury patients. *Appl. Sci.* **2020**, *10*, 963. [CrossRef]
13. Proença, J.P.; Quaresma, C.; Vieira, P. Serious games for upper limb rehabilitation: A systematic review. *Disabil. Rehabil. Assist. Technol.* **2018**, *13*, 95–100. [CrossRef] [PubMed]
14. Frolov, A.A.; Mokienko, O.; Lyukmanov, R.; Biryukova, E.; Kotov, S.; Turbina, L.; Nadareyshvily, G.; Bushkova, Y. Post-stroke rehabilitation training with a motor-imagery-based brain-computer interface (bci)-controlled hand exoskeleton: A randomized controlled multicenter trial. *Front. Neurol.* **2017**, *11*, 400. [CrossRef]
15. Pereira, J.; Ofner, P.; Schwarz, A.; Sburlea, A.I.; Müller-Putz, G.R. EEG neural correlates of goal-directed movement intention. *Neuroimage* **2017**, *149*, 129–140. [CrossRef] [PubMed]
16. Wang, K.; Xu, M.; Wang, Y.; Zhang, S.; Chen, L.; Ming, D. Enhance decoding of pre-movement EEG patterns for brain-computer interfaces. *J. Neural. Eng.* **2020**, *17*, 016033. [CrossRef]

17. Dehem, S.; Montedoro, V.; Edwards, M.G.; Detrembleur, C.; Stoquart, G.; Renders, A.; Heins, S.; Dehez, B.; Lejeune, T. Development of a robotic upper limb assessment to configure a serious game. *NeuroRehabilitation* **2019**, *44*, 263–274. [CrossRef]
18. Zhang, L.; Guo, S.; Sun, Q. Development and assist-as-needed control of an end-effector upper limb rehabilitation robot. *Appl. Sci.* **2020**, *10*, 6684. [CrossRef]
19. Mekbib, D.B.; Han, J.; Zhang, L.; Fang, S.; Jiang, H.; Zhu, J.; Roe, A.W.; Xu, D. Virtual reality therapy for upper limb rehabilitation in patients with stroke: A meta-analysis of randomized clinical trials. *Brain Inj.* **2020**, *34*, 445–465. [CrossRef]
20. Hughes, C.M.L.; Padilla, A.; Hintze, A.; Raymundo, T.M.; Sera, M.; Weidner, S.; Ontiveros, J.; Peng, T.; Encarcion, A.; Cruz, Z.A.; et al. Developing an mHealth app for post-stroke upper limb rehabilitation: Feedback from US and Ethiopian clinicians. *Health Inform. J.* **2020**, *26*, 1104–1117. [CrossRef]
21. Maier, M.; Ballester, B.R.; Verschure, P.F. Principles of neurorehabilitation after stroke based on motor learning and brain plasticity mechanisms. *Front. Syst. Neurosci.* **2019**, *13*, 74. [CrossRef] [PubMed]
22. Spüler, M.; López-Larraz, E.; Ramos-Murguialday, A. On the design of EEG-based movement decoders for completely paralyzed stroke patients. *J. Neuroeng. Rehabil.* **2018**, *15*, 110. [CrossRef]
23. Trigili, E.; Grazi, L.; Crea, S.; Accogli, A.; Carpaneto, J.; Micera, S.; Vitiello, N.; Panarese, A. Detection of movement onset using EMG signals for upper-limb exoskeletons in reaching tasks. *J. Neuroeng. Rehabil.* **2019**, *16*, 45. [CrossRef]
24. Choi, M.H.; Kim, B.; Kim, H.S.; Gim, S.Y.; Kim, W.R.; Chung, S.C. Perceptual threshold level for the tactile stimulation and response features of ERD/ERS-based specific indices upon changes in high-frequency vibrations. *Front. Hum. Neurosci.* **2017**, *11*, 207. [CrossRef] [PubMed]
25. Wilson, R.; Mullinger, K.J.; Francis, S.T.; Mayhew, S.D. The relationship between negative BOLD responses and ERS and ERD of alpha/beta oscillations in visual and motor cortex. *Neuroimage* **2019**, *199*, 635–650. [CrossRef] [PubMed]
26. Lotze, M.; Ladda, A.M.; Stephan, K.M. Cerebral plasticity as the basis for upper limb recovery following brain damage. *Neurosci. Biobehav. Rev.* **2019**, *99*, 49–58. [CrossRef]
27. Alcover, E.A.; Jaume-i-Capó, A.; Moyà-Alcover, B. PROGame: A process framework for serious game development for motor rehabilitation therapy. *PLoS ONE* **2018**, *13*, e0197383.
28. Angelova, S.; Ribagin, S.; Raikova, R.; Veneva, I. Power frequency spectrum analysis of surface EMG signals of upper limb muscles during elbow flexion-A comparison between healthy subjects and stroke survivors. *J. Electromyogr. Kinesiol.* **2018**, *38*, 7–16. [CrossRef]
29. Jia, T.; Liu, K.; Qian, C.; Li, C.; Ji, L. Denoising algorithm for event-related desynchronization-based motor intention recognition in robot-assisted stroke rehabilitation training with brain-machine interaction. *J. Neurosci. Methods* **2020**, *346*, 108909. [CrossRef]
30. Little, S.; Bonaiuto, J.; Barnes, G.; Bestmann, S. Human motor cortical beta bursts relate to movement planning and response errors. *PLoS ONE* **2019**, *17*, e3000479. [CrossRef]
31. Weersink, J.B.; Maurits, N.M.; de Jong, B.M. EEG time-frequency analysis provides arguments for arm swing support in human gait control. *Gait. Posture* **2019**, *70*, 71–78. [CrossRef] [PubMed]
32. Wairagkar, M.; Hayashi, Y.; Nasuto, S.J. Exploration of neural correlates of movement intention based on characterisation of temporal dependencies in electroencephalography. *PLoS ONE* **2018**, *13*, e0193722. [CrossRef] [PubMed]

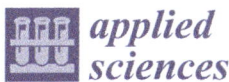

Article

Comparison of Endurance Time Prediction of Biceps Brachii Using Logarithmic Parameters of a Surface Electromyogram during Low-Moderate Level Isotonic Contractions

Chang-ok Cho [1], Jin-Hyoung Jeong [2], Yun-jeong Kim [3], Jee Hun Jang [3], Sang-Sik Lee [4,*] and Ki-young Lee [4,*]

[1] Korea Paralympic Committee, Seoul 05540, Korea; cco7171@hanmail.net
[2] Department of Biomedical IT, Catholic Kwandong University, Gangneung-si 25601, Korea; jjh830813@naver.com
[3] Department of Sport and Leisure Studies, Catholic Kwandong University, Gangneung-si 25601, Korea; yunjeong45@naver.com (Y.-j.K.); jjh@cku.ac.kr (J.H.J.)
[4] Department of Biomedical Engineering, Catholic Kwandong University, Gangneung-si 25601, Korea
* Correspondence: lsskyj@cku.ac.kr (S.-S.L.); kylee@cku.ac.kr (K.-y.L.)

Abstract: At relatively low effort level tasks, surface electromyogram (sEMG) spectral parameters have demonstrated an inconsistent ability to monitor localized muscle fatigue and predict endurance capacity. The main purpose of this study was to assess the potential of the endurance time (T_{end}) prediction using logarithmic parameters compared to raw data. Ten healthy subjects performed five sets of voluntary isotonic contractions until their exhaustion at 20% of their maximum voluntary contraction (MVC) level. We extracted five sEMG spectral parameters namely the power in the low frequency band (LFB), the mean power frequency (MPF), the high-to-low ratio between two frequency bands (H/L-FB), the Dimitrov spectral index (DSI), and the high-to-low ratio between two spectral moments (H/L-SM), and then converted them to logarithms. Changes in these ten parameters were monitored using area ratio and linear regressive slope as statistical predictors and estimating from onset at every 10% of T_{end}. Significant correlations ($r > 0.5$) were found between $\log(T_{end})$ and the linear regressive slopes in the logarithmic H/L-SM at every 10% of T_{end}. In conclusion, logarithmic parameters can be used to describe changes in the fatigue content of sEMG and can be employed as a better predictor of T_{end} in comparison to the raw parameters.

Keywords: electromyography; muscle; endurance capacity; isotonic; prediction capability

1. Introduction

In everyday life, low-moderate level isotonic exercise is the natural way of human activity and includes a concentric contraction and an eccentric contraction. Concentric contractions are the primary functions of biceps brachii muscles, and endurance contractions primarily work to slow twitch fibers and develop such fibers in their efficiency and resistance to fatigue [1]. Fatigue can be defined as the exercise-induced decrease in the ability to produce force [2] and has been measured by using surface electromyography (sEMG) as an assessment tool in prevention, monitoring, and rehabilitation fields [3].

Endurance capacity is the ability to sustain a given force over time, while measurement of the endurance time (T_{end}) is an indicator of the muscle resistance to fatigue [4–6]. Although widely used in clinical practice, it is problematic to measure the effect of physical and psychological factors such as pain and motivation [7,8]. Thus, methods that enable reliable estimates of muscle endurance time during the time shorter than the endurance time are of great importance for studying muscle function and motor control. A lot of researchers have studied endurance time prediction due to the fact that firing statistics of the active motor units (MU) were shown to affect the sEMG power spectrum toward lower frequencies as spectral compression [9–12]. In addition, sEMG has been shown to be a more objective approach to measuring muscle fatigue which is generally accompanied by an

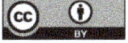

increase in amplitude of the sEMG signal because of the firing rates of increased motor unit recruitment [13,14]. Badier et al. (1993) found a significant relationship between T_{end} and the time-constant of a high-to-low ratio with the fixed frequency band as computed within the first 10–20 s of contraction [15]. Hanayama (1994) found no significant correlation beween T_{end} and the decreasing changes of muscle fiber conduction velocity (MFCV) [16]. After that, extrapolation of T_{end} based on linear regressive slopes of sEMG power spectrum has been reliable when computed over submaximal durations more than 50% T_{end} whatever the level of contraction considered [17–20]. In addition, Maïsetti et al. (2002) demonstrated that the area ratio which was proposed by Merletti et al. (1991) as changes of the low frequency band (LFB), as estimated around the first 25% of T_{end}, were significantly correlated with T_{end}. Lee et al. (2011) found the sustained times around 31% of T_{end}, when the Dimitrov spectral index (DSI) (Dimitrov et al. 2006) was above 130% of the first value, were significantly correlated with T_{end}. Lee et al. (2017) proposed high-to-low ratio between two signal spectral moments without choosing the optimal border frequencies of the low and high bands (H/L-SM). The experimental result obtained showed that linear regressive slopes of H/L-SM over the first 30% of T_{end} were significantly correlated with T_{end} [21–23].

Mean power frequency (MPF), median frequency (MDF), and high-to-low ratio with fixed frequency band (H/L-FB) are proposed as the spectral parameters related to the spectral compression of the sEMG signal, which decline throughout fatigue trials [24–26]. However, their consistent changes have been documented especially for relative high effort levels [27]. In contrast, these parameters have yielded an inconsistent pattern during sustained contractions at low level efforts. González-Izal et al. (2010) employed the logarithmic transformation of DSI as a predictor of the performance change in muscle power to reduce the large variability [28]. Lee et al. (2017; 2019) proposed the H/L-SM and converted it to logarithms to monitor the more sensitive activity of biceps femoris muscles during treadmill walking [23,29]. Yassierli and Nussbaum (2003; 2008) demonstrated that the Poisson-fit model using the logarithmic transformation could be more sensitive in localized muscle fatigue in sEMG-based assessments [30,31]. In myoelectric pattern recognition, logarithmic parameters in sEMG are especially useful to decode limb movements regarding the control of powered prostheses [32]. To our knowledge, the ability to predict T_{end} using logarithmic parameters at submaximal time periods shorter than T_{end} during the isotonic contraction test is limited.

Our study was designed to test whether changes in the logarithmic parameters calculated over a shorter duration than T_{end} could predict the endurance time of the biceps brachii muscle. Thus, sEMG parameters such as LFB, MPF, H/L-FB, DSI, and H/L-SM were converted to logarithms, and two types of changes were calculated by using the area ratio and the slope of linear regression model as predictors of T_{end}. Subsequently, the relationships between T_{end} and predictors were analyzed and evaluated.

2. Materials and Methods

2.1. Subjects

Ten healthy subjects (5 males and 5 females) with no history of cardiovascular, neurological, and musculoskeletal disorders, volunteered for this study. Their demographics (age, height, and mass) were measured and are described in Table 1. The subjects were informed of the purpose of the study before their consent was obtained. This study was approved by the Institutional Bioethics Committee of the Catholic Kwandong University, South Korea.

Table 1. Subject demographics data.

Variable	Mean	Standard Deviation
Age (yrs)	26.0	2.7
Height (cm)	165.4	6.2
Weight (kg)	63.7	12.5

2.2. Apparatus

2.2.1. MMT

The manual muscle tester (MMT) (Model: 01163, Manufacture: Lafayette Instrument Company, Sagamore Pkwy, IN, USA) was used to measure the maximal voluntary contraction (MVC) in accordance with the manufacture's manual (Figure 1).

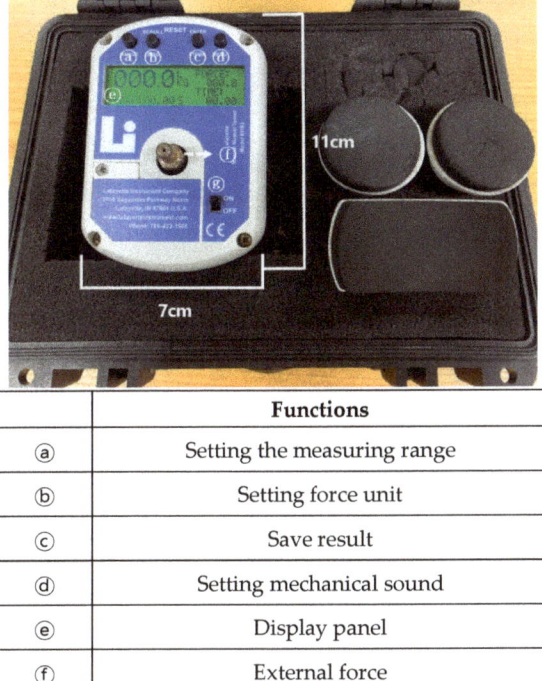

	Functions
ⓐ	Setting the measuring range
ⓑ	Setting force unit
ⓒ	Save result
ⓓ	Setting mechanical sound
ⓔ	Display panel
ⓕ	External force
ⓖ	Power button

Figure 1. Manual muscle tester.

The arm was at 110° flexion under the forearm in neutral position to measure the MVC of the subject using the MMT. The subject performed three maximal contractions 3 s long with 3 min rest period between them. The MVC was determined as the highest measured value.

2.2.2. Electromyography (EMG)

Surface EMG recordings were obtained from the biceps brachii muscles using bipolar surface electrodes (2 cm apart), which were connected to the measuring apparatus MyoTrace 400 with MyoResearch 3.6 software (Noraxon, AZ, USA). The sampling frequency was set at 1 kHz and boundaries of the band pass filter were set at 6 and 500 Hz (Figure 2). The electrodes were placed on the skin with anti-allergic tape after the skin was cleaned with alcohol and placed on the area of greatest muscle bulk along the longitudinal midline of the muscle [33,34].

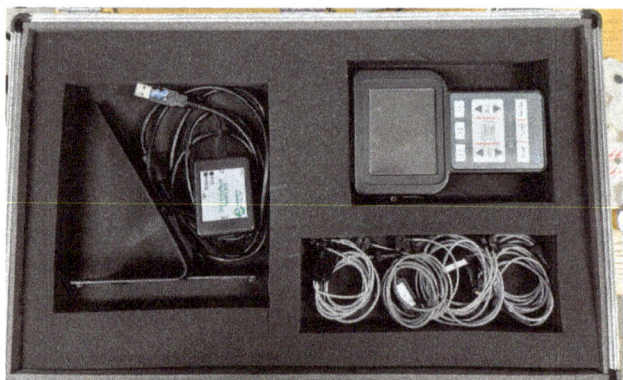

Figure 2. Surface EMG 4-channel wired instrument (MyoTrace 400).

2.3. Experimental Protocol

A schematic diagram of isotonic contraction of the biceps brachii muscles is shown in Figure 3. The subjects were asked to stand erect with their upper arm fixed and to move their lower arm through a range of motion from full extension to 110° flexion at a speed of 25 repetitions per minute using a metronome. Each repeated contraction was observed by an investigator and was considered successful if performed with the full range of motion within the metronome-guided time interval (2.4 s). During one set of the isotonic contraction trials, the subject was asked to continue repetitive contractions until exhaustion. The time of termination was determined when the participant indicated that they could no longer continue the full range of motion with the metronome speed for more than two repetitions, despite verbal encouragement without threats. This time point was noted as the T_{end} for each subject. Ten subjects completed five sets of the isotonic contraction trials until their exhaustion at 20% MVC. Two hours of rest was provided between three sets of trials conducted over 1 day, and the subsequent two sets of trials were conducted after 3 days to avoid fatigue.

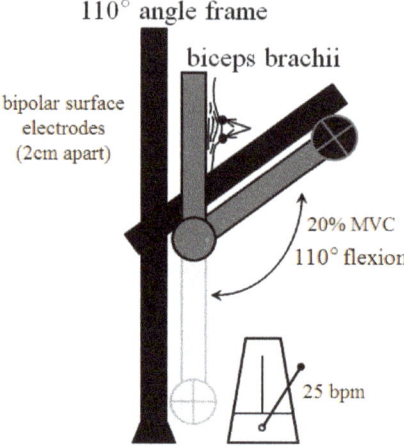

Figure 3. A schematic diagram of the isotonic contraction of the biceps brachii muscles.

2.4. Surface EMG Signal Acquisition

Surface EMG signals were collected using MyoResearch 3.6 software which guided the data acquisition steps. Figures 4 and 5 show the initial screen using this software, and the time-based graphic screen in the real-time progress, respectively.

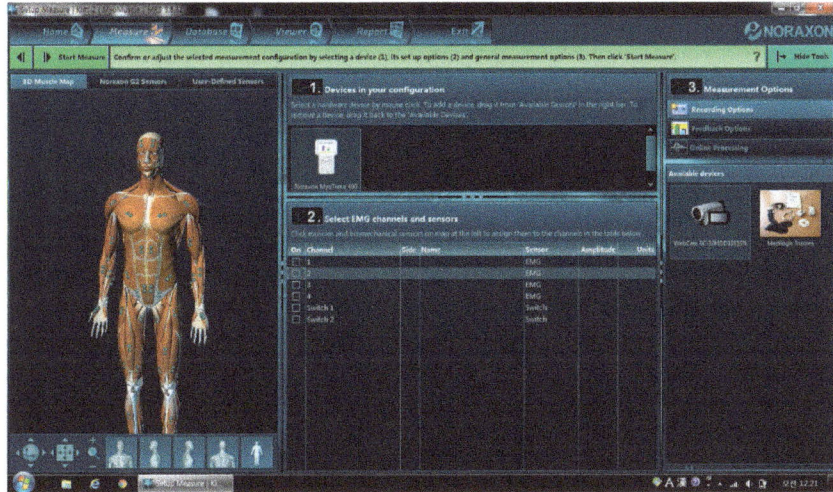

Figure 4. The initial screen.

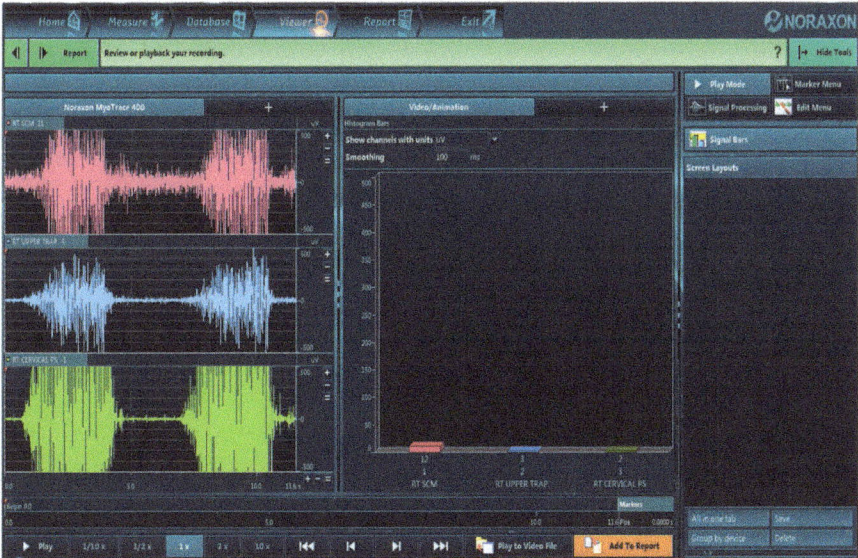

Figure 5. Surface EMG signal screen.

2.5. Mathematical Models

In this study, we used the five raw parameters from the sEMG power spectrum namely LFB, MPF, H/L-FB, DSI, and H/L-SM, and then converted these parameters to logarithms. The definitions of these logarithmic parameters are as follows [35].

$$\log\text{LFB} = \log\left\{\sum_{f=f_{L1}}^{f_{L2}} P(f)\right\} \quad (1)$$

$$\log\text{MPF} = \log\left\{\frac{\sum_{f=f_0}^{f_s/2} fP(f)}{\sum_{f=f_0}^{f_s/2} P(f)}\right\} \quad (2)$$

$$\log\text{H/L} - \text{FB} = \log\left\{\frac{\sum_{f=f_{H1}}^{f_{H2}} P(f)}{\sum_{f=f_{L1}}^{f_{L2}} P(f)}\right\} \quad (3)$$

$$\log\text{DSI} = \log\left\{\frac{\sum_{f=f_0}^{f_s/2} f^{-1}P(f)}{\sum_{f=f_0}^{f_s/2} f^5 P(f)}\right\} \quad (4)$$

$$\log\text{H/L} - \text{SM} = \log\left\{\frac{\sum_{f=f_0}^{f_s/2} f^5 P(f)}{\sum_{f=f_0}^{f_s/2} f^{-1}P(f)}\right\} \quad (5)$$

Here,

$f_{L1} = 15$ Hz, $f_{L2} = 45$ Hz and (f): power spectrum in expression (1);
$f_0 = 6$ Hz and $\frac{f_s}{2} = 500$ Hz in expression (2), (4) and (5);
$f_{H1} = 95$ Hz, $f_{H2} = 500$ Hz, $f_{L1} = 15$ Hz, $f_{L2} = 45$ Hz in expression (3).

In the curly brackets of Expressions (1)–(5), first, LFB in expression (1) is the power in the low frequency band of the sEMG power spectrum. MPF in expression (2) refers to the high-to-low ratio between the order 1 and the order 0 spectral moments as a measure of the change in muscle fiber propagation velocity. H/L-FB in expression (3) is the high-to-low ratio between two high and low bands with fixed border frequencies, whereas, DSI in expression (4) is the order (−1) spectral moment normalized by the order 5 moment, while DSI revealed a more notable change in muscle fatigue than MPF. Lastly, in expression (5), H/L-SM is similar to H/L-FB, and could be calculated without the fixed border frequencies. Following the definitions in expressions (1)–(5), these five sEMG spectral parameters were converted to logarithms. Logarithmic transformation has been widely used in biomedical and psychosocial research to deal with inconsistent data [36].

2.6. Data Analysis

Data analysis was performed using personal computer. For accurate spectral analysis of the sEMG signals (Figure 6) in isotonic contraction cycles (2.4 s), we used a 1 s time Hamming window every 0.3 s. Short-time Fourier transformation was conducted on each windowed segment to calculate the power spectrum, which was used to estimate the raw parameters such as LFB, MPF, H/L-FB, DSI, and H/L-SM in the curly brackets of expression (1)–(5). These parameters except MPF were normalized and expressed as percentages of initial values, and converted to logarithms. The coefficient of variation (CV) is known as the relative standard deviation and defined as the ratio of the standard deviation to the mean [37]. We used the CV to compare variability between the five raw and the five logarithmic parameters.

The T_{end} of each subject was divided into 10 equal intervals at every 10% of T_{end} to evaluate the relationships between T_{end} and the statistical predictors such as the area ratio and the slope of linear regression model as estimated over the shorter periods than the T_{end} [38]. For this purpose, we used the predictors as follows.

1. The area ratios in the five raw parameters
2. The area ratios in the five logarithmic parameters
3. The slopes in the five raw parameters
4. The slopes in the five logarithmic parameters

These four predictors were estimated over the periods from the onset to every 10% of T_{end}. The one-way ANOVA was used to compare the changes of each predictor according to the 10 periods. Pearson's correlation coefficient was used to quantify the performance of the relationships between T_{end} and these values. The level of significance was set at $p < 0.05$.

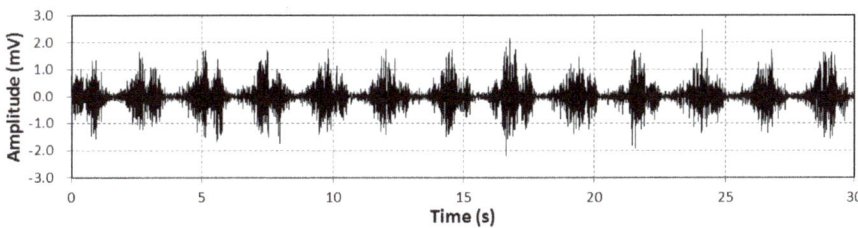

Figure 6. An example of the sEMG signal during isotonic contraction.

3. Results

3.1. MVC and T_{end}

MVC was 19.1 (5.9) kgf and T_{end} was 53.7 (19.6) s during isotonic contractions at 20% MVC. Endurance times were sorted in descending order and displayed according to the isotonic contraction sets of the 10 subjects in Figure 7.

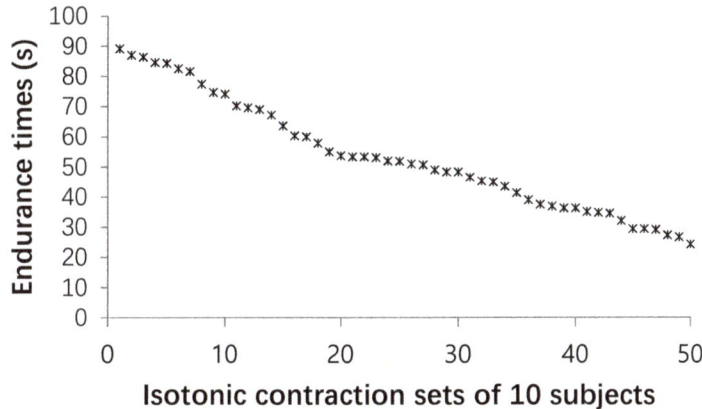

Figure 7. Endurance times in descending order.

3.2. Changes in sEMG Parameters and Predictors

Figure 8 showed the five raw and the five logarithmic parameters over the whole endurance time (T_{end}) for the subject whose T_{end} was almost the same as the mean of the endurance times of all subjects. The left column (a) displays the five raw parameters, and the right column (b) displays the five logarithmic ones with respect to time. The ripple period in LFB and logLFB time series in Figure 8a,b is 2.4 s which can be calculated as 50 s divided by 21 ripples, and the same as the repeated period during the isotonic contractions.

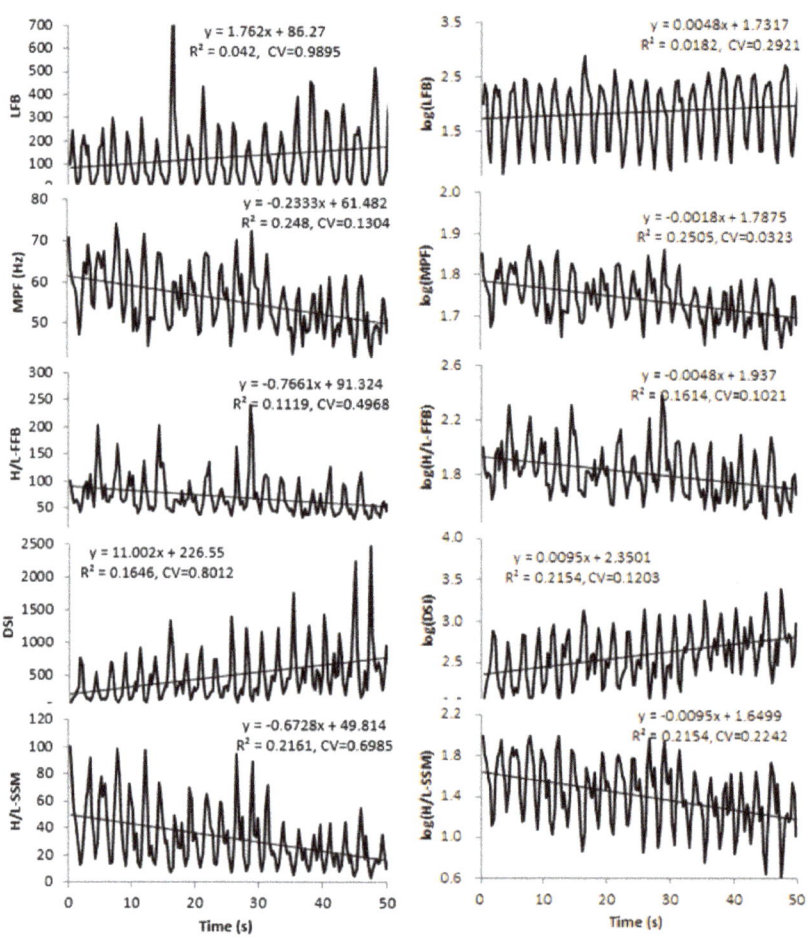

(a) The five raw parameters (b) The five logarithmic parameters

Figure 8. The time series of sEMG parameters during the endurance time (T_{end}) for the subject whose T_{end} was almost the same as the mean for all measured sEMG of all subjects. The left column (**a**): the five raw parameters; the right column (**b**): the five logarithmic parameters; R2: coefficient of determination; CV: coefficient of variation.

The time series of LFB, DSI, logLFB, and logDSI increased, and those of the other parameters decreased during the endurance contractions, because muscle fatigue is generally accompanied by an increased firing rate of motor unit recruitment and spectral parameters related to spectral compression during static and dynamic contractions [39]. Similar results were reported in previous studies [9,23,27].

The CVs of the five raw and the five logarithmic parameters are compared in Table 2 which shows that the CV of the logarithmic parameter is less than that of the raw one. These results revealed that the logarithmic transformation could reduce the large variability in the raw parameter.

Figures 9 and 10 with Tables 3 and 4 show the time series of two predictors namely the area ratio and the slope in the raw and the logarithmic parameters as estimated over every period of 10% of T_{end}, respectively. In Figure 9 and Table 3, the area ratios in LFB, DSI, logLFB, and logDSI decreased linearly, and those in the others increased linearly, because the definition varied between 0 and 1 for decreasing patterns and is negative for increasing patterns. In contrast, slopes in LFB, DSI, logLFB, and logD SI decayed exponentially, and those in the others rose exponentially as shown in Figure 10 and Table 4. One-way ANOVA was conducted on changes with respect to every period of 10% T_{end} in each parameter. There were significant differences for the two predictors of all parameters ($p < 0.05$). Thus, these results showed that the time series of the area ratios and the slopes of the raw and the logarithmic parameters varied independently.

Table 2. Mean and standard deviation of coefficient of variation (CV) of all parameters.

-	LFB	MPF	H/L-FB	DSI	H/L-SM
Raw	0.27 ± 0.51	0.19 ± 0.11	0.20 ± 0.15	0.26 ± 0.24	0.20 ± 0.18
Logarithm	0.12 ± 0.04	0.17 ± 0.13	0.12 ± 0.05	0.14 ± 0.08	0.17 ± 0.09

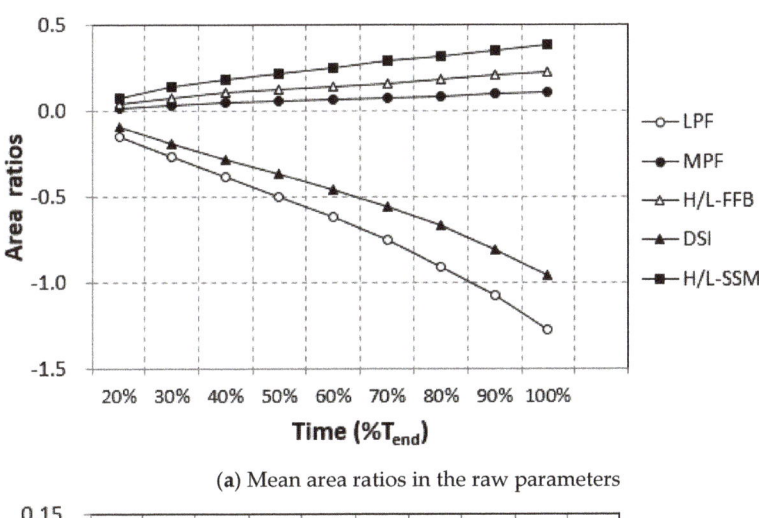

(a) Mean area ratios in the raw parameters

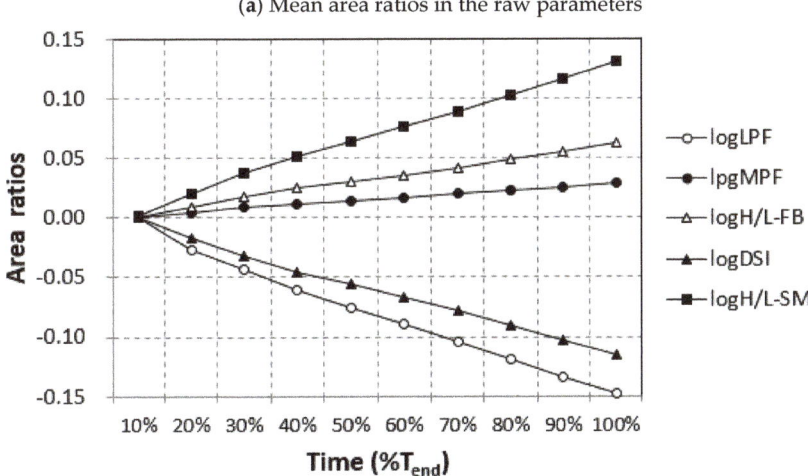

(b) Mean area ratios in the logarithmic parameters

Figure 9. The time series of area ratios in the sEMG raw parameters (a) and logarithmic ones (b) with respect to time as estimated over every 10% of T_{end} (White circle: LFB and logLFB; Black circle: MPF and logMPF; White triangle: H/L-FB and logH/L-FB; Black triangle: DSI and logDSI; Black square: H/L-SM and logH/L-SM).

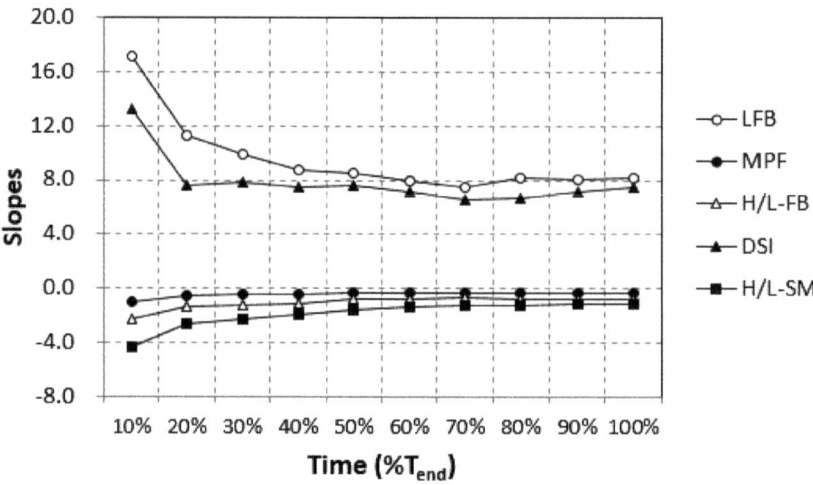

(a) Mean slopes in the raw parameters

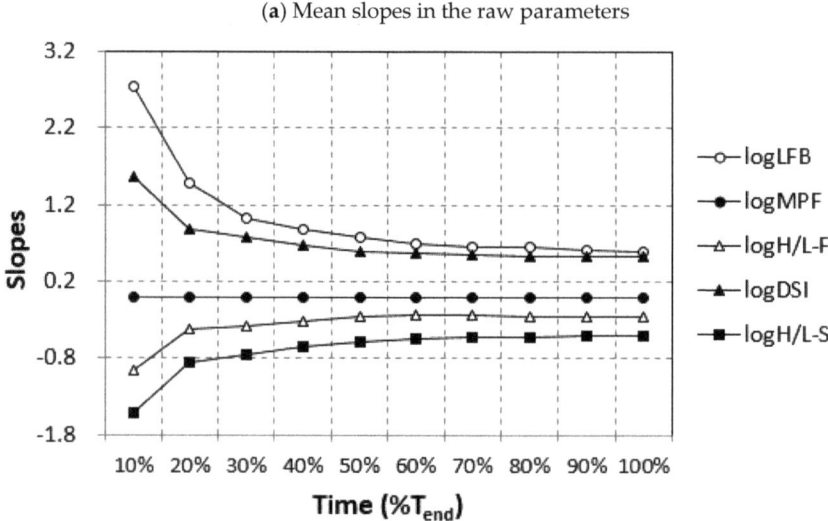

(b) Mean slopes in the logarithmic parameters

Figure 10. The time series of slopes in the sEMG raw parameters (**a**) and logarithmic ones (**b**) with respect to time as estimated over every 10% of T_{end} (White circle: LFB and logLFB; Black circle: MPF and logMPF; White triangle: H/L-FB and logH/L-FB; Black triangle: DSI and logDSI; Black square: H/L-SM and logH/L-SM).

Table 3. Area ratios (mean and S.D.) in the sEMG raw parameters (a) and logarithmic ones (b) with respect to time as estimated over every 10% of T_{end} (S.D.: standard deviation).

	(a) Mean area ratios in the raw parameters									
	%Tend	10%	20%	30%	40%	50%	60%	70%	80%	90%	100%
LFB	Mean	0.00	−0.15	−0.27	−0.39	−0.50	−0.62	−0.75	−0.91	−1.07	−1.27
	S.D.	0.00	0.17	0.23	0.26	0.31	0.36	0.41	0.48	0.57	0.71
MPF	Mean	0.00	0.02	0.03	0.05	0.05	0.06	0.08	0.09	0.10	0.11
	S.D.	0.00	0.02	0.03	0.03	0.04	0.04	0.04	0.04	0.04	0.04
H/L-FB	Mean	0.00	0.04	0.08	0.10	0.12	0.14	0.16	0.18	0.21	0.23
	S.D.	0.00	0.07	0.09	0.09	0.10	0.10	0.11	0.11	0.11	0.10
DSI	Mean	0.00	−0.09	−0.19	−0.28	−0.37	−0.46	−0.56	−0.67	−0.81	−0.96
	S.D.	0.00	0.10	0.16	0.24	0.33	0.34	0.36	0.38	0.46	0.49
H/L-SM	Mean	0.00	0.07	0.14	0.18	0.22	0.25	0.29	0.32	0.35	0.38
	S.D.	0.00	0.06	0.08	0.10	0.10	0.11	0.11	0.12	0.11	0.11
	(b) Mean area ratios in the logarithmic parameters									
	%Tend	10%	20%	30%	40%	50%	60%	70%	80%	90%	100%
logLFB	Mean	0.00	−0.03	−0.04	−0.06	−0.08	−0.09	−0.10	−0.12	−0.13	−0.15
	S.D.	0.00	0.03	0.04	0.04	0.05	0.05	0.05	0.05	0.05	0.06
logMPF	Mean	0.000	0.004	0.009	0.012	0.014	0.017	0.020	0.023	0.026	0.029
	S.D.	0.000	0.006	0.008	0.009	0.011	0.011	0.011	0.011	0.012	0.012
logH/L-FB	Mean	0.00	0.01	0.02	0.02	0.03	0.03	0.04	0.05	0.06	0.06
	S.D.	0.00	0.02	0.02	0.02	0.02	0.03	0.03	0.03	0.03	0.03
logDSI	Mean	0.00	−0.02	−0.03	−0.05	−0.06	−0.07	−0.08	−0.09	−0.10	−0.12
	S.D.	0.00	0.01	0.02	0.03	0.03	0.03	0.04	0.04	0.04	0.04
logH/L-SM	Mean	0.00	0.02	0.04	0.05	0.06	0.08	0.09	0.10	0.12	0.13
	S.D.	0.00	0.02	0.02	0.03	0.04	0.04	0.04	0.04	0.04	0.05

Table 4. Slopes (mean and S.D.) in the sEMG raw parameters (a) and logarithmic ones (b) with respect to time as estimated over every 10% of T_{end} (S.D.: standard deviation).

	(a) Mean slopes in the raw parameters									
	%T_{end}	10	20	30	40	50	60	70	80	90	100
LFB	Mean	17.09	11.25	9.90	8.79	8.48	7.99	7.54	8.18	8.10	8.21
	S.D.	28.55	14.74	13.83	13.15	11.72	11.01	8.70	9.46	8.90	8.02
MPF	Mean	−1.02	−0.55	−0.49	−0.39	−0.32	−0.30	−0.29	−0.28	−0.28	−0.27
	S.D.	1.82	0.63	0.39	0.31	0.27	0.22	0.18	0.16	0.15	0.13
H/L-FB	Mean	−2.27	−1.35	−1.25	−1.11	−0.83	−0.73	−0.72	−0.76	−0.76	−0.76
	S.D.	8.36	2.48	1.20	0.78	0.67	0.58	0.52	0.49	0.46	0.40
DSI	Mean	13.24	7.65	7.82	7.51	7.62	7.09	6.55	6.67	7.17	7.45
	S.D.	20.77	8.53	10.01	11.32	12.19	7.77	5.28	4.89	5.80	5.21
H/L-SM	Mean	−4.30	−2.64	−2.33	−1.93	−1.53	−1.39	−1.30	−1.23	−1.17	−1.12
	S.D.	8.63	2.42	1.44	1.29	0.84	0.78	0.71	0.65	0.61	0.58
	(b) Mean slopes in the logarithmic parameters									
	%Tend	10%	20%	30%	40%	50%	60%	70%	80%	90%	100%
logLFB	Mean	2.74	1.48	1.04	0.88	0.77	0.69	0.66	0.65	0.61	0.59
	S.D.	5.70	2.01	1.10	0.74	0.69	0.52	0.44	0.37	0.30	0.25
logMPF	Mean	−0.007	−0.004	−0.004	−0.003	−0.002	−0.002	−0.002	−0.002	−0.002	−0.002
	S.D.	0.013	0.005	0.003	0.003	0.002	0.002	0.001	0.001	0.001	0.001
logH/L-FB	Mean	−0.95	−0.43	−0.38	−0.32	−0.26	−0.23	−0.24	−0.25	−0.26	−0.26
	S.D.	2.59	0.79	0.39	0.25	0.20	0.18	0.17	0.17	0.16	0.14

Table 4. Cont.

logDSI	Mean	1.57	0.88	0.78	0.68	0.60	0.57	0.54	0.54	0.53	0.53
	S.D.	2.39	0.77	0.54	0.49	0.44	0.39	0.34	0.32	0.30	0.26
logH/L-SM	Mean	−1.52	−0.85	−0.75	−0.66	−0.58	−0.54	−0.52	−0.52	−0.51	−0.51
	S.D.	2.44	0.77	0.55	0.49	0.42	0.36	0.30	0.27	0.25	0.21

3.3. Relationships between T_{end} and Predictors

The correlation coefficients between T_{end} and the changes in the raw and the logarithmic parameters as computed over every 10% of T_{end} are shown in Tables 5 and 6. When the changes were estimated using the area ratio, no significant correlations between the endurance time and the changes in the raw and logarithmic parameters were found (Table 5).

On the other hand, there were significant correlations between T_{end} and the changes in the raw and the logarithmic parameters as estimated using the slope, except for LFB slopes estimated over longer periods than 50% of T_{end} and DSI slopes over 100% T_{end} (Table 6).

These results showed that the slopes in the logarithmic parameters correlated significantly with T_{end}. Table 6 shows that mean correlation coefficient of the raw parameters is 0.44 and that of the logarithmic ones 0.56, while the percentage increase was 26.3%. The predictor whose significant correlation was larger than 0.50 was the slope in logH/L-SM. Scatter plots of two predictors using the area ratio and the slope against T_{end} and log(T_{end}) are shown in Figures 11 and 12, comparing the two predictors using the raw and the logarithmic parameters. Mean correlation coefficients between T_{end} and the slopes in the raw and the logarithmic parameters are shown in Figure 13 In a recent study, logH/L-SM was found to be more sensitive to muscle fatigue than the existing sEMG parameters such as RMS (root mean square), MPF and H/L-FB. It could be speculated that the more sensitive the parameter to muscle fatigue the better the correlation with endurance capacity.

Table 5. Correlation coefficients between the endurance times and area ratios as predictors estimated over the time periods of every 10% of T_{end}.

(a) Raw parameter slopes v.s. T_{end}											
%T_{end}	10	20	30	40	50	60	70	80	90	100	Mean
LFB	n.s.	n.s.	n.s.	n.s.	n.s.	n.s.	n.s.	n.s.	0.44 [a]	0.60 [b]	n.s.
MPF	n.s.	n.s.	n.s.	n.s.	n.s.	n.s.	n.s.	n.s.	n.s.	n.s.	n.s.
H/L-FB	n.s.	n.s.	n.s.	n.s.	n.s.	n.s.	n.s.	n.s.	n.s.	n.s.	n.s.
DSI	n.s.	n.s.	n.s.	n.s.	n.s.	n.s.	n.s.	n.s.	n.s.	n.s.	n.s.
H/L-SM	n.s.	n.s.	n.s.	n.s.	n.s.	n.s.	n.s.	n.s.	n.s.	n.s.	n.s.
Mean	n.s.	n.s.	n.s.	n.s.	n.s.	n.s.	n.s.	n.s.	n.s.	n.s.	n.s.
(b) Logarithmic parameter slopes v.s. log(Tend)											
%T_{end}	10	20	30	40	50	60	70	80	90	100	Mean
logLFB	n.s.	n.s.	n.s.	n.s.	n.s.	n.s.	n.s.	n.s.	n.s.	n.s.	n.s.
logMPF	n.s.	n.s.	n.s.	n.s.	n.s.	n.s.	n.s.	n.s.	n.s.	n.s.	n.s.
logH/L-FB	n.s.	n.s.	n.s.	n.s.	n.s.	n.s.	n.s.	n.s.	n.s.	n.s.	n.s.
logDSI	n.s.	n.s.	n.s.	n.s.	n.s.	n.s.	n.s.	n.s.	n.s.	n.s.	n.s.
logH/L-SM	n.s.	n.s.	n.s.	n.s.	n.s.	n.s.	n.s.	n.s.	n.s.	n.s.	n.s.
Mean	n.s.	n.s.	n.s.	n.s.	n.s.	n.s.	n.s.	n.s.	n.s.	n.s.	n.s.

n.s.: non-significant; [a]: $p < 0.05$ indicates that the correlation coefficient is significant; [b]: $p < 0.05$ indicates that the correlation coefficient is significant and larger than 0.5.

Table 6. Correlation coefficients between the endurance times and slopes as predictors estimated over the time periods of every 10% of T_{end}.

	(a) Raw parameters slopes v.s. T_{end}										
%T_{end}	10	20	30	40	50	60	70	80	90	100	Mean
LFB	0.42 [a]	0.34 [a]	0.36 [a]	0.31 [a]	0.31 [a]	n.s.	n.s.	n.s.	n.s.	n.s.	n.s.
MPF	0.50 [b]	0.43 [a]	0.58 [b]	0.56 [b]	0.54 [b]	0.60 [b]	0.59 [b]	0.60 [b]	0.53 [b]	0.50 [b]	0.54
H/L-FB	0.42 [a]	0.32 [a]	0.44 [a]	0.59 [b]	0.45 [a]	0.48 [a]	0.38 [a]	0.45 [a]	0.48 [a]	0.49 [a]	0.45
DSI	0.43 [a]	0.42 [a]	0.42 [a]	0.39 [a]	0.41 [a]	0.52 [b]	0.53 [b]	0.47 [a]	0.32 [a]	n.s.	0.41
H/L-SM	0.43 [a]	0.45 [a]	0.58 [b]	0.54 [b]	0.68 [b]	0.69 [b]	0.63 [b]	0.64 [b]	0.56 [b]	0.47 [a]	0.57
Mean	0.44	0.39	0.48	0.48	0.48	0.51	0.46	0.45	0.38	n.s.	0.44
	(b) Logarithmic parameters slopes v.s. log(T_{end})										
%T_{end}	10	20	30	40	50	60	70	80	90	100	Mean
logLFB	0.49 [a]	0.48 [a]	0.57 [b]	0.69 [b]	0.62 [b]	0.65 [b]	0.65 [b]	0.64 [b]	0.55 [b]	0.47 [a]	0.58
logMPF	0.57 [b]	0.49 [a]	0.62 [b]	0.58 [b]	0.57 [b]	0.63 [b]	0.57 [b]	0.56 [b]	0.45 [a]	0.40 [a]	0.54
logH/L-FB	0.52 [b]	0.39 [a]	0.47 [a]	0.59 [b]	0.59 [b]	0.57 [b]	0.41 [a]	0.45 [a]	0.45 [a]	0.46 [a]	0.49
logDSI	0.57 [b]	0.53 [b]	0.60 [b]	0.60 [b]	0.64 [b]	0.66 [b]	0.60 [b]	0.58 [b]	0.51 [b]	0.45 [a]	0.58
logH/L-SM	0.57 [b]	0.55 [b]	0.59 [b]	0.60 [b]	0.66 [b]	0.70 [b]	0.66 [b]	0.65 [b]	0.57 [b]	0.51 [b]	0.61
Mean	0.54	0.49	0.57	0.61	0.61	0.64	0.58	0.58	0.51	0.46	0.56

n.s.: non-significant; [a]: $p < 0.05$ indicates that the correlation coefficient is significant; [b]: $p < 0.05$ indicates that the correlation coefficient is significant and larger than 0.5.

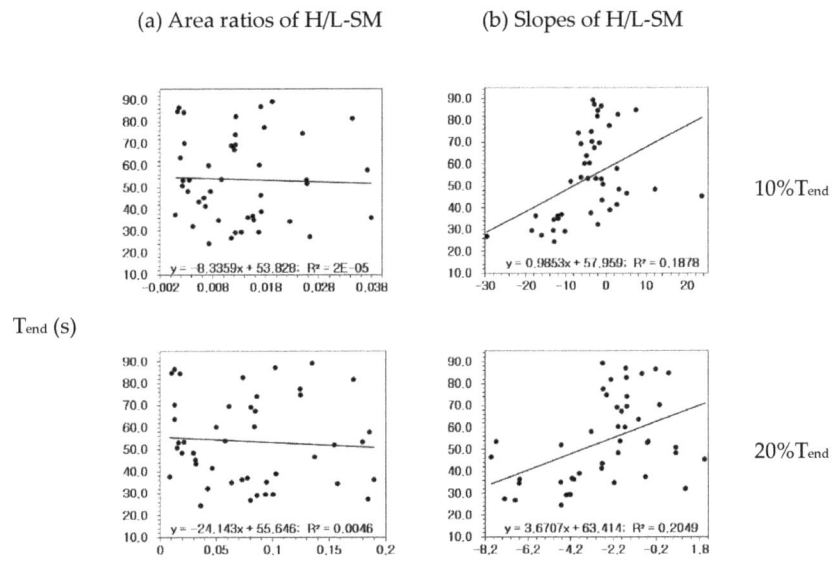

Figure 11. Cont.

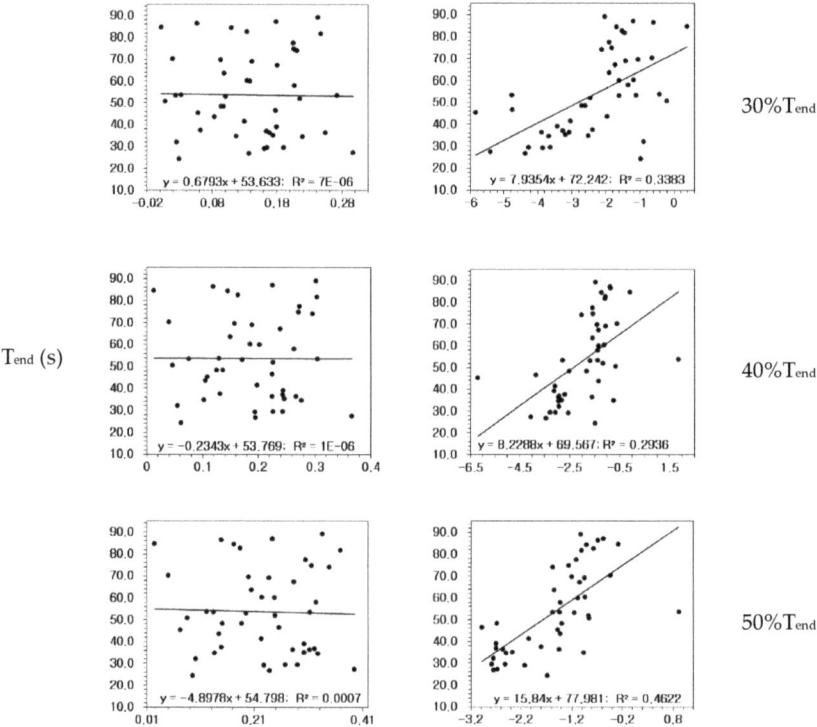

Figure 11. Scatter plots of the area ratio in the column (**a**) and the slope in the column (**b**) of the H/L-SM against T_{end}.

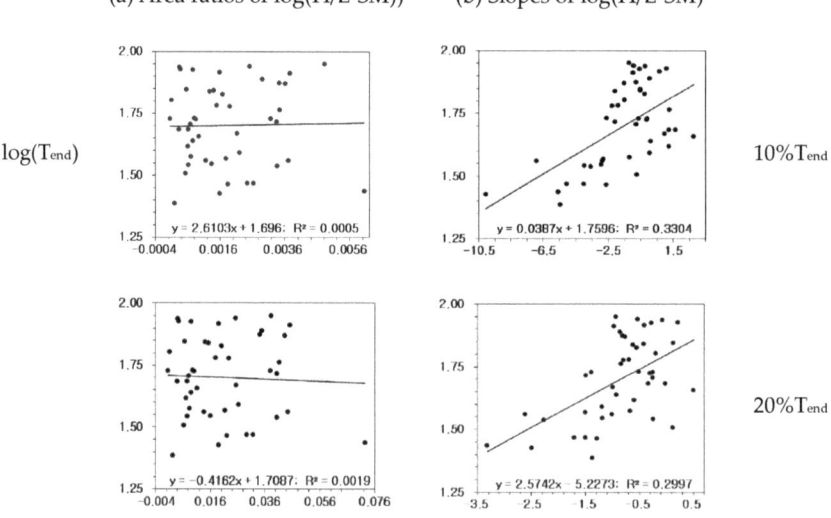

Figure 12. *Cont.*

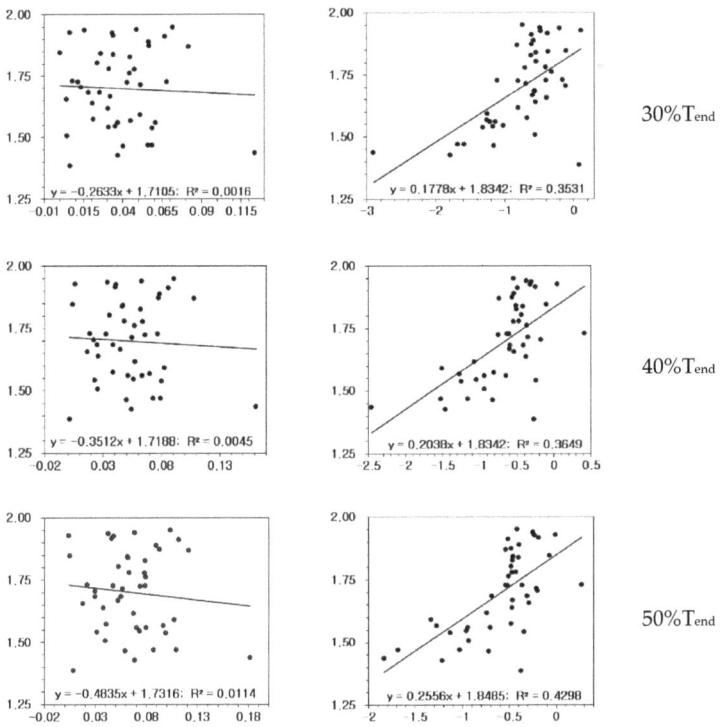

Figure 12. Scatter plots of the area ratio in the column (**a**) and the slope in the column (**b**) of logH/L-SM against log (T_{end}).

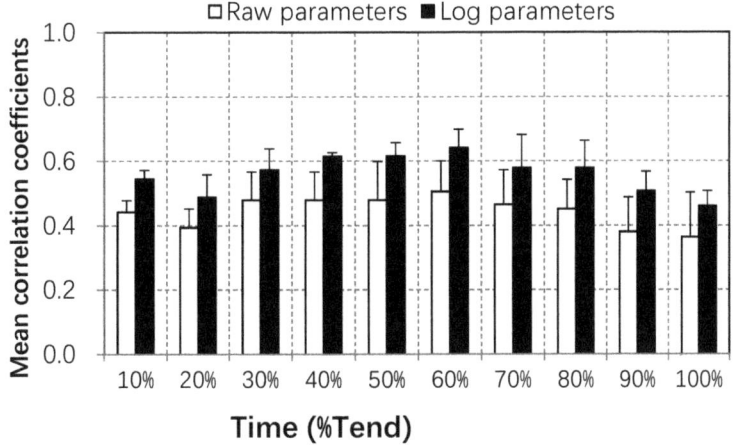

Figure 13. Comparison of mean and standard deviation of the correlation coefficients of raw and logarithmic parameters as described in Table 6 (a) and (b).

4. Discussion

The main object of this study was to assess the predictability of the endurance time using logarithmic parameters during isotonic contractions at low-moderate intensity. Previous studies had only focused on relatively high contraction levels which are generally uncommon in daily activities. In the present study, at 20% MVC the predictors such as the area ratio and the slope using the raw and the logarithmic sEMG parameters were estimated from the onset to every 10% of T_{end}, and their relationships with T_{end} were evaluated.

4.1. Changes in sEMG Parameters

The area ratio and the linear regressive slope as two statistical predictors of T_{end} were used to estimate T_{end} in this study. The area ratios varied linearly with respect to time (Figure 9). Maïsetti et al. (2002) obtained similar results showing that the area ratios in sEMG parameters were statistically linear with respect to time [8]. In contrast, the slopes varied exponentially with respect to time (Figure 10) in MPF and H/L-FB, while H/L-SM increased during the first part of the low-moderate level endurance test, probably because the behavior of the time series of the sEMG signal might be related to additional recruitment of motor units which occurred throughout sustained contractions at low contraction levels [40]. Similar results were obtained in the isometric endurance test of Van Dieën et al. (1998) and in the isotonic test of Lee et al. (2017) [20,23].

4.2. Comparison of Relationships

There were no significant correlations between T_{end} and the predictor using the area ratio (Table 3), and scatter plots showed that the coefficients of determination were not enough to have significant correlation with T_{end} (the column (a) in Figures 11 and 12). Maïsetti et al. (2002) also reported no correlations between T_{end} and the area ratio in MPF, MDF, and MFCV with the exception of the highestt area ratio of LFB (6–30 Hz) observed for quadriceps muscles at 50% MVC [8]. In addition, Boyas et al. (2009) demonstrated that no correlations between T_{end} and the changes in MPF using the area ratio were found, but there were significant correlations between T_{end} and the changes in MPF using the linear regressive slope [38]. In the present study, when using the slope, we also found significant correlations between T_{end} and the changes in the raw and the logarithmic parameters (Table 6), and the scatter plots showed their relationships (the column (b) in Figures 11 and 12), although spectral parameters have produced inconsistent trends during sustained contractions at low level.

As shown in Table 6, the mean correlation coefficient using the logarithmic parameters was increased by 26.3% compared to that using the raw parameters, and significant correlations larger than 0.50 were found between $\log(T_{end})$ and the slopes in logH/L-SM over the duration periods of every 10% of T_{end}. Previous studies showed that the slope in the spectral parameters as estimated over a shorter period than T_{end} could be a suitable predictor and correlated with T_{end} significantly. The logarithmic transformations were used to reduce the large variability in the raw parameters, and to show more sensitivity in localized muscle fatigue in sEMG-based assessments.

4.3. Limitations

The spectral parameters namely LFB, MPF, H/L-FB, DSI, and H/L-SM were extracted from the sEMG signal which, however, was non-stationary during the test, and wasaffected by many confounding factors [41], including electrode location, thickness of the subcutaneous tissues, the detection system used to obtain the recording, changes in the transmembrane action potential, and cross-talk from nearby muscles.

Due to all these confounding factors, caution is needed when using changes in the sEMG parameter as a predictor of the level of muscle fatigue. Although these factors could not be entirely excluded and do affect the estimated spectral parameters, we followed the recommendations that the careful placement of the electrodes between the innervation zone and the tendon and the normalized amplitudes should minimize the influence on the results.

The logarithmic transformation was used to convert the sEMG spectral parameters during the endurance dynamic contractions to minimize the effects of these factors [42]. MacIsaac et al. (2001) demonstrated that muscle fatigue could be assessed during dynamic contractions using a short-term Fourier transformation [43]. Some authors extracted the signal spectral moments as spectral parameters using Fourier transformation [44]. Coorevits et al. (2008) found that continuous wavelet transformation and traditional Fourier transformation are generally reliable to assess muscle fatigue [45].

As mentioned in the introduction, the endurance capacity is problematic in measuring the effect of physical and psychological factors such as pain and motivation. Because many factors can influence sEMG spectral parameters, the correlation of their changes with endurance might be lower than expected.

5. Conclusions

The present study demonstrated that the slope of the logarithmic parameter was a suitable predictor for monitoring biceps brachii muscle fatigue and for predicting T_{end}, even when it was estimated over every 10% of T_{end} during isotonic fatiguing contractions at a low-moderate level. The main conclusions of this study can be stated as follows:

(1) The linear regressive slope was a more suitable predictor of T_{end} than the area ratio.
(2) Significant correlations using the logarithmic parameters were about 26.3% higher than those using the raw ones.
(3) Significant correlations larger than 0.5 were found between $\log(T_{end})$ and the slopes of logH/L-SM over a duration time of every 10% of T_{end}.

From a clinical perspective, this sEMG method is useful to predict T_{end} compared to the mechanical method of measuring T_{end}, in reducing the length of the endurance test and in minimizing the influence of physical and psychological factors. Further studies are needed to evaluate this method for the muscles of the lower limbs and to develop the predictability using a combination of the parameters.

Author Contributions: Conceptualization, S.-S.L.; Formal analysis, J.-H.J.; Methodology, J.H.J.; Resources, Y.-j.K.; Visualization, C.-o.C.; Writing—review & editing, K.-y.L. All authors have read and agreed to the published version of the manuscript.

Funding: This study was supported by the Catholic Kwandong University (202001900001).

Institutional Review Board Statement: Approved by the Ethics Committee.

Informed Consent Statement: Informed consent was obtained from all subjects involved in the study.

Data Availability Statement: MDPI Research Data Policies.

Conflicts of Interest: The authors declare no conflict of interest.

References

1. Merletti, R.; Parker, P. *Electromyography: Physiology, Engineering and Non-Invasive Applications*; Wiley-IEEE Press: New York, NY, USA, 2004; ISBN 978-0-471-67580-8.
2. Wan, J.-J.; Qin, Z.; Wang, P.-Y.; Sun, Y.; Liu, X. Muscle fatigue: General understanding and treatment. *Exp. Mol. Med.* **2017**, *49*, e384. [CrossRef]
3. Merletti, R.; Muceli, S. Tutorial. Surface EMG detection in space and time: Best practices. *J. Electromyogr. Kinesiol.* **2019**, *49*, 102363. [CrossRef] [PubMed]
4. Bigland-Ritchie, B.; Donovan, E.; Roussos, C. Conduction velocity and EMG power spectrum changes in fatigue of sustained maximal efforts. *J. Appl. Physiol.* **1981**, *51*, 1300–1305. [CrossRef] [PubMed]
5. Gandevia, S.C. Spinal and Supraspinal Factors in Human Muscle Fatigue. *Physiol. Rev.* **2001**, *81*, 1725–1789. [CrossRef]
6. Bazzucchi, I.; Marchetti, M.; Rosponi, A.; Fattorini, L.; Castellano, V.; Sbriccoli, P.; Felici, F. Differences in the force/endurance relationship between young and older men. *Graefe's Arch. Clin. Exp. Ophthalmol.* **2004**, *93*, 390–397. [CrossRef] [PubMed]
7. Enoka, R.M.; Stuart, D.G. Neurobiology of muscle fatigue. *J. Appl. Physiol.* **1992**, *72*, 1631–1648. [CrossRef] [PubMed]
8. Maïsetti, O.; Guével, A.; Legros, P.; Hogrel, J.Y. Prediction of endurance capacity of quadriceps muscles in humans using surface electromyogram spectrum analysis during submaximal voluntary isometric Contraction. *Eur. J. Appl. Physiol.* **2002**, *87*, 509–519. [PubMed]
9. Petrofsky, J.S.; Glaser, R.M.; Phillips, C.A.; Lind, A.R.; Williams, C. Evaluation of the amplitude and frequency components of the surface EMG as an index of muscle fatigue. *Ergonomics* **1982**, *25*, 213–223. [CrossRef]
10. Basmajian, J.; De Luca, C.J. *Muscle Alive; Their Functions Revealed by Electromyography*, 5th ed.; Williams and Wilkins: Baltimore, MD, USA, 1985.

11. Duchêne, J.; Goubel, F. EMG spectral shift as an indicator of fatigability in an heterogeneous muscle group. *Eur. J. Appl. Physiol. Occup. Physiol.* **1990**, *61*, 81–87. [CrossRef]
12. Potvin, J.R. Effect of Muscle Kinematics on surface EMG Amplitude and Frequency during Fatiguing Dynamic Contrac-tions. *J. Appl. Physiol.* **1997**, *82*, 144–151. [CrossRef] [PubMed]
13. Merletti, R.; Lo Conte, L.; Orizio, C. Indices of muscle fatigue. *J. Electromyogr. Kinesiol.* **1991**, *1*, 22–33. [CrossRef]
14. De Luca, C.J. The Use of Surface Electromyography in Biomechanics. *J. Appl. Biomech.* **1997**, *13*, 135–163. [CrossRef]
15. Badier, M.; Guillot, C.; Burnet, H.; Jammes, Y. EMG power spectrum of respiratory and skeletal muscles during static contraction in healthy man. *Muscle Nerve* **1993**, *16*, 601–609. [CrossRef]
16. Hanayama, K. Recovery of Conduction Velocity of Muscle Fiber Action Potential after Strenuous Isometric Contraction. *Jpn. J. Physiol.* **1994**, *44*, 75–88. [CrossRef] [PubMed]
17. Mannion, A.F.; Dolan, P. Electromyographic Median Frequency Changes During Isometric Contraction of the Back Extensors to Fatigue. *Spine* **1994**, *19*, 1223–1229. [CrossRef]
18. Dollan, P.; Mannio, A.F.; Adam, M.A. Fatigue of the erector spinae muscles. A quantative assessment using frequency banding of the surface electromyography signal. *Spine* **1995**, *20*, 149–159. [CrossRef]
19. Merletti, R.; Roy, S. Myoelectric and Mechanical Manifestations of Muscle Fatigue in Voluntary Contractions. *J. Orthop. Sports Phys. Ther.* **1996**, *24*, 342–353. [CrossRef]
20. Van Dieën, J.H.; Heijblom, P.; Bunkens, H. Extrapolation of Time Series of EMG Power Spectrum Parameters in Isometric Endurance Tests of Trunk Extensor Muscles. *J. Electromyogr. Kinesiol.* **1998**, *8*, 35–44. [CrossRef]
21. Lee, K.Y.; Lee, S.; Choi, A.R.; Choi, C.-H.; Mun, J.H. Endurance time prediction of biceps brachii muscle using Dimitrov spectral index of surface electromyogram during isotonic contractions. *Int. J. Precis. Eng. Manuf.* **2011**, *12*, 711–717. [CrossRef]
22. Dimitrov, G.V.; Arabadzhiev, T.I.; Mileva, K.N.; Bowtell, J.L.; Crichton, N.; Dimitrova, N.A. Muscle Fatigue during Dynamic Contractions Assessed by New Spectral Indices. *Med. Sci. Sports Exerc.* **2006**, *38*, 1971–1979. [CrossRef]
23. Lee, S.; Jang, J.; Cho, C.; Kim, D.; Moon, G.; Kim, B.; Choi, A.; Lee, K. Endurance capacity of the biceps brachaii using the high-to-low ratio between two signal spectral moments of surface EMG signals during isotonic contractions. *J. Electr. Eng. Technol.* **2017**, *12*, 1641–1648.
24. Lindstrom, L.; Kadefors, R.; Petersén, I. An electromyographic index for localized muscle fatigue. *J. Appl. Physiol.* **1977**, *43*, 750–754. [CrossRef]
25. Stulen, F.B.; De Luca, C.J. Frequency Parameters of the Myoelectric Signal as a Measure of Muscle Conduction Velocity. *IEEE Trans. Biomed. Eng.* **1981**, *28*, 515–523. [CrossRef]
26. Moxham, J.; Edward, R.H.; Aubier, M.; De Troy, A.; Farkas, G.; Macklem, P.T.; Rousses, C. Changes in EMG Power Spectrum (high-to-low ratio) with Force Fatigue in Humans. *J. Appl. Physiol.* **1982**, *53*, 1094–1099. [CrossRef]
27. Dunchene, J.; Goubel, F. Surface electromyogram during voluntary contraction: Processing tools and relation to physio-logical events. *Clitical Rev. Biomed. Eng.* **1993**, *21*, 313–397.
28. González-Izal, M.; Malanda, A.; Navarro-Amézqueta, I.; Gorostiaga, E.M.; Mallor, F.; Ibañez, J.; Izquierdo, M. EMG spectral indices and muscle power fatigue during dynamic contractions. *J. Electromyogr. Kinesiol.* **2010**, *20*, 233–240. [CrossRef] [PubMed]
29. Lee, S.; Choi, A.; Kim, S.; Won, J.; Lee, K. Comparison of EMG activity using spectrum indices from biceps femoris muscle during treadmill walking. *Int. J. Adv. Sci. Technol.* **2019**, *28*, 33–39.
30. Yassierli, Y.; Nussbaum, M.A. Logarithmic Power-Frequency: An Alternative Method for Emg-Based Fatigue Assessment. *Hum. Fact. Ergon. Soc. Annu. Meet. Proc.* **2003**, *47*, 1184–1188. [CrossRef]
31. Nussbaum, M.A. Utility of traditional and alternative EMG-based measures of fatigue during low-moderate level isometric efforts. *J. Electromyogr. Kinesiol.* **2008**, *18*, 44–53. [CrossRef]
32. Abbaspour, S.; Lindén, M.; GholamHosseini, H.; Naber, A.; Ortiz-Catalan, M. Evaluation of surface EMG-based recognition algorithms for decoding hand movements. *Med. Biol. Eng. Comput.* **2020**, *58*, 83–100. [CrossRef]
33. Hermens, H.J.; Freriks, B.; Disselhorst-Klug, C.; Rau, G. Development of recommendations for SEMG sensors and sensor placement procedures. *J. Electromyogr. Kinesiol.* **2000**, *10*, 361–374. [CrossRef]
34. Lim, S.K. An electromyographic analysis of muscle activation in the latissimus dorsi, pectoralis major, deltoid, trapezius, and biceps brachii muscles according to the type of lat pull down exercise. *Off. J. Korean Acad. Kinesiol.* **2017**, *19*, 55–62.
35. Allison, G.T.; Fujiwara, T. The relationship between EMG median frequency and low frequency band amplitude chages at different levels of muscle capacity. *Clin. Biomech.* **2002**, *17*, 464–469. [CrossRef]
36. Feng, C.; Wang, H.; Lu, N.; Tu, X.M. Log transformation: Application and interpretation in biomedical research. *Stat. Med.* **2012**, *32*, 230–239. [CrossRef] [PubMed]
37. Krishnamoorthy, K.; Lee, M. Improved tests for the equality of normal coefficients of variation. *Comput. Stat.* **2014**, *29*, 215–232. [CrossRef]
38. Boyas, S.; Maïsetti, O.; Guével, A. Changes in sEMG parameters among trunk and thigh muscles during a fatiguing bilat-eral isometric multi-joint task in trained and untrained participants. *J. Electromyogr. Kinesiol.* **2009**, *19*, 259–268. [CrossRef]
39. Masuda, K.; Masuda, T.; Sadoyama, T.; Inaki, M.; Katsuta, S. Changes in Surface EMG Parameters during Static and Dy-namic Fatiguing Contractions. *J. Electromyogr. Kinesiol.* **1999**, *9*, 39–46. [CrossRef]
40. Fallentin, N.; Simonsen, E.B. Motor unit recruitment during prolonged isometric contractions. *Graefe's Arch. Clin. Exp. Ophthalmol.* **1993**, *67*, 335–341. [CrossRef]

41. Farina, D. Interpretation of the Surface Electromyogram in Dynamic Contractions. *Exerc. Sport Sci. Rev.* **2006**, *34*, 121–127. [CrossRef]
42. González-Izal, M.; Rodríguez-Carreño, I.; Mallor-Giménez, F.; Malanda, A.; Izquierdo, M. New Wavelet Indices to Assess Muscle Fatigue during Dynamic Contractions. *World Acad. Sci. Eng. Technol.* **2009**, *55*, 480–485.
43. MacIssac, D.; Parker, P.A.; Scott, R.N. The Short time Fourier Transform and Muscle Fatigue Assessment in Dynamic Con-tractions. *J. Electromyogr. Kinesiol.* **2001**, *11*, 439–449. [CrossRef]
44. Dimitrova, N.A.; Arabadzhiev, T.I.; Hogrel, J.-Y.; Dimitrov, G.V. Fatigue analysis of interference EMG signals obtained from biceps brachii during isometric voluntary contraction at various force levels. *J. Electromyogr. Kinesiol.* **2009**, *19*, 252–258. [CrossRef]
45. Coorevits, P.; Danneels, L.; Cambier, D.; Ramon, H.; Druyts, H.; Karlsson, J.S.; De Moor, G.; Vanderstraeten, G. Test–retest reliability of wavelet—And Fourier based EMG (instantaneous) median frequencies in the evaluation of back and hip muscle fatigue during isometric back extensions. *J. Electromyogr. Kinesiol.* **2008**, *18*, 798–806. [CrossRef] [PubMed]

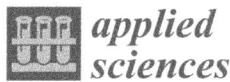

Article

Effect of the Location of Strut Chordae Insertion on Computational Modeling and Biomechanical Evaluation of Mitral Valve Dynamics

Woojae Hong, Soohwan Jeong, Minsung Ko, Hyun Hak Kim and Hyunggun Kim *

Department of Biomechatronic Engineering, Sungkyunkwan University, Suwon 16419, Korea; woojaehong94@gmail.com (W.H.); jeongsoohwan92@gmail.com (S.J.); minsungko413@gmail.com (M.K.); kim.hyun.hak95@gmail.com (H.H.K.)
* Correspondence: hkim.bme@skku.edu; Tel.: +82-31-290-7821

Abstract: The strut chordae (SC) have a unique structure and play an important role in reinforcing the tunnel-shaped configuration of the mitral valve (MV) at the inflow and outflow tracts. We investigated the effect of varying the SC insertion location on normal MV function and dynamics to better understand the complex MV structures. A virtual parametric MV model was designed to replicate a normal human MV, and a total of nine MV modes were created from combinations of apical and lateral displacements of the SC insertion location. MV function throughout the full cardiac cycle was simulated using dynamic finite element analysis for all MV models. While the leaflet stress distribution and coaptation showed similar patterns in all nine MV models, the maximum leaflet stress values increased in proportion to the width of the SC insertion locations. A narrower SC insertion location resulted in a longer coaptation length and a smaller anterior coaptation angle. The top-narrow MV model demonstrated the shortest anterior leaflet bulging distance, lower stresses across the anterior leaflet, and the lowest maximum stresses. This biomechanical evaluation strategy can help us better understand the effect of the SC insertion locations on mechanism, function, and pathophysiology of the MV.

Keywords: mitral valve; strut chordae; strut chordae insertion location; finite element; computational simulation

1. Introduction

An intricate tissue structure, the mitral valve (MV), regulates blood flow between the left atrium and the left ventricle (LV), and the components of the MV apparatus play complex roles to properly maintain normal MV function. The MV apparatus is composed of the mitral annulus, two (anterior and posterior) leaflets, chordae tendineae, and papillary muscles. While LV pressure increases during systole, the circumferential size of the mitral annulus decreases. This facilitates leaflet contact and closes the mitral orifice. The papillary muscles contract and hold the chordae tendineae to prevent the leaflets from prolapsing towards the left atrium.

The chordae tendineae play an important role in maintaining the ventricular architecture and ensuring an efficient cardiac output [1,2]. It acts like a parachute cord that holds the leaflets at a high pressure to prevent blood from back-flowing towards the left atrium during systole. Hence, the chordae tendineae must have a high degree of elasticity, strength, and resistance to traction to support the heart of an average adult with an approximate load of 75 tons a day [1]. The chordae tendineae have been classified according to their site of insertion on the leaflets, yet their morphology and distribution on the leaflets result in a wide variety of distribution, form, and configuration for which there is no clear consensus on terminology [3].

Three types of chordae tendineae can be described according to their attachment on the leaflets. The (1) basal (or tertiary) chordae branch out from the papillary muscles and/or directly from the LV wall and are tied to the basal regions of the posterior leaflets; the (2) marginal (or primary) chordae are attached to the margin of the leaflets, and the space between the two marginal chordae is known to not exceed 3 mm with an attachment to the leaflet that is often bifurcated or trifurcated; and the (3) intermediary (or secondary) chordae extend from the papillary muscles and are attached to the LV side of the leaflets. The present study focuses on the intermediary chordae, which are also known as the strut chordae (SC).

In the anterior leaflets, the two thick and resistant SC are located originating in the medial aspect of the ventricular side of the leaflet and provide resistance to the leaflet at closing during systole to thus avoid a prolapse [4–6]. As the LV pressure increases, the tension along the SC raises rapidly, and the maximum SC tension value becomes three times larger than the surrounding chordae in the anterior leaflet [3,7,8]. Although the SC do not show much direct impact on leaflet coaptation, they play a vital role in creating a tunnel-shaped morphology of the MV throughout the cardiac cycle and maintaining MV function [5,9–11]. The large leaflet stress distribution over the anterior leaflet spreads from the fibrous trigone across the anterior central region towards the zone where the SC are connected [2,6,12]. All of these studies have emphasized the SC are critical to maintaining the long-term function of the MV.

Recent excellent studies have revealed diverse advancement in computational MV modeling, more specifically in terms of modeling of the chordae tendineae [13–16]. Moreover, solid mechanical evaluation of the chordae tissue and improved mathematical modeling of the chordae tendineae [17–21] as well as experimental and computational blood flow studies with respect to the chordae structure [22–24] have revealed the importance of chordae tendineae studies. However, there is still a lack of biomechanical information of the role of the SC; therefore, it is important to investigate the biomechanical effects of the insertion location of the SC in computational MV evaluations.

We employed our previously developed and validated computational MV modeling and evaluation protocols [25–31] to investigate the effect of varying the SC insertion location on normal MV function and dynamics to better understand the complex MV structures. Computational evaluations were conducted to assess the physiologic and biomechanical features of nine types of MVs with various insertion locations of the SC. Detailed information of the leaflet coaptation, stress distribution, coaptation length, coaptation angle, bulging height, and bulging distance with respect to the SC insertion location were investigated.

2. Materials and Methods

Figure 1 provides a brief demonstration of the virtual MV modeling and simulation procedures to assess the effect of altering the SC insertion location. A virtual parametric MV model was created to replicate a geometric 3D model for a normal human MV that can be easily transformed to investigate the effect of morphologic alteration by modifying several key geometric parameters. MATLAB (Mathworks Inc., Natick, MA, USA) was primarily utilized to produce the virtual parametric MVs and SC modeling, and ABAQUS (SIMULIA, Providence, RI, USA) was used to perform the computational simulations and evaluate the functional and biomechanical characteristics of MV function with respect to various insertion locations of the SC. A series of alterations were made in the SC insertion location for the parametric MVs, and computational simulations of MV function were performed to compare the MV models.

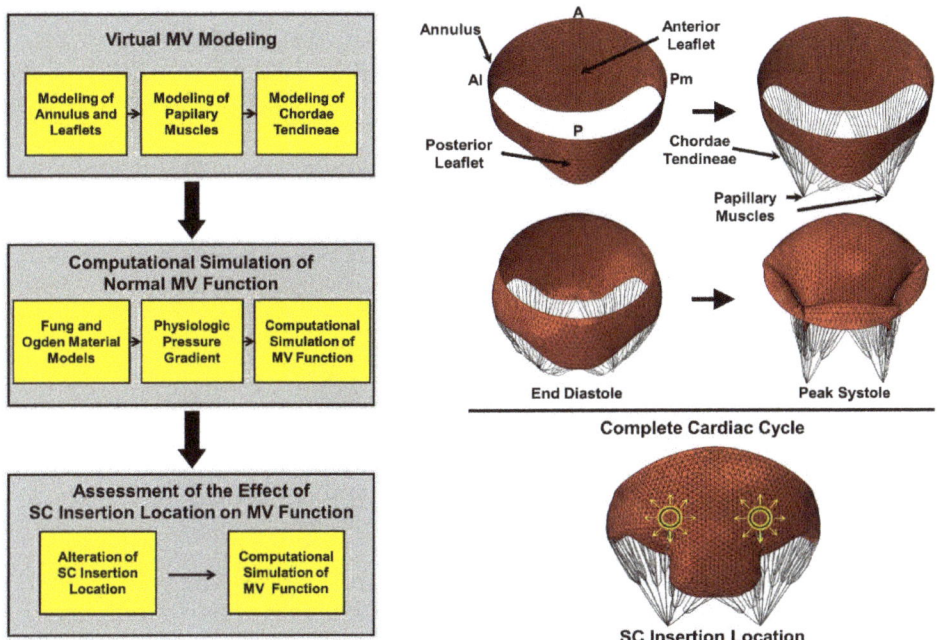

Figure 1. Study protocol for virtual parametric MV modeling and computational simulation of MV function to determine the effect of altering the SC insertion location. A—anterior; Al—anterolateral; P—posterior; Pm—posteromedial.

2.1. Virtual Parametric MV Modeling

A normal parametric MV geometry at end diastole was designed to conduct a mechanistic study of the SC insertion location as described in our previous studies [25,26]. The representative structural dimensions of the mitral annulus, the anterior leaflet (a single cusp), the posterior leaflet (three cusps), the marginal chordae tendineae, and the papillary muscle tips were utilized in the present study. Briefly, the entire MV model was designed to be symmetric with respect to the center of the mitral orifice and aligned to the anterior-posterior (AP) plane of the annulus. The mitral annulus was created by implementing four primary landmark information with the cubic spline interpolation methods. The marginal leaflet boundary was created using a combination of sinusoidal functions, and a number of three-dimensional (3D) lines linking the mitral annulus and the free leaflet margin were constructed [25,32]. The non-uniform rational B-spline (NURBs) surface model was employed to generate a 3D surface model of the MV leaflets.

This MV leaflet model was meshed using triangular shell elements and imported into ABAQUS. The papillary muscle tips were placed 22 mm from the mid-annular plane positioning the two papillary muscle tips 24 mm apart to each other [33]. The marginal chordae tendineae were designed linking the leaflet free margin and the papillary muscle tips, and the chordal insertion was spread around the papillary muscle tips.

2.2. SC Modeling and Alteration of SC Insertion Location

The two SC were modeled by connecting the central region of the anterior leaflet (from the top portion of the rough zone to the medial portion of the atrial zone) and the papillary muscles [34]. The position of the SC is set as the ratio of the distance in the apical and lateral directions. Figure 2 presents the nine different SC insertion locations on the anterior leaflet. In the apical direction, the anterior leaflet centerline connecting the center point of the anterior annulus and anterior leaflet free margin served as reference for the position of the SC. With the center point of the free margin of the anterior leaflet set to zero, the center point of anterior annulus is set to one. The lateral location of the SC in the anterior view is set by the intercommissural line that connects the anterolateral (Al) and posteromedial (Pm) points. The half point of the intercommissural line located on the anterior leaflet centerline was set to zero, and the Al and Pm points were set to one.

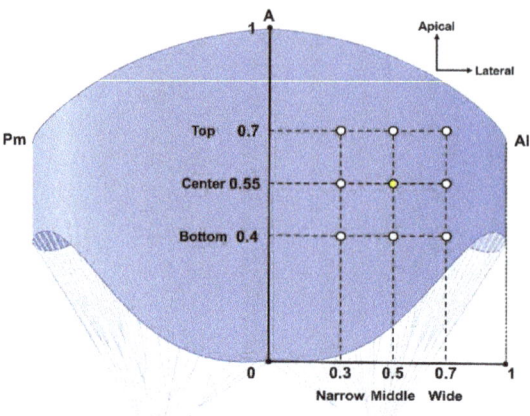

Figure 2. A schematic of anatomical alteration of the SC insertion location (anterior viewpoint). The yellow point indicates the normal SC insertion location. A—anterior; Al—anterolateral; Pm—posteromedial.

Several SC insertion locations were determined according to the ratio of the centerline of the anterior leaflet and half of the intercommissural line. All insertion locations of the SC were connected to the nearest node where the ratios were selected. The standard SC insertion location was set to the coordinates of 0.55 in the apical direction and 0.5 in the lateral direction. The displacement threshold for the SC insertion location (apical ± 0.15, lateral ± 0.2) along each anatomical direction was determined according to the normal range of the SC insertion location based on previous clinical studies [35]. A total of nine MV modes were created from combinations of apical and lateral displacements of the SC insertion location. They are named as top, center, and bottom according to the ratios (0.7, 0.55, and 0.4) in the apical direction and as narrow, middle, and wide at ratios of 0.3, 0.5, and 0.7 in the lateral direction. The SC lengths were determined according to the distance from the papillary muscle tips to the selected SC insertion nodes, with the shortest being 2.35 cm and the longest being 2.98 cm. The altered SC insertion locations were implemented to the MV models, and the corresponding MV function was computationally analyzed using our dynamic finite element analysis protocol [25–27,31,32].

2.3. Dynamic Finite Element Simulation of MV Function

The Ogden model was employed to define the nonlinear material behaviors of the marginal and SC tendineae. The cross-sectional areas of 0.29 mm^2 and 0.27 mm^2 were applied to the anterior and posterior marginal chordae, and 0.61 mm^2 was set for the SC [36]. A Fung-type elastic material model was utilized to describe the anisotropic hyperelastic material behavior of the MV leaflets [31]. The principal material directions were defined along the circumferential (σ_c) and radial (σ_t) directions, and the material parameters of the anterior and posterior leaflet tissue were obtained from biaxial mechanical test data that were experimentally determined in a previous study [37]. The Fung-type elastic material model was then implemented in ABAQUS. The leaflet thicknesses of the anterior and posterior leaflets were set to 0.69 and 0.51 mm, respectively [38]. The Poisson's ratio and density of the leaflets and chordae tissue were set to 0.48 and 1100 kg/m^3, respectively. A physiologic pressure gradient over the MV leaflet surface in the normal direction was incorporated throughout the full cardiac cycle. The maximum systolic ventricular pressure was 126 mmHg (16.8 kPa) [39]. Specific contact interactions for leaflet-to-leaflet and leaflet-to-chordae with the friction coefficient of 0.05 were taken into consideration for leaflet coaptation [40]. Detailed protocols of our finite element MV evaluation are demonstrated in our previous studies [25–27,31,32].

2.4. Evaluation of the Effect of the Alteration of SC Insertion Location

Distributions of stress and coaptation across the leaflets over the full cardiac cycle were collected to investigate the effect of the different SC insertion locations. Biomechanical characteristics of the MV models at peak systole were evaluated. The structural and physiologic features of the MV models were qualitatively and quantitatively evaluated. Several geometric indices including coaptation length, coaptation angle, anterior bulging height at peak systole, and anterior leaflet bulging distance at end diastole were calculated and compared. The coaptation length refers to the distance between the free margin of the leaflet and the highest position of the leaflet coaptation. The anterior coaptation angle was defined by the angle between the A–P line and the line positioning between the anterior annular point and the highest position of the leaflet coaptation. The anterior bulging height indicates the distance between the A–P plane and the highest position of each leaflet toward the aorta. The anterior leaflet bulging distance was measured to evaluate how much blood flow was obstructed from the LV to the aorta during the diastole. The anterior leaflet bulging distance was determined using the length between the plane including the anterior annular point and two papillary muscles and the furthest anterior leaflet node.

3. Results
3.1. Coaptation Distribution and Leaflet Stress Distribution

Figure 3 demonstrates the MV configuration and MV leaflet contact distributions at peak systole from the anterior viewpoint. Nine MV models with different SC insertion locations were visualized and qualitatively compared. All nine MV models revealed appropriate leaflet coaptation while exhibiting the largest contact between the two leaflets in the center-narrow MV model. As the SC insertion location became wider, the contact distribution between the leaflets flattened more.

Figure 4 shows the leaflet stress distributions at peak systole of the MVs with nine different insertion locations of the SC from the atrial viewpoint. A threshold (at 0.4 MP in red) of stress value was assigned to display the leaflet stress distributions so that larger stresses (>0.4 MPa) than the threshold were presented in red while aiding in the comparison of the leaflet stress distributions among the MV models. As the SC insertion was located further toward the mitral annulus (apical) or wider (lateral), the leaflet stresses near the saddle-horn region of the anterior leaflet increased. The maximum stresses increased in accordance with the width of the SC insertion location (Figure 5). In all nine MV models, a similar stress distribution pattern was found in the anterior leaflet, demonstrating large stress values around the trigone region regardless of the differences in the SC insertion location. The top-narrow MV model showed the lowest maximum stress value, and the bottom-wide MV model revealed the largest maximum stress value.

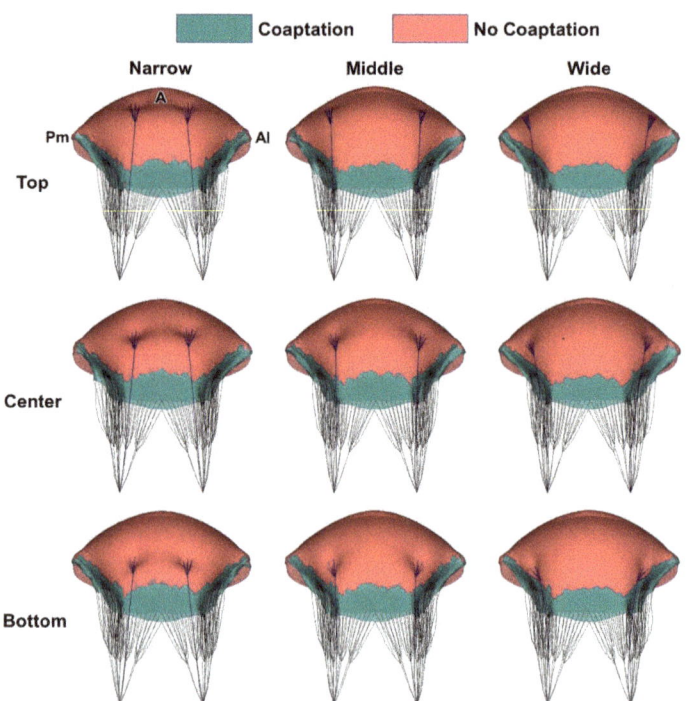

Figure 3. Leaflet coaptation distributions at peak systole with respect to alteration of the SC insertion location (anterior viewpoint). A—anterior; Al—anterolateral; Pm—posteromedial.

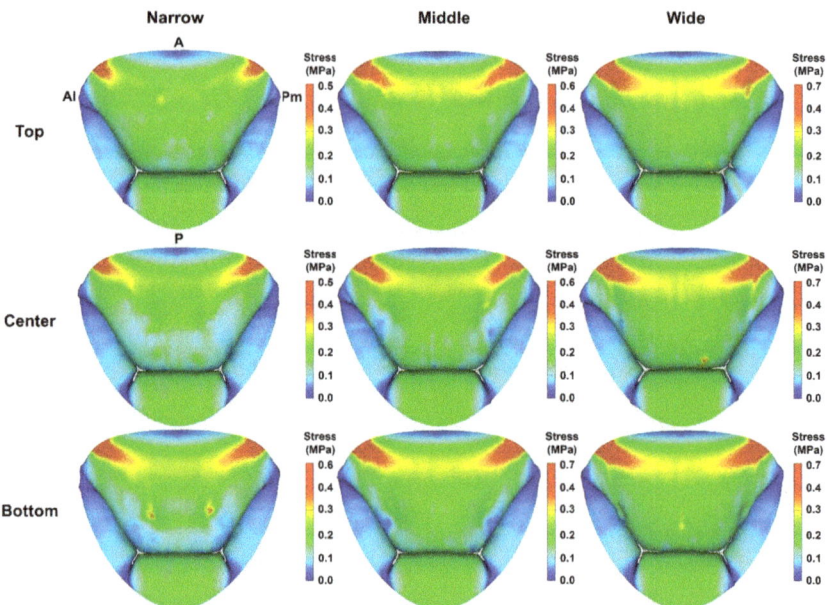

Figure 4. Stress distributions on the MV leaflets at peak systole with respect to alteration of the SC insertion location (atrial viewpoint). A—anterior; Al—anterolateral; P—posterior; Pm—posteromedial.

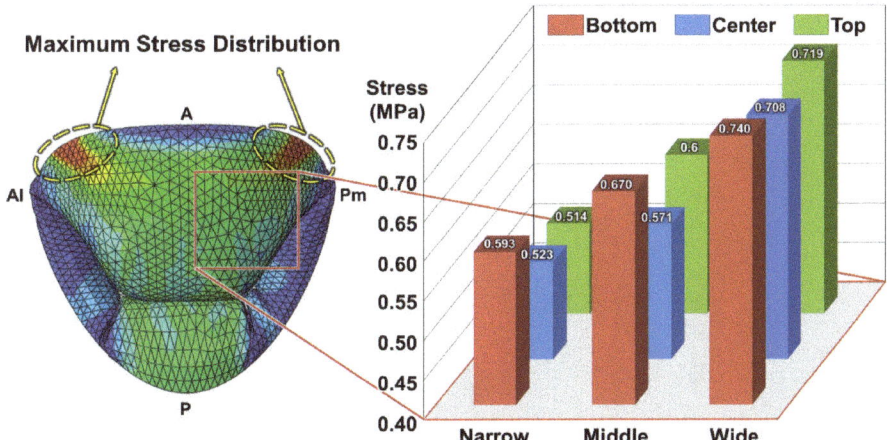

Figure 5. Maximum stress values in the annular trigone. The yellow circles represent the sites having the maximum stress values (atrial viewpoint). The red box indicates the leaflet region where the SC was inserted. A—anterior; Al—anterolateral; P—posterior; Pm—posteromedial.

3.2. Leaflet Morphology and Mobility

The morphologic features of the nine MV models with different SC insertion locations at peak systole were quantitated to assess the structure and mobility of the anterior leaflet (Figure 6). The cross-sectional views of the anteroposterior (A–P) leaflet edges are presented as blue (anterior leaflet) and red (posterior leaflet) lines to visualize and quantitate the coaptation lengths, coaptation angles, and anterior bulging heights. Dividing the nine MV models into three groups (top, center, and bottom), the center (narrow = 7.03 mm, middle = 5.93 mm, wide = 4.77 mm) and bottom (narrow = 6.86 mm, middle = 5.94 mm, wide = 4.79 mm) groups demonstrated decreased coaptation lengths in proportion to the width of the SC insertion location. The center and bottom groups also displayed an increase in coaptation angles in proportion to the width of the insertion location (center: narrow = 7.71°, middle = 8.63°, wide = 11.91°; bottom: narrow = 6.19°, middle = 8.66°, wide = 11.97°). In the top group, the middle and wide MV models showed similar coaptation lengths and coaptation angles (coaptation length: middle = 4.78 mm, wide = 4.79 mm; coaptation angle: middle = 11.91°, wide = 12.09°). The top-wide MV model demonstrated the greatest anterior bulging height (4.13 mm), and the bottom-middle MV model showed the minimum anterior bulging height (3.88 mm). In the wide group, all three MV models had similar bulging heights (top = 4.13 mm, center = 4.09 mm, bottom = 4.1 mm). In the middle group, the bulging heights decreased markedly when the SC insertion location moved from the top to the middle and bottom.

3.3. Anterior Leaflet Bulging Distance

The anterior leaflet bulging distances of the nine MV models with different types of SC insertion location at end diastole are shown in Figure 7. While similar bulging distances were observed in eight MV models (11.12–11.42 mm), a much smaller bulging distance was found in the top-narrow MV model (0.74 mm).

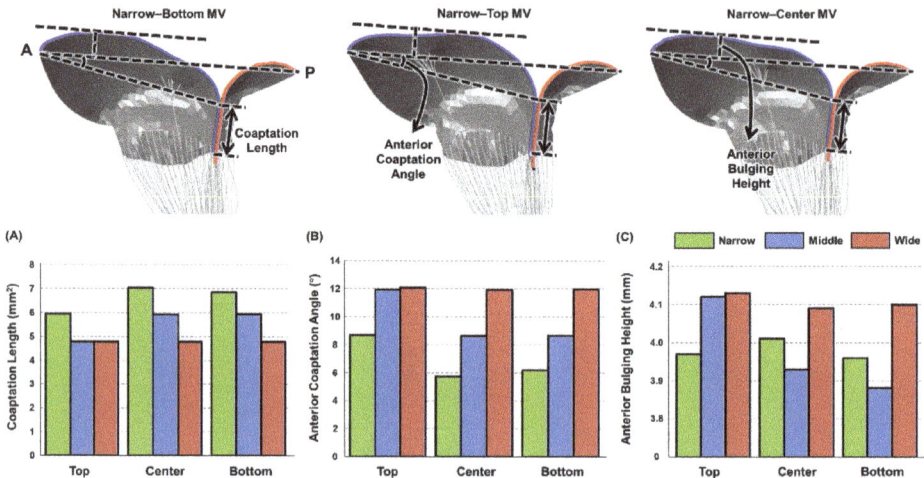

Figure 6. Morphologic features and quantitative assessment of the MV leaflets at peak systole. For the narrow MV group, the cross-sectional views of the A2-P2 leaflet edges are presented in blue (anterior leaflet) and red (posterior leaflet) lines. Quantitative morphologic assessment includes (**A**) coaptation lengths, (**B**) coaptation angles, and (**C**) anterior bulging heights. A—anterior; P—posterior.

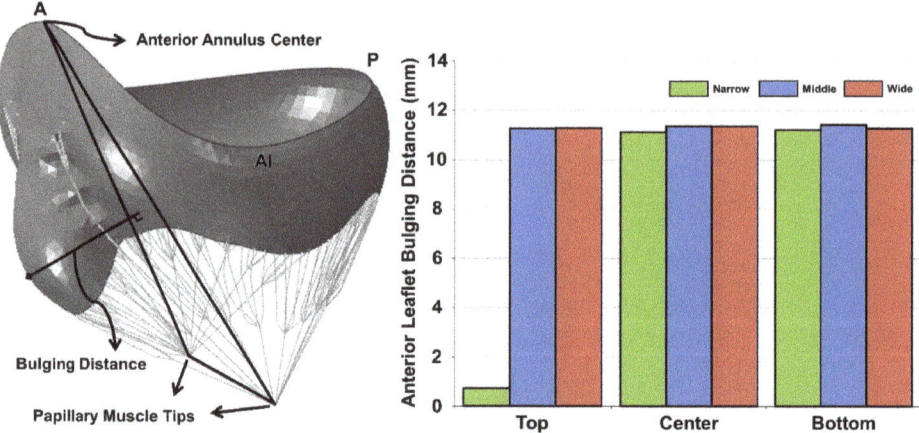

Figure 7. Anterior leaflet bulging distance with respect to alteration of the SC insertion location during the diastolic phase. The shortest distance is found in the narrow–top MV model. A—anterior; Al—anterolateral; P—posterior.

4. Discussion

Two tendon-like SCs, particularly strong and thick, are inserted in a fanlike manner into the ventricular side of the anterior MV leaflet and stretched toward the annulus. The importance of the roles of the SC in maintaining an appropriate anatomical valvular shape is obviously inferred from their anatomical location and bigger size when compared to other chordae. The SC endure tensional stresses three times larger than the marginal chordae but do not affect the existence of mitral regurgitation. Removing the SC tethering would cause the central region of the anterior leaflet to extend further towards the mitral annulus, resulting in flexible leaflet tissue around the coaptating leaflet margin [6,34]. In the present study, we utilized parametric MV modeling and finite element simulation to evaluate the biomechanics and function of the anatomical alteration of the SC insertion location based on clinical data.

Alteration of the SC insertion location demonstrated the smallest maximum leaflet stress (0.514 MPa) in the top-narrow MV model and the largest maximum leaflet stress (0.740 MPa) in the bottom-wide MV model at peak systole (Figures 4 and 5). The overall pattern of leaflet stress distribution was similar for all nine MV models, and large stresses near the anterior annular saddle-horn region increased in proportion to the width of the SC insertion location. In all nine MV models, the maximum stresses were found in the anterior annular trigone region. It is speculated that a wide width of the SC insertion location would not provide the central area of the anterior leaflet with sufficient tensional support, resulting in increased leaflet stresses near the anterior annular saddle-horn region. In addition, the maximum stress value was found to decrease as the SC insertion location was close to the mitral annulus. With the SC insertion location close to the annulus, the anterior leaflet displayed more leaflet bulging, indicating increased stresses in the central and marginal zone of the anterior leaflet. As the SC can maintain three times larger chordal stresses than the marginal chordae, lower leaflet stress values were observed in the region from the central to marginal zone when the SC was inserted far from the mitral annulus, reducing a considerable amount of overall leaflet stresses in the zone.

Consistent with previous studies suggesting that the presence of the SC does not affect coaptation, all nine MV models exhibited full coaptation and similar leaflet contact distribution (Figure 3). The MV models with a wider SC insertion location displayed further spread distribution of leaflet coaptation. A narrower SC insertion location resulted in a longer coaptation length and hence a smaller anterior coaptation angle (Figure 6). In the center and bottom groups, as the width increased, the coaptation length decreased proportionally while the coaptation angle increased. However, in the top group, the middle and wide MV models revealed similar values of the coaptation length and anterior coaptation angle. In the wide group, all three locations along the apical direction showed comparable coaptation lengths, anterior coaptation angles, and anterior bulging heights. Particularly in the wide group, little difference was found in the leaflet stress and contact distributions (coaptation length and coaptation angle) as well as the anterior bulging height and bulging distance.

The anterior leaflet bulging distance indicates how the SC influence the blood outflow from the left ventricle. Systolic anterior motion (SAM) refers to the clinical observation such that the distal portion of the anterior leaflet is placed obstructing the left ventricular outflow area. When the SC restrict the anterior leaflet mobility, SAM can occur [6]. The SC prevent the lateral portion of the anterior leaflet from bulging toward the left ventricular outflow tract (LVOT) by acting like a sail. The top-narrow MV model demonstrated the shortest anterior leaflet bulging distance, indicating that the SC prevent the entire anterior leaflet bulging toward the LVOT to develop an orifice area at diastole smaller than the others (Figure 7). The top-narrow MV model also showed lower stresses across the anterior leaflet (Figure 4) and the lowest maximum stresses (Figure 5). Therefore, in principle, this top-narrow MC model could be assumed to have the most suitable SC insertion location from the valvular functional perspective. However, in the case of functional mitral regurgitation accompanied by distal displacement of the papillary muscles, the tethering force in the SC increases; this could result in tenting and regurgitation [35].

The parametric MV modeling strategy employed in the present study has several limitations. Although recent studies demonstrated and emphasized the importance of patient-specific chordae modeling [41–43], true geometric configurations of the complete chordae tendineae structure are still not available from 3D echocardiographic data due to the restricted spatial and temporal resolution issue of the currently available clinical imaging modality. The parametric MV model was created based on the average dimensions of normal human MVs. The key focus of the present study is to evaluate the effect of varying the SC insertion location on normal MV function and dynamics to better understand the complex MV structures from the biomechanical perspectives. The length of the SC is not directly configured but determined by quantitating the distance between the papillary muscle tips and the locations where the SC were inserted in this study. Therefore, the simulated variations of the SC insertion location may not implement directly on evaluation of patient MV models. Nevertheless, valuable information can be obtained from assessing the relative dimensional comparisons of these MV apparatus deformations to better understand the effect of the SC insertion locations on MV function.

5. Conclusions

We conducted computational evaluations to examine the effect of the SC insertion location on the function and dynamics a normal MV. Alterations of the SC insertion locations demonstrated differences in the biomechanical measurements and functional indices throughout the cardiac cycle. The SC have a unique structure and play a key role in reinforcing the tunnel-shape of the MV throughout the cardiac cycle and ensuring mobility of the anterior leaflet. While the leaflet stress distribution and coaptation showed similar patterns in all nine MV models, the maximum leaflet stresses increased in accordance with the width of the SC insertion locations. This computational MV evaluation can aid in understanding the effect of the SC insertion locations on mechanism, function, and pathophysiology of the MV.

Author Contributions: Conceptualization, W.H. and H.K.; methodology, W.H. and S.J.; validation, W.H. and S.J.; investigation, W.H., S.J., M.K. and H.H.K.; resources, H.K.; writing—original draft preparation, W.H.; writing—review and editing, H.K.; visualization, M.K. and H.H.K.; supervision, H.K. All authors have read and agreed to the published version of the manuscript.

Funding: This research was supported by the National Research Foundation of Korea (NRF) through the Ministry of Science and ICT (NRF-2019R1A2C1005094).

Institutional Review Board Statement: Not applicable.

Informed Consent Statement: Not applicable.

Data Availability Statement: The datasets generated during this study are available from the corresponding author on reasonable request.

Conflicts of Interest: The authors declare no conflict of interest.

References

1. Mestres, C.A.; Bernal, J.M. Mitral valve repair: The chordae tendineae. *J. Tehran Heart Cent.* **2012**, *7*, 92–99.
2. Chen, L.; Yin, F.C.; May-Newman, K. The structure and mechanical properties of the mitral valve leaflet-strut chordae transition zone. *J. Biomech. Eng.* **2004**, *126*, 244–251. [CrossRef]
3. Degandt, A.A.; Weber, P.A.; Saber, H.A.; Duran, C.M. Mitral valve basal chordae: Comparative anatomy and terminology. *Ann. Thorac. Surg.* **2007**, *84*, 1250–1255. [CrossRef]
4. Goetz, W.A.; Lim, H.S.; Lansac, E.; Saber, H.A.; Pekar, F.; Weber, P.A.; Duran, C.M. Anterior mitral basal 'stay' chords are essential for left ventricular geometry and function. *J. Heart Valve Dis.* **2005**, *14*, 195–202. [PubMed]
5. Goetz, W.A.; Lim, H.S.; Pekar, F.; Saber, H.A.; Weber, P.A.; Lansac, E.; Birnbaum, D.E.; Duran, C.M. Anterior mitral leaflet mobility is limited by the basal stay chords. *Circulation* **2003**, *107*, 2969–2974. [CrossRef] [PubMed]
6. Chen, L.; May-Newman, K. Effect of strut chordae transection on mitral valve leaflet biomechanics. *Ann. Biomed. Eng.* **2006**, *34*, 917–926. [CrossRef] [PubMed]
7. Marcus, R.H.; Sareli, P.; Pocock, W.A.; Meyer, T.E.; Magalhaes, M.P.; Grieve, T.; Antunes, M.J.; Barlow, J.B. Functional anatomy of severe mitral regurgitation in active rheumatic carditis. *Am. J. Cardiol.* **1989**, *63*, 577–584. [CrossRef]
8. van Rijk-Zwikker, G.L.; Delemarre, B.J.; Huysmans, H.A. Mitral valve anatomy and morphology: Relevance to mitral valve replacement and valve reconstruction. *J. Card. Surg.* **1994**, *9*, 255–261. [CrossRef]
9. Obadia, J.F.; Casali, C.; Chassignolle, J.F.; Janier, M. Mitral subvalvular apparatus: Different functions of primary and secondary chordae. *Circulation* **1997**, *96*, 3124–3128. [CrossRef] [PubMed]
10. Obadia, J.F.; Janier, M. Second order anterior mitral leaflets play a role in preventing systolic anterior motion. *Ann. Thorac. Surg.* **2002**, *73*, 1689–1690. [CrossRef]
11. Kunzelman, K.S.; Cochran, R.P.; Chuong, C.; Ring, W.S.; Verrier, E.D.; Eberhart, R.D. Finite element analysis of the mitral valve. *J. Heart Valve Dis.* **1993**, *2*, 326–340. [PubMed]
12. Padala, M.; Gyoneva, L.; Yoganathan, A.P. Effect of anterior strut chordal transection on the force distribution on the marginal chordae of the mitral valve. *J. Thorac. Cardiovasc. Surg.* **2012**, *144*, 624–633.e2. [CrossRef]
13. Feng, L.; Qi, N.; Gao, H.; Sun, W.; Vazquez, M.; Griffith, B.E.; Luo, X. On the chordae structure and dynamic behaviour of the mitral valve. *IMA J. Appl. Math.* **2018**, *83*, 1066–1091. [CrossRef]

14. Khalighi, A.H.; Rego, B.V.; Drach, A.; Gorman, R.C.; Gorman, J.H., 3rd; Sacks, M.S. Development of a functionally equivalent model of the mitral valve chordae tendineae through topology optimization. *Ann. Biomed. Eng.* **2019**, *47*, 60–74. [CrossRef]
15. Panicheva, D.; Villard, P.F.; Hammer, P.E.; Perrin, D.; Berger, M.O. Automatic extraction of the mitral valve chordae geometry for biomechanical simulation. *Int. J. Comput. Assist. Radiol Surg.* **2021**, *16*, 709–720. [CrossRef]
16. Marom, G.; Plitman Mayo, R.; Again, N.; Raanani, E. Numerical biomechanics models of the interaction between a novel transcatheter mitral valve device and the subvalvular apparatus. *Innovations* **2021**, 1556984521999362, Online ahead of print.
17. Chen, S.; Sari, C.R.; Gao, H.; Lei, Y.; Segers, P.; De Beule, M.; Wang, G.; Ma, X. Mechanical and morphometric study of mitral valve chordae tendineae and related papillary muscle. *J. Mech. Behav. Biomed. Mater.* **2020**, *111*, 104011. [CrossRef] [PubMed]
18. Kaiser, A.D.; McQueen, D.M.; Peskin, C.S. Modeling the mitral valve. *Int. J. Numer. Method. Biomed. Eng.* **2019**, *35*, e3240. [CrossRef]
19. Paulsen, M.J.; Imbrie-Moore, A.M.; Wang, H.; Bae, J.H.; Hironaka, C.E.; Farry, J.M.; Lucian, H.J.; Thakore, A.D.; MacArthur, J.W.; Cutkosky, M.R.; et al. Mitral chordae tendineae force profile characterization using a posterior ventricular anchoring neochordal repair model for mitral regurgitation in a three-dimensional-printed ex vivo left heart simulator. *Eur. J. Cardiothorac. Surg.* **2020**, *57*, 535–544. [CrossRef]
20. Ross, C.J.; Laurence, D.W.; Hsu, M.C.; Baumwart, R.; Zhao, Y.D.; Mir, A.; Burkhart, H.M.; Holzapfel, G.A.; Wu, Y.; Lee, C.H. Mechanics of porcine heart valves' strut chordae tendineae investigated as a leaflet-chordae-papillary muscle entity. *Ann. Biomed. Eng.* **2020**, *48*, 1463–1474. [CrossRef] [PubMed]
21. Shen, X.; Wang, T.; Cao, X.; Cai, L. The geometric model of the human mitral valve. *PLoS ONE* **2017**, *12*, e0183362. [CrossRef]
22. Meschini, V.; de Tullio, M.D.; Verzicco, R. Effects of mitral chordae tendineae on the flow in the left heart ventricle. *Eur. Phys. J. E Soft Matter* **2018**, *41*, 27. [CrossRef]
23. Papolla, C.; Darwish, A.; Kadem, L.; Rieu, R. Impact of mitral regurgitation on the flow in a model of a left ventricle. *Cardiovasc. Eng. Technol.* **2020**, *11*, 708–718. [CrossRef] [PubMed]
24. Toma, M.; Einstein, D.R.; Bloodworth, C.H.t.; Cochran, R.P.; Yoganathan, A.P.; Kunzelman, K.S. Fluid-structure interaction and structural analyses using a comprehensive mitral valve model with 3d chordal structure. *Int. J. Numer. Method. Biomed. Eng.* **2017**, *33*, e2815. [CrossRef]
25. Choi, A.; McPherson, D.D.; Kim, H. Biomechanical evaluation of the pathophysiologic developmental mechanisms of mitral valve prolapse: Effect of valvular morphologic alteration. *Med. Biol. Eng. Comput.* **2016**, *54*, 799–809. [CrossRef]
26. Choi, A.; McPherson, D.D.; Kim, H. Neochordoplasty versus leaflet resection for ruptured mitral chordae treatment: Virtual mitral valve repair. *Comput. Biol. Med.* **2017**, *90*, 50–58. [CrossRef]
27. Choi, A.; McPherson, D.D.; Kim, H. Computational virtual evaluation of the effect of annuloplasty ring shape. *Int. J. Numer. Method. Biomed. Eng.* **2017**, *33*, e2831. [CrossRef] [PubMed]
28. Rim, Y.; Chandran, K.B.; Laing, S.T.; Kee, P.; McPherson, D.D.; Kim, H. Can computational simulation quantitatively determine mitral valve abnormalities? *JACC Cardiovasc. Imaging* **2015**, *8*, 1112–1114. [CrossRef] [PubMed]
29. Rim, Y.; Choi, A.; Laing, S.T.; McPherson, D.D.; Kim, H. Three-dimensional echocardiography-based prediction of posterior leaflet resection. *Echocardiography* **2014**, *31*, E300–E303. [CrossRef]
30. Rim, Y.; Laing, S.T.; Kee, P.; McPherson, D.D.; Kim, H. Evaluation of mitral valve dynamics. *JACC Cardiovasc. Imaging* **2013**, *6*, 263–268. [CrossRef]
31. Rim, Y.; McPherson, D.D.; Chandran, K.B.; Kim, H. The effect of patient-specific annular motion on dynamic simulation of mitral valve function. *J. Biomech.* **2013**, *46*, 1104–1112. [CrossRef] [PubMed]
32. Rim, Y.; Choi, A.; McPherson, D.D.; Kim, H. Personalized computational modeling of mitral valve prolapse: Virtual leaflet resection. *PLoS ONE* **2015**, *10*, e0130906. [CrossRef] [PubMed]
33. Sonne, C.; Sugeng, L.; Watanabe, N.; Weinert, L.; Saito, K.; Tsukiji, M.; Yoshida, K.; Takeuchi, M.; Mor-Avi, V.; Lang, R.M. Age and body surface area dependency of mitral valve and papillary apparatus parameters: Assessment by real-time three-dimensional echocardiography. *Eur. J. Echocardiogr.* **2009**, *10*, 287–294. [CrossRef] [PubMed]
34. Lam, J.H.; Ranganathan, N.; Wigle, E.D.; Silver, M.D. Morphology of the human mitral valve. I. Chordae tendineae: A new classification. *Circulation* **1970**, *41*, 449–458. [CrossRef] [PubMed]
35. Song, J.M.; Kim, J.J.; Ha, T.Y.; Lee, J.W.; Jung, S.H.; Hwang, I.S.; Lee, I.; Sun, B.J.; Kim, D.H.; Kang, D.H.; et al. Basal chordae sites on the mitral valve determine the severity of secondary mitral regurgitation. *Heart* **2015**, *101*, 1024–1031. [CrossRef]
36. Prot, V.; Skallerud, B.; Sommer, G.; Holzapfel, G.A. On modelling and analysis of healthy and pathological human mitral valves: Two case studies. *J. Mech. Behav. Biomed. Mater.* **2010**, *3*, 167–177. [CrossRef]
37. May-Newman, K.; Yin, F.C. A constitutive law for mitral valve tissue. *J. Biomech. Eng.* **1998**, *120*, 38–47. [CrossRef]
38. May-Newman, K.; Yin, F.C. Biaxial mechanical behavior of excised porcine mitral valve leaflets. *Am. J. Physiol.* **1995**, *269*, H1319–H1327. [CrossRef]
39. Mitchell, J.R.; Wang, J.J. Expanding application of the wiggers diagram to teach cardiovascular physiology. *Adv. Physiol. Educ.* **2014**, *38*, 170–175. [CrossRef]
40. Stevanella, M.; Votta, E.; Redaelli, A. Mitral valve finite element modeling: Implications of tissues' nonlinear response and annular motion. *J. Biomech. Eng.* **2009**, *131*, 121010. [CrossRef]
41. Khalighi, A.H.; Drach, A.; Bloodworth, C.H.; Pierce, E.L.; Yoganathan, A.P.; Gorman, R.C.; Gorman, J.H., 3rd; Sacks, M.S. Mitral valve chordae tendineae: Topological and geometrical characterization. *Ann. Biomed. Eng.* **2017**, *45*, 378–393. [CrossRef] [PubMed]

42. Sacks, M.; Drach, A.; Lee, C.H.; Khalighi, A.; Rego, B.; Zhang, W.; Ayoub, S.; Yoganathan, A.; Gorman, R.C.; Gorman Iii, J.H. On the simulation of mitral valve function in health, disease, and treatment. *J. Biomech. Eng.* **2019**, *141*, 0708041. [CrossRef] [PubMed]
43. Zuo, K.; Pham, T.; Li, K.; Martin, C.; He, Z.; Sun, W. Characterization of biomechanical properties of aged human and ovine mitral valve chordae tendineae. *J. Mech. Behav. Biomed. Mater.* **2016**, *62*, 607–618. [CrossRef] [PubMed]

Article

Changes in Fatigue Recovery and Muscle Damage Enzymes after Deep-Sea Water Thalassotherapy

Nam-Ik Kim [1], Sagn-Jin Kim [1], Jee-Hun Jang [2], Woon-seob Shin [3], Hyok-ju Eum [4], Buom Kim [5], Ahnryul Choi [6] and Sang-Sik Lee [6],*

1. Department of Physical Education, College of Education, Catholic Kwandong University, Gangneung-si 25601, Korea; kni8993@cku.ac.kr (N.-I.K.); Chuna2258@naver.com (S.-J.K.)
2. Department of Sports Leisure, College of Tourism and Sports, Catholic Kwandong University, Gangneung-si 25601, Korea; jjh@cku.ac.kr
3. Department of Microbiology, College of Medicine, Catholic Kwandong University, Gangneung-si 25601, Korea; shinws@cku.ac.kr
4. Gyeonggido Ujeongbu Office of Education, Uijeongbu-si 11690, Korea; polight@daum.net
5. Department of Physical Education, Kyungdong University, Yangju-si 11458, Korea; Kbswim2442@kduniv.ac.kr
6. Department of Biomedical Engineering, College of Medical Convergence, Catholic Kwandong University, Gangneung-si 25601, Korea; achoi@cku.ac.kr
* Correspondence: lsskyj@cku.ac.kr

Received: 22 September 2020; Accepted: 23 November 2020; Published: 25 November 2020

Abstract: The purpose of this study was to verify the effect of deep-sea water thalassotherapy (DSWTT) on recovery from fatigue and muscle damage. The same exercise program is conducted in general underwater and deep-sea water to confirm the characteristics of deep-sea water through fatigue recovery and muscle damage enzymes. A total of 30 male college students were studied, including 10 belonging to the control group (CG), 10 in the water exercise group (WEG), and 10 in the deep-sea water exercise group (DSWEG). The DSWTT treatment consists of three components—preheating, treatment, and cooling—and the DSWTT program stretches and massages the entire upper body, lower body, back, and the entire body for a total of 25 min in a deep-sea tank. After the DSWTT program, blood tests were conducted to confirm the level of fatigue-related parameters and muscle damage enzymes. Fatigue-related parameters including glucose, lactate, ammonia, and lactate dehydrogenase (LDH), and the levels of muscle damage enzymes such as creatinine kinase (CK) and aspartate aminotransferase (AST) were measured. The results revealed that fatigue had a primary effect ($p < 0.001$) and exhibited strongly significant interaction ($p < 0.001$) with lactate, ammonia, and LDH levels, whereas the glucose level remained unchanged. The post hoc results showed a significant decrease in these parameters among DSWEG compared to CG and WEG ($p < 0.01$). Muscle damage enzymes showed a main effect ($p < 0.001$) and significant interaction ($p < 0.001$) with CK and AST ($p < 0.001$). The post hoc results showed a significant decrease in DSWEG compared with CG and WEG ($p < 0.01$). In conclusion, the DSWTT program applied to this study showed significant effects on muscle fatigue and muscle damage recovery. When the DSWTT program is applied in hot springs, it can have a positive effect on muscle fatigue and muscle damage recovery and can contribute to improving national health and quality of life. Further studies are needed to investigate DSWTT programs with various research subjects at different program temperatures, exercise times, and frequencies of treatment and exercise.

Keywords: fatigue rehabilitation; thalassotherapy adverse effects; blood test; lactate dehydrogenase; creatinine kinase

1. Introduction

In recent years, both men and women have become interested in effective physical activity and healing while pursuing a healthy life. As a result of the increase in interest, studies on physical recovery programs such as fatigue recovery and muscle damage due to various sports and physical activities are actively being conducted [1,2]. Fatigue is a decline in mental and physical functions that occur accompanied by continuous or repeated mental and physical work and is an indicator of physiological stress, defensive response, or pathological precursor [3]. Therefore, fatigue and muscle damage caused by physical and mental activity are common early symptoms of many diseases [4]. In addition, fatigue may degrade the quality of life of daily life [5], cause physiological homeostasis disorder, and develop into a disease or a chronic disease, which may result in decreased physical and mental functions [6].

Fatigue is triggered by a peripheral signal from the brain, which inhibits the motor system, and thereby the mobilization of exercise units, and it is controlled by accumulation of metabolites or energy depletion [7]. The accumulation of these fatigue substances is important to prevent exercise-related injuries caused by fatigue, depending on the intensity, time, shape, and environment [8,9].

Methods to promote recovery from fatigue include static measures such as rest or sleep and dynamic elements such as bathing, massage, and gymnastics. Among the bathing methods performed underwater, the recovery in hot water (37~38 °C) is known to activate blood circulation by reducing the imbalance of the upper and lower limbs of the body [10]. It can also increase muscle fatigue and resilience to muscle damage by not only adding pressure to the muscles but also carrying heat to the muscle tissue [11]. Ice fomentation at low temperature (15 °C) is known to relieve excitement of the central nervous system and promote the removal of metabolites [12,13]. The detailed mechanism underlying recovery from fatigue using water therapy has yet to be reported.

However, regular exercise has a positive effect on prevention and treatment of lifestyle diseases by decreasing the risk factors of cardiovascular disease and metabolic syndrome, but it also has a negative effect depending on exercise intensity. In particular, high-intensity exercise causes muscle damage and damage to human tissues due to upper respiratory tract infection, inhibition of immune system function, increased lipid peroxidation, and reduction in antioxidant enzymes [14].

The exercise-induced muscle damage is caused by one-time or long-term muscle cell and tissue damage, which can be indirectly predicted by the blood concentration of enzymes such as creatinine kinase (CK) and lactate dehydrogenase (LDH) released from muscle tissue following exercise [15,16]. According to Yeom's [17] study, treadmill exercise was performed until the time when the exercise intensity consumed energy of 40, 60, and 80% to 200, 400, and 600 kcal of VO2max, and all creatine phosphokinase(CPK) was significantly higher; the CPK concentration changed according to the exercise intensity and momentum.

These changes in CPK serve as biochemical variables of exercise and physical strength. They are used as indirect indicators of muscle damage and inflammation such as cell membrane destruction and tissue necrosis in long-term exercise or high-intensity exercise. The increase in LDH and CPK levels in the blood is attributed to damaged muscle fibers due to excessive exercise, resulting in muscle pain and muscle fatigue, which can lead to declining performance and exercise-related injuries.

The underwater treatment program reduces the load on the body weight and leads to greater joint movement than the ground treatment program [18], which is predicted to improve the range of motion (ROM) quickly and effectively [19] by promoting recovering from muscle damage after vigorous exercise. In recent years, the application of thalassotherapy (TT; derivation of Greek Thalassa, which means the sea) using deep-sea water (DSW), characterized by low temperature stability, eutrophic, clean, and anti-aging properties [20], has become a hot topic in the field of water therapy.

The progress of the study, which restores fatigue and muscle damage quickly after physical activity, can be a great help in restoring physical condition and improving exercise ability. The underwater treatment program increases blood flow to the muscle, which leads to recovery from muscle tension [21] and facilitates the elimination of metabolic byproducts by improving venous reflux rate [22]. However, most studies have shown that there are treatments in the water, but the treatments using hot spring water have not been reported yet [23], and the effect of DSW-based fatigue and muscle injury recovery programs on exercise physiology has yet to be demonstrated.

Therefore, this study is to verify the effect on fatigue and muscle damage recovery through an exercise program based on deep-sea water thalassotherapy (DSWTT) and to confirm the characteristics of DSW.

2. Materials and Methods

2.1. Subjects

The subjects of this study were a selected group of Korean male college students in their 20s. Subjects with a history of neurosurgical and orthopedic issues within 6 months of the measurement date were excluded from the study if they were associated with musculoskeletal problems interfering with the water treatment and DSWTT programs. In addition, participants were randomly selected from numbers 1 to 30, and participants were randomly assigned to each group, and the experiment was conducted in compliance with the ethical principles of the Helsinki Declaration. During the DSWTT program, the participants were photographed, and the photographs taken were agreed to be used in the thesis. A total of 30 participants were classified equally as 10 as control group (CG), 10 as water exercise group (WEG), and 10 as deep-sea water exercise group (DSWEG). The general physical characteristics of the subjects are shown in Table 1.

Table 1. General characteristics of subjects.

Groups (n)	Age (year)	Height (cm)	Weight (kg)	Body Fat (%)	SBP (mmHg)	DBP (mmHg)	Shuttle Run Round Trip Times (time)
CG (n = 10)	20.50 ± 2.01	173.31 ± 2.97	71.52 ± 10.16	16.46 ± 3.49	121.50 ± 3.37	81.00 ± 6.14	83.80 ± 7.00
WEG (n = 10)	20.09 ± 2.07	174.61 ± 6.39	73.25 ± 10.46	17.25 ± 2.96	122.00 ± 3.49	80.50 ± 5.98	88.10 ± 7.82
DSWEG (n = 10)	20.70 ± 2.11	173.94 ± 2.74	73.42 ± 9.59	18.42 ± 2.89	122.50 ± 3.53	79.50 ± 7.24	88.80 ± 7.13

Means ± S.D. SBP: systolic blood pressure, DBP: diastolic blood pressure, CG: control group, WEG: water exercise group, DSWEG: deep-sea water exercise group.

2.2. DSWTT Treatment Program

The water therapy and DSWTT programs administered in this study are presented in Table 2. After fatigue induced by exercise program progression, the subjects were asked to identify the effects of DSWTT program on fatigue recovery and muscle damage enzymes.

The subjects in WEG actively participated in a water treatment program involving a tap-water bath (standard 3 × 3 × 1.5 m, horizontal × vertical × height) maintained at 34 ± 1 °C. The subjects in the DSWEG actively performed the same DSWTT program similar to the WEG but in a deep-sea water bath, which was maintained at 34 ± 1 °C (Figure 1). The subjects in the CG underwent dynamic recovery on the ground. The subjects of the study, which were first conducted by research director by group, were thoroughly educated in advance to perform the program with an accurate attitude on the DSWTT program (lower body, upper body, back body, whole body).

The DSWTT program was used by reconstructing the items used by Kim et al. The program was organized in the order of warm-up, treatment (lower body, upper body, back, body stretching and massage treatment), and cool-down phases. The time required for each phase was 2~5 min, lasting a total of 25 min. The DSWTT program consists of 7 lower body exercises, 8 upper body exercises, and 2 full body exercises. Each action was performed by an expert. The composition of the DSWTT program, treatment sites, and the time are shown in Table 2.

Table 2. Thalassotherapy using deep-sea water.

Stage	Treatment Method	Time (min)
Warm-up	Floating (floating belts on wrists and ankles)	2
Lower body	Ankle stretch (left, right) Toe stretching (left, right) Foot pressure (left, right) Knee stretching (left, right)	5
	Gastrocnemius massage Hamstring massage Holding your feet and rock them up and down	5
Upper body	Wrist stretch (left, right) Finger stretch (left, right) Palm pressure (left, right) Arm stretch (left, right) Shoulder stretch (left, right)	3
	Fore-arm massage Upper arm massage Holding your arms and rocking them up and down	3
Back	Neck massage Back massage	2
Body as a whole	Stimulation of arms, legs, and sides (left, right) Keeping your back up	2
Cool-down	Floating (floating belts on wrists and ankles)	3
Total		25

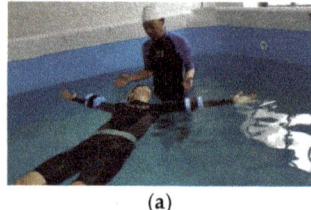 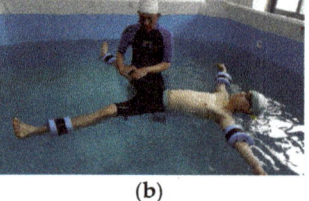

(a) (b)

Figure 1. Deep-sea water thalassotherapy (DSWTT) treatment program: (a) floating; (b) lower body.

In the DSWTT program environment, DSWEG was warmly heated with a regenerative boiler using the unique characteristics and properties of DSW with 34.03% salinity and pH 7.81 water depth of 0.5 m. The main elements included magnesium 1270 mg/L, calcium 367 mg/L, potassium 357 mg/L, sodium 11,033 mg/L, manganese 1.9 mg/L, zinc 0.68 mg/L, and iron 018 mg/L. WEG used tap water supplied by K-water to warm up. Considering the characteristics of this study, a special bathtub was installed in the room $3 \times 3 \times 1.5$ m (horizontal × vertical × height), and the program was applied while maintaining a depth of 1.2 ± 0.1 m.

2.3. Measurement Parameters and Method

2.3.1. Fatigue Inducement Test

The fatigue inducement test was conducted using the 20 m shuttle run test (20 m multi-shuttle run test; 20 m-MST) designed by Leger and Lambert [24] and conducted by the "National Fitness Award 100 Center" of Korea, C university. The 20 m-MST method involves long-distance driving at a length of 20 m and speeds up every minute. The 20 m section was initially measured using a cassette that started to walk at a speed of 8.5 km/h and was set to increase the beep interval by 0.5 km/h every minute.

The subjects were started by a beep. It was impossible to continue running according to the beep after running for 20 m based on a regularly accelerating audio rhythm, and when the rhythm could not be followed more than twice (about 3 m behind), the shuttle run test was completed for each individual (Figure 2). After the shuttle run, the recovery program started immediately without a time interval. The number of round trips to and from the finished 20 m section was recorded, and the number of recorded numbers is in Table 3 [25]. The data designed by the study were used, and using Table 3, we calculated the acceleration by section, and the performance ability of the subjects was the difference according to individual difference; so, when the two times did not follow the standard, it was selected as the maximum exercise.

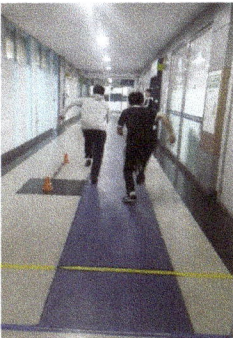

Figure 2. Fatigue inducement test (20 m shuttle run).

Table 3. Sectional acceleration of shuttle run test.

Stage (Numbers)	Period (s)	Speed (km/h)
Level 1 (7)	9.0	8.5
Level 2 (7)	8.5	9.0
Level 3 (8)	8.0	9.5
Level 4 (8)	7.6	10.0
Level 5 (8)	7.2	10.5
Level 6 (9)	6.9	11.0
Level 7 (9)	6.6	11.5
Level 8 (10)	6.3	12.0
Level 9 (10)	6.0	12.5
Level 10 (10)	5.8	13.0
Level 11 (11)	5.5	13.5
Level 12 (12)	5.3	14.0
Level 13 (13)	5.1	14.5
Level 14 (14)	5.0	15.0
Level 15 (15)	4.8	15.5
Level 16 (16)	4.7	16.0
Level 17 (17)	4.5	16.5
Level 18 (18)	4.4	17.0
Level 19 (19)	4.2	17.5
Level 20 (20)	4.1	18.0

2.3.2. Blood Test

Blood tests were performed to ensure the reliability of the test data, and blood was collected by clinical pathologists 3 times in total (Figure 3). The first test was conducted at the laboratory 30 min before the start of the experiment and was collected under a stable time. The second test was performed immediately after the artificial fatigue inducement exercise (20 m shuttle run test). The third test was performed after 25 min of treatment program.

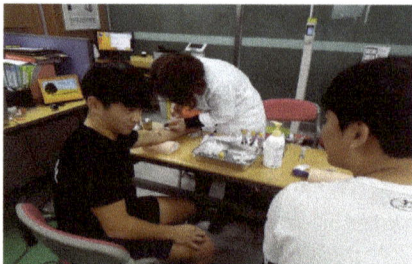

Figure 3. Blood test.

Blood samples (10 mL each) were collected from the subjects' upper veins and were centrifuged at 3000 rpm for 5 min and stored at −70 °C until analysis. The samples were collected by the Clinical Pathology Department of the E Medical Foundation (Seoul, Korea), and the fatigue parameters and muscle damage enzymes were analyzed. The fatigue parameters included lactate, ammonia, glucose, and LDH. The muscle damage enzymes included CK and aspartate aminotransferase (AST).

2.3.3. Statistical Analysis

The statistical differences were calculated using the SPSS Version 18.0 program, and the average difference between groups was measured by 3 × 3 repeated measurements of the group and the measurement time as independent variables (two-way ANOVA with the measurements). Measurements were taken three times pre-exercise, post-exercise, and post-treatment. A two-way repeated measures ANOVA was performed when the main effect and the interaction effects between the group and the measurement time were significant. The significance level of statistical analysis was set to α = 0.05.

3. Results

3.1. Fatigue Recovery

The changes in fatigue recovery after the DSWTT program are shown in Table 4.

Table 4. Changes in fatigue recovery parameters.

Item	Groups	Test			Source	F-Value	
		Pre-Exercise	Post-Exercise	Post-Treatment			
Glucose (mg/dL)	CG	95.30±10.49	102.20 ± 15.99	101.50 ± 12.40	Test	2.132	
	WEG	96.50 ± 9.05	103.00 ± 18.79	99.30 ± 13.40	Group	0.917	
	DWEG	91.70 ± 9.92	98.70 ± 13.46	95.23 ± 15.13 $	Group × Test	0.130	
Lactate acid (mmol/L)	CG	1.93 ± 0.35	14.29 ± 2.26	10.09 ± 2.34	Test	163.629	***
	WEG	1.83 ± 0.40	13.85 ± 1.09	8.69 ± 2.65 $	Group	1.031	
	DWEG	2.11 ± 0.39	17.44 ± 3.93	4.72 ± 2.57 #	Group × Test	13.307	***
Ammonia (umol/L)	CG	23.20 ± 2.78	53.30 ± 6.07	44.30 ± 4.62	Test	176.681	***
	WEG	21.50 ± 3.37	50.70 ± 6.94	39.60 ± 7.64 $	Group	3.383	*
	DWEG	24.50 ± 4.67	52.82 ± 5.65	28.80 ± 4.58 #	Group × Test	22.487	***
LDH (U/L)	CG	199.50 ± 32.22	258.20 ± 29.93	247.50 ± 35.69	Test	12.196	**
	WEG	189.80 ± 34.38	249.50 ± 31.92	234.30 ± 33.92	Group	6.390	**
	DWEG	178.40 ± 34.81	252.30 ± 21.83	158.80 ± 31.77 #	Group × Test	9.972	***

Means ± S.D., *: $p < 0.05$, **: $p < 0.01$, ***: $p < 0.001$, $: significantly different from CG, #: significantly different from within the group, LDH: lactate dehydrogenase, CG: control group, WEG: water exercise group, DWEG: deep-sea water exercise group.

Glucose was not significantly different in the analysis of interaction effects between the groups and the measurement time, the main effect according to the measurement time. Lactic acid showed a significant difference in the interaction ($p < 0.001$) between the group and the measurement time

($p < 0.01$). However, there was no difference between the groups at the time of measurement. The post hoc analysis showed that DSWEG significantly decreased after program following maximum exercise ($p < 0.01$), and WEG significantly decreased after CG ($p < 0.05$).

Ammonia showed a significant difference in the main effect of measurement ($p < 0.001$) between groups within the measurement time ($p < 0.05$), and the interaction effect ($p < 0.01$) between the group and the measurement time. The post hoc analysis showed that DSWEG significantly decreased after the program following maximum exercise ($p < 0.01$), and WEG significantly decreased after CG ($p < 0.05$). LDH showed a significant difference in the main effect of measurement ($p < 0.001$) between groups within the measurement time ($p < 0.01$), and the interaction ($p < 0.01$) between the group and the measurement time. The post hoc analysis revealed that DSWEG significantly decreased after the maximum exercise program in the CG and WEG ($p < 0.01$).

3.2. Enzymes Released in Muscle Damage

The changes in enzymes released in muscle damage following the DSWTT program are shown in Table 5.

Table 5. Changes in enzyme levels during exercise-induced muscle damage.

Item	Groups	Test			Source	F-Value	
		Pre-Exercise	Post-Exercise	Post-Treatment			
CK(U/L)	CG	175.00 ± 37.16	236.80 ± 62.58	231.90 ± 61.00	Test	14.867	***
	WEG	185.60 ± 35.31	251.00 ± 31.36	210.90 ± 18.08 $	Group	0.208	
	DWEG	180.00 ± 33.71	267.80 ± 37.50	171.90 ± 28.51 #	Group × Test	8.582	***
AST(U/L)	CG	20.10 ± 3.72	24.90 ± 5.23	28.10 ± 5.87	Test	25.793	***
	WEG	19.30 ± 4.11	27.20 ± 3.35	25.20 ± 3.25 $	Group	1.547	
	DWEG	20.30 ± 4.05	28.50 ± 4.14	16.80 ± 2.44 #	Group × Test	26.831	***

Means ± S.D., *: $p < 0.05$, **: $p < 0.01$, ***: $p < 0.001$, $: significantly different from CG, #: significantly different from within the group, CK: creatinine kinase, AST: aspartate aminotransferase, CG: control group, WEG: water exercise group, DWEG: deep-sea water exercise group.

CK showed a significant difference in the interaction ($p < 0.001$) between the groups and the measurement time ($p < 0.001$). However, there was no difference between the groups at the time of measurement. The post hoc analysis showed that DSWEG significantly decreased after program following maximum exercise ($p < 0.01$), and WEG significantly decreased after CG ($p < 0.05$). AST showed a significant difference in the interaction ($p < 0.001$) between the group and the measurement time ($p < 0.001$). However, there was no difference between the groups at the time of measurement. The post hoc analysis showed that DSWEG significantly decreased after program-induced loss after maximum exercise ($p < 0.01$), and WEG significantly decreased after CG ($p < 0.05$). In this study, subjects in the DSWEG recovered significantly faster than those of the WEG and CG, suggesting that DSW was effective in ameliorating muscle damage as well as promoting fatigue recovery. Thus, the DSWTT program was found to be relevant and necessary not only in elite sports but also to enhance the performance of sports activity.

Elevated serum AST level is a marker of liver or cardiac muscle damage. AST is also known as glutamic oxaloacetic transaminase (GOT), an enzyme present in various cells of the living body facilitating synthesis of amino acids. It increases after drinking or exercising, and it is one of the enzymes associated with muscle damage, which increases in liver disease or muscle disease [26]. AST is present not only in the liver but also in the muscles. It increases when the muscles are damaged after exercise and, therefore, can be used to evaluate exercise-induced stress. The concentration of AST is proportional to exercise intensity or exercise duration [27]. Therefore, DSWEG showed a significant recovery compared to WEG and CG, which may have facilitated the recovery of muscle damage by promoting relaxation of the body through floating, stretching, and massage during the DSWTT program and gently coordinating various movements.

4. Discussion

This study demonstrates that fatigue and muscle damage are induced by a shuttle run test, and following the DSWTT program, the DSWEG showed a significant decrease in lactate, ammonia, LDH, CK, and AST compared to WEG and CG. WEG showed a significant decrease in lactate, ammonia, CK, and AST compared to CG, but CG did not show any difference compared to other groups.

Recently, DSW treatment was used to demonstrate recovery from fatigue and muscle damage using hot spring water [28]. DSW is a resource that maintains a cold temperature at seabeds below a depth of 200 m. DSW is clean seawater that is not contaminated by Escherichia coli or common bacteria. When DSW is applied as an underwater motion, DSW shows buoyancy and water pressure higher than normal water due to eutrophication and salt concentration, and it acts on the human body in a more favorable environment than the general water in the floating posture. Therefore, in this study, DSWTT was applied to the exercise environment in the floating posture and the recovery of fatigue and muscle damage was verified.

Fatigue, a physiological phenomenon that is induced by high-intensity training and long-term exercise, significantly reduces muscle glycogen and blood glucose, which reduces the function of organs and tissues in the human body [29]. In general, the blood–glucose concentration is 80~110 mL/dL when the adult is stabilized. During the exercise, the muscle glycogen is rapidly depleted, resulting in fatigue. If exercise reduces blood sugar, insulin secretion is reduced and blood–glucose level is maintained [30]. In order to determine the changes in the secretion of glucose concentration, this study compared the glucose concentration before, immediately after exercise, and 30 min of exercise. Based on the results of group comparison, the effects were significantly higher in DWEG than in CG.

These results attributed to a decrease in blood sugar level due to the increased demand for energy sources during the one-time exercise. The muscle glycogen levels depleted immediately after exercise reduced the blood–glucose level, as the glucose entered the muscle to supplement the glycogen reserves [31]. Boer and Armstrong [32] reported an increase in the use of blood sugar immediately after exercise, and this study was consistent. Another study [33] showed that the underwater environment strongly facilitated blood flow, human body metabolism, and fatigue parameters by inducing changes in the physiology of the human body depending on the differences between water temperature, water viscosity, density, depth, body parts, and individual. This study also showed that the effect of DSW on fatigue recovery was highly favorable. These results suggest that DSWTT can prevent glycogen depletion in the body and lower the blood lactate acid and ammonia concentration, which are private fatigue substances when recovering and have a positive effect on the improvement of recovery ability after high-intensity fatigue induction training. Recovery from muscle fatigue to improve physical activity quickly eliminates lactate accumulated by energy metabolism and enzyme action in muscles and plays a very important role in improving activities of daily life and control conditions [34]. The accumulation and elimination of blood lactate determines the limitations of muscle movement directly linked to muscle fatigue [35]. Among them, the weight load is reduced due to buoyancy and water pressure. During the underwater exercise, the movement of the joints is larger than on the land, and the effect of stability and stretching is increased [19]. Based on this principle, this study, which verified the effectiveness of DSW, showed that the DSWTT program was effective in eliminating lactate. DSWTT may have increased blood flow to the muscle and improved muscle function. Especially, in the recovery process, it was found that DSWTT was very effective in the recovery of muscle tension and the removal of byproducts of metabolic processes through improvement of varicose reflux rate.

Water therapy has various effects on the physiology of the human body by providing an environment different from the atmosphere such as buoyancy, resistance, water pressure, and water temperature [33]. The results of this study, compared with previous studies [28,36], suggest that the underwater treatment facilitates circulation of blood and lymph to the skin or damaged muscle tissue and ameliorated the pain by relieving muscle spasms. In addition, DSW promotes metabolism and helps blood circulation, such that lactate or waste is discharged more quickly to the outside of the body, and the body is replenished with the required oxygen or nutrients.

Ammonia, one of the fatigue-inducing substances, increases the central fatigue and motor coordination [37]. However, the supply of proteins as energy supplements has been shown to inhibit serotonin production, thereby reducing central fatigue and improving endurance performance [38]. In this study, subjects in the WEG recovered faster than those of the CG group, and the DSWG recovered significantly faster than the WEG and CG. In accordance with Marybetts' [39] findings that heat takes 15 min to transfer to the muscles, the exposure to 25 min of underwater flooding at 34 ± 1 °C in this study is likely to induce muscle relaxation and eliminate lactate and ammonia. In this study, we discussed the impact of DSWTT program on ammonia level, which is a strong exercise-induced fatigue substance, known to decrease the exercise performance. Participation in the DSWTT program led to rapid excretion of accumulated ammonia. Studies on DSWTT and energy supplementation are needed when BCAA intake induced by fatigue and OKG or albumin are reported to inhibit ammonia accumulation [40].

LDH regulates the formation and conversion of lactate in muscle cells during muscle activity. LDH regulates the formation of lactate by reducing polysaccharide synthesis during anoxic metabolism in muscles and liver [41]. LDH activity in the blood is very low at rest, but if muscle cells are damaged by high-intensity exercise, LDH in the cell is released out of the cell, and LDH activity in the blood is high. Muscle LDH catalyzes the reduction of pyruvate into lactate, which occurs at higher rates when the glycolysis flux increases, such as during muscle contraction. LDH is an intra-blood specific enzyme that can be used to evaluate the energy system in various exercise situations. It represents the degree of adaptation of metabolic function during energy metabolism, exercise intensity, muscle stiffness, fatigue recovery, and excessive training and histological damage analysis [42,43]. In this study, the subjects in DSWEG recovered significantly faster than those in WEG and CG, which confirmed that the DSWTT program using DSW resolved fatigue. When high-intensity fatigue-induced exercise is performed, the muscle is overloaded and affected by cell membrane destruction or tissue necrosis, which increases blood CK and LDH concentrations. LDH is mainly present in red cell and muscle cells, and it is an essential enzyme that produces ATP via the lactic acid system. It plays a role of balancing glucose physicochemical and assimilation by using pyruvate at the final stage of the lactic acid system.

However, an appropriate level of physical activity in various exercises improves performance, but excessive physical activity has a negative effect [44,45]. Typical negative effects include muscle damage due structural damage of muscle fiber [46], followed by protein leakage in muscle tissue [47], and acute inflammation reaction [48]. Muscle damage is accompanied by a decrease in maximum strength, delayed onset muscle soreness (DOMS) [49], and leakage of muscle proteins such as CK, myoglobin (Mb), and AST into the blood [50].

CPK is a non-platelet-specific enzyme that affects muscle damage and inflammation rather than muscle metabolism. CPK concentration increases proportionally as muscle damage increases after high-intensity exercise [51]. Therefore, rapid recovery from accumulated fatigue and muscle damage is an important factor in exercise performance. Body changes due to muscle damage have a negative effect on the participation of the general public in exercise programs and increase psychological discomfort. In order to recover muscle damage quickly, this study is consistent with previous studies [28,33,36], suggesting that water treatment was effective in inducing a psychological sense of stability and a refreshing mood.

In this study, subjects in the DSWEG recovered significantly faster than those of the WEG and CG, suggesting that DSW was effective in ameliorating muscle damage as well as promoting fatigue recovery. Thus, the DSWTT program was found to be relevant and necessary not only in elite sports but also to enhance the performance of sports activity. In the fatigue-inducing 20 m-MST test, the mobilization of the type I was greater, and the expression of the type II was greater in the weight test. Based on this, it can be explained that if the mobilization of the type II is greater than the mobilization of the type I, the fatigue induction and the muscle itself are more damaged.

Elevated serum AST level is a marker of liver or cardiac muscle damage. AST is also known as glutamic oxaloacetic transaminase (GOT), an enzyme present in various cells of the living body facilitating synthesis of amino acids. It increases after drinking or exercising, and it is one of the enzymes associated with muscle damage, which increases in liver disease or muscle disease [26]. AST is present not only in the liver but also in the muscles. It increases when the muscles are damaged after exercise and, therefore, can be used to evaluate exercise-induced stress. The concentration of AST is proportional to exercise intensity or exercise duration [27]. Therefore, DSWEG showed a significant recovery compared to WEG and CG, which may have facilitated the recovery of muscle damage by promoting relaxation of the body through floating, stretching, and massage during the DSWTT program and gently coordinating various movements.

In conclusion, the DSWTT program had a significant effect on fatigue and muscle damage recovery, suggesting that application of the program in hot springs can contribute to national health care and promotion and quality of life. Further studies are needed to investigate DSWTT programs with various research subjects at different program temperatures, exercise times, and frequencies of treatment and exercise. In addition, it is necessary to analyze the effects of DSWTT program to maintain the refreshing state of various classes, especially the weak and the elderly.

DSWTT application is a useful seawater resource with low temperature, cleanliness, stability, eutrophicity, minerality, and aging properties in the mechanism that affects the recovery of fatigue of human body. It is a huge clean resource that is generated from the material circulation system with solar energy as a source of energy and is produced as seawater and recycled as sea water. These DSW show higher buoyancy and hydrostatic pressure than normal water due to eutrophicity and salinity concentration, and stretching and massage performance in underwater floating posture can be interpreted as more effective in restoring human fatigue than normal water. In addition, when stretching or massage activities in DSW compared to the normal water, it means that the fatigue material generated in the muscle recovered more quickly.

The most important characteristic of DSW in the mechanism that DSWTT application affects the recovery of muscle damage in human body is that it maintains stable low temperature and has little organic matter such as bacteria and pathogens, and it is applied to the treatment of muscle damage by applying artificial heat, as sea water is rich in minerals such as nutrients and minerals essential for the growth of marine plants. This suggests that warm DSW is more stable than normal water in DSWTT program, and that the relaxation of the body through stretching and muscle massage provides conditions for muscle damage recovery.

There is a limitation of not comparing other evaluation parameters in this study. However, in this study, a study was conducted to evaluate factors such as glucose, lactate acid, ammonia, LDH, CK, and AST, which are very important for physiological fatigue. It is considered to require a study to evaluate the different parameters mentioned later.

Author Contributions: Conceptualization, W.-s.S.; Data curation, S.-J.K.; Formal analysis, A.-R.C.; Investigation, J.-H.J. and H.-j.E.; Methodology, B.K.; Writing—original draft, N.-I.K.; Writing—review & editing, S.-S.L. All authors have read and agreed to the published version of the manuscript.

Funding: This paper was funded by the Ministry of Oceans and Fisheries in 2016 and supported by the Korea Institute of Marine Science & Technology Promotion (Task Number: 20160300).

Conflicts of Interest: The authors declare no conflict of interest.

References

1. Kang, S.R.; Jeong, G.Y.; Bae, J.J.; Min, J.Y.; Yu, C.H.; Kim, J.J.; Kwon, T.K. Effect of muscle function and muscular reaction of knee joint in the twenties on the whole body vibration exercise. *J. Korean Soc. Precis. Eng.* **2013**, *30*, 762–768. [CrossRef]
2. Cho, J.S.; Kwon, T.K.; Hong, J.P. A study of evaluation index development of healthcare rehabilitation device design. *Korea Soc. Emot. Sensib.* **2014**, *17*, 129–142. [CrossRef]
3. Kathryu, A.; Lentz, M.J.; Taylor, D.L. Fatigue as a response to environmental demands in women's lives image. *J. Nurs. Scholarsh.* **1994**, *26*, 149–154.

4. Blesch, K.S.; Paice, J.A.; Wickham, R.; Harte, N.; Schnoor, D.K.; Purl, S.; Rehwal, T.M.; Kopp, P.L.; Manson, S.; Coveny, S.B. Correlates of fatigue in people with breast or lung cancer. *Oncol. Nurs. Forum* **1991**, *18*, 81–87.
5. Youn, B.B.; Kang, H.C.; Shin, K.K.; Lee, K.S. An analysis of fatigue among outpatients. *Korean J. Fam. Med.* **1999**, *20*, 978–990.
6. Larun, L.; Brurberg, K.G.; Odgaard-Jensen, J.; Price, J.R. Exercise therapy for chronic fatigue syndrome. *Cochrane Database Syst. Rev.* **2017**, *25*, 1–4.
7. Kay, D.; Marino, F.E.; Cannon, J.; Gibson, A.S.C.; Lambert, M.I.; Noakes, T.D. Evidence for neuromuscular fatigue during high-intensity cycling in warm, humid conditions. *Eur. J. Appl. Physiol.* **2001**, *84*, 115–121. [CrossRef] [PubMed]
8. Ohkuwa, T.; Miyamura, M. Plasma LDH activity and LDH isozymes after 400m and 3,000m runs in sprint and long distance runners. *J. Sports Med. Phys. Fit.* **1986**, *26*, 362–368.
9. Kim, J.K.; Moon, H.W. Effect of Blood fatigue factors following eccentric exercise on delayed muscle damage. *Exerc. Sci.* **2004**, *13*, 251–262.
10. Kim, I.G. The effect of sauna and half-bath participation on systolic blood pressure, heart rate and vascular elasticity of middle-aged men. *Korean Sports Res.* **2006**, *17*, 319–327.
11. Cha, S.W.; Shin, S.K.; Lim, I.S. The effect of passive recovery, massage, cold & hot bath and aroma therapy on fatigue metabolic substrate after 10km running. *J. Exerc. Nutr. Biochem.* **2006**, *10*, 37–42.
12. Darryl, J. Alternating hot and cold water immersion for athlete recovery: A review. *Phys. Ther. Sports* **2004**, *5*, 26–32.
13. Mang, H.J. Cortisol and testosterone changes in cold therapy after muscle fatigue induced. *Korean J. Phys. Educ.* **2002**, *41*, 317–323.
14. Pedersen, B.K.; Hoffman-Goetz, L. Exercise and the immune system regulation, integration, and adaptation. *Physiol. Rev.* **2000**, *80*, 1055–1081. [CrossRef]
15. Brancaccio, P.; Maffulli, N.; Buonauro, R.; Limongelli, F.M. Serum enzyme monitoring in sports medicine. *Clin. Sports Med.* **2008**, *27*, 1–18. [CrossRef]
16. Lippi, G.; Schena, F.; Salvagno, G.L.; Montagnana, M.; Gelati, M.; Tarper, I.C.; Banfi, G.; Guidi, G.C. Acute variation of biochemical markers of muscle damage following a 21-km, half-marathon run. *Scand. J. Clin. Lab. Investig.* **2008**, *68*, 667–672. [CrossRef]
17. Yeom, I.H. Effect of Exercise Intensity on Inflammatory Marker and Immunoglobulin. Master's Thesis, Incheon National University, Incheon, Korea, 2011. Unpublished.
18. Lee, S.K.; Chung, E.Y. The effect of Ai Chi aquatic exercise to the level of human stress and muscle activities. *Korean J. Wellness* **2014**, *9*, 131–137.
19. Hay, L.; Wylie, K. Towards evidence-based emergency medicine: Best BETs from the Manchester Royal Infirmary. BET 4: Hydrotherapy following rotator cuff repair. *Emerg. Med. J.* **2011**, *28*, 634–635.
20. Jun, S.Y.; Lee, K.S.; Nam, K.S. Efficacy testing for tarasotherapy in deep sea water. In Proceedings of the Korean Marine Environmental Engineering Society, Seoul, Korea, 21 May 2017.
21. Weinberg, R.; Jackson, A. The relationship of massage and exercise to mood enhancement. *Sports Psychol.* **1988**, *2*, 202–211. [CrossRef]
22. Dubrovsky, V.I. Changes in muscle and venous blood flow after massage. *Sov. Sports Rev.* **1982**, *4*, 56–57.
23. Mooenthan, A.; Nivethitha, L. Scientific evidence-based effects of hydrotherapy on various systems of the body. *N. Am. J. Med. Sci.* **2014**, *6*, 199–209. [CrossRef]
24. Leger, L.A.; Lambert, J. A maximal multistage 20m shuttle run test to predict VO2max. *Eur. J. Appl. Physiol.* **1982**, *49*, 1–12. [CrossRef]
25. Brewer, J.; Ramsbottom, R.; Williams, C. *Multistage Fitness Test*; National Coaching Foundation: Leeds, UK, 1988.
26. Armstrong, R.B. Initial event in exercise induced muscular injury. *Med. Sci. Sport Exerc.* **1990**, *22*, 429–435.
27. Barranco, T.; Tvarijonaviciute, A.; Tecles, F.; Carrillo, J.M.; Sánchez-Resalt, C.; Jimenez-Reyes, P.; Rubio, M.; García-Balletbó, M.; Cerón, J.J.; Cugat, R. Changes in CK, LDH and AST in saliva samples after an intense exercise: A pilot study. *J. Sports Med. Phys. Fit.* **2017**, *5*, 2441–2455.
28. Lee, S.S.; Kim, J.T.; Shin, W.S.; Kim, N.I.; Ryu, O.S.; Jang, J.H. Changes of trunk ROM and maximal muscular strength after deep sea water thalassotherapy. *Korean Soc. Growth Dev.* **2017**, *25*, 353–361.
29. Gibson, H.; Edwards, R.H.T. Muscular exercise and fatigue. *Sports Med.* **1985**, *2*, 120–132. [CrossRef]
30. Heath, G.W.; Gavin, J.R., III; Hinderliter, J.M.; Hagberg, J.M.; Bloomfield, S.A.; Hollozy, J.O. Effect of exercise and lack of exercise on glucose tolerance and insulin sensitivity. *J. Appl. Physiol.* **1983**, *55*, 512–517. [CrossRef]

31. Praet, S.F.; van Loon, L.J. Exercise therapy in type 2 diabetes. *Acta Diabetol.* **2009**, *46*, 263–278. [CrossRef]
32. Borer, J.; Armstrong, P. Proceedings of the 99th meeting of the Food and Drug Administration Cardiovascular and Renal Drugs Advisory Committee. *Circulation* **2003**, *107*, e9052. [CrossRef]
33. Jung, B.K. Understanding of aquatic rehabilitation movement. *Korean Assoc. Certif. Exerc. Prof. Annu. Meet.* **2002**, *1*, 13–17.
34. Aslan, A.; Acikada, C.; Güvenç, A.; Gören, H.; Hazir, T.; Ozkara, A. Metabolic demands of match performance in young soccer players. *J. Sports Sci. Med.* **2012**, *11*, 170–179.
35. Park, H.S.; Kim, M.K.; Shim, B.C.; Chae, J.R.; Cho, S.C.; Jun, H.Y.; Kim, H.J. A comparative analysis of blood lactate, LDH, and glucose before and after treadmill exercise in athletics. *J. Dongui Physiol.* **2006**, *20*, 1254–1260.
36. Park, J.O. The Effect of Sports Massage on the Recovery of Fatigue and Injury Prevention of Dancers. Master's Thesis, Kyungseung University, Busan, Korea, 2001. Unpublished.
37. Meneguello, M.O.; Mendonca, J.R.; Lancha, A.H., Jr.; Costa Rosa, L.F. Effect of arginine, ornithine and citrulline supplementation upon performance and metabolism of trained rats. *Cell Biochem. Funct.* **2003**, *21*, 85–91. [CrossRef]
38. Blomstrand, E.; Celsing, F.; Newshorme, E.A. Changes in concentration of aromatic and branched chain amino acid during sustained exercise in man and their possible role in fatigue. *Acta Physiol. Scand.* **1998**, *33*, 115–121. [CrossRef]
39. Marybetts, S. *Modern Hydrotherapy for the Massage Therapist*; Lippincott Williams & Wilkins, Inc.: Philadelphia, PA, USA, 2008.
40. Cho, S.Y.; Paik, I.Y.; Woo, J.H.; Kim, K.S. The effects of BCAA and additional OKG or albumin supplements on blood fatigue factors and energy substrates. *Korean J. Sport Sci.* **2004**, *15*, 1–10.
41. Everse, J.; Kaplan, N.O. Mechanism a of action and biological function of various dehydrogenease isozymes. In *Isozymes Physiological Function*; Markert, C.L., Ed.; Academic Press: New York, NY, USA, 1975; pp. 29–44.
42. Hooloszy, J.O.; Booth, F.W. Biochemical adaptation to endurance exercise in muscle. *Ann. Rev. Physiol.* **1976**, *22*, 623–627. [CrossRef]
43. Apple, P.F.; Rogers, M.A. Skeletal muscle lactate dehydrogenase isozyme alterations in men and women marathon runners. *J. Applex Physiol.* **1986**, *61*, 477–481. [CrossRef]
44. Reznick, A.Z.; Witt, E.; Matsumoto, M.; Packer, L. Vitamin E inhibits protein oxidation in skeletal muscle of resting and exercise rats. *Biochem. Biophys. Res. Commun.* **1992**, *189*, 801–806. [CrossRef]
45. Jun, Y.K.; Lee, K.H. Effect of different methods of recovery after high strength aerobic exercise on antioxidant enzymes. *Korean J. Phys. Educ. Sci.* **2014**, *23*, 1127–1135.
46. Jaworski, C.A. Medical concerns of marathons. *Curr. Sports Med. Rep.* **2005**, *4*, 137–143. [CrossRef]
47. Sorichter, S.; Puschendorf, B.; Mair, J. Skeletal muscle injury induced by eccentric muscle action: Muscle proteins as markers of muscle fiber injury. *Exerc. Immunol. Rev.* **1999**, *5*, 5–21.
48. McIntyre, K.W.; Shuster, D.J.; Gillooly, K.M.; Warrier, R.R.; Connaughton, S.E.; Hall, L.B.; Arp, L.H.; Gately, M.K.; Magram, J. Reduced incidence and severity of collagen-induced arthritis in interleukin-12-deficient mice. *Eur. J. Immunol.* **1996**, *26*, 2933–2938. [CrossRef]
49. Howatson, G.; Hoad, M.; Goodall, S.; Tallent, J.; Bell, P.G.; French, D.N. Exercise-induced muscle damage is reduced in resistance-trained males by branched chain amino acids: A randomized, double-blind, placebo controlled study. *J. Int. Soc. Sports Nutr.* **2013**, *9*, 20. [CrossRef]
50. Matsumoto, K.; Koba, T.; Hamada, K.; Sakurai, M.; Higuchi, T.; Miyata, H. Branched-chain amino acid supplementation attenuates muscle soreness, muscle damage and inflammation during an intensive training program. *J. Sports Med. Phys. Fit.* **2009**, *49*, 424–431.
51. Brancaccio, P.; Lippi, G.; Maffulli, N. Biochemical markers of muscular damage. *Clin. Chem. Lab. Med.* **2010**, *48*, 757–767. [CrossRef]

Publisher's Note: MDPI stays neutral with regard to jurisdictional claims in published maps and institutional affiliations.

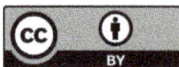

© 2020 by the authors. Licensee MDPI, Basel, Switzerland. This article is an open access article distributed under the terms and conditions of the Creative Commons Attribution (CC BY) license (http://creativecommons.org/licenses/by/4.0/).

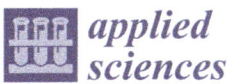

Article

Cold-Water Immersion Promotes Antioxidant Enzyme Activation in Elite Taekwondo Athletes

Eun-Hee Park, Seung-Wook Choi * and Yoon-Kwon Yang *

Department of sports Leisure, Sungshin Women's University, Seoul 02844, Korea; peh7904@gmail.com
* Correspondence: swchoi@sungshin.ac.kr (S.-W.C.); yangyk@sungshin.ac.kr (Y.-K.Y.)

Abstract: The aim of this study was to investigate the effect of cold-water immersion (CWI) on lipid peroxides and antioxidant enzymes in adult Taekwondo athletes after a match. A cross-sectional study was performed. After a Taekwondo match, the control group remained seated passively, while the treatment group immersed their legs below the knee joint in cold water at 10 °C. Blood samples were taken at pre-match, post-match, post-treatment, and post-rest, and changes in malondialdehyde (MDA), superoxide dismutase (SOD), and glutathione peroxidase (GPx) concentrations were analyzed. The results showed that there was a significant difference in MDA between the two groups, and while the CWI group had 19% lower SOD concentration compared to the control group, and the difference was not significant. However, in case of interaction for GPx concentration ($p < 0.001$), a statistically significant difference was found between the two groups ($p < 0.05$). In conclusion, CWI after a Taekwondo match elevates the concentration of antioxidant enzymes.

Keywords: cold-water immersion; malondialdehyde; antioxidant enzyme; Taekwondo athletes; recovery

Citation: Park, E.-H.; Choi, S.-W.; Yang, Y.-K. Cold-Water Immersion Promotes Antioxidant Enzyme Activation in Elite Taekwondo Athletes. *Appl. Sci.* **2021**, *11*, 2855. https://doi.org/10.3390/app11062855

Academic Editor: Leonel Pereira

Received: 19 February 2021
Accepted: 19 March 2021
Published: 23 March 2021

Publisher's Note: MDPI stays neutral with regard to jurisdictional claims in published maps and institutional affiliations.

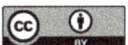

Copyright: © 2021 by the authors. Licensee MDPI, Basel, Switzerland. This article is an open access article distributed under the terms and conditions of the Creative Commons Attribution (CC BY) license (https://creativecommons.org/licenses/by/4.0/).

1. Introduction

It is well known that free radicals and reactive oxygen species (ROS) produced in the human body cause cellular damage as well as aging and various chronic disease [1]. However, from a physiological perspective, enzymatic and non-enzymatic systems (antioxidant system) neutralize the harmful effects of ROS [2].

Unlike normal oxygen, ROS are free radicals containing oxygen that are highly reactive. They contain an unpaired electron and have a strong tendency to achieve a stable state, by either taking or giving up an electron. Therefore, when ROS is produced in the body, they easily react with lipids, proteins and DNA, and can cause functional impairments. When ROS attacks cellular membranes, they oxidize unsaturated fatty acids and form lipid peroxides; furthermore, malondialdehyde (MDA) is used as a marker of lipid peroxide [3]. However, ROS are suppressed by antioxidant enzymes, such as superoxide dis-mutase (SOD), glutathione peroxidase (GPX), and catalase (CAT) [4].

Antioxidant enzymes play an important role in defending cells against oxidative damage caused by free radicals [5] that are generated through physical activity through various pathways [6]. Regular and appropriate exercise promotes metabolism, prevents disease, helps with weight management, and strengthens immune function. However, strenuous exercise, such as that performed by well-trained athletes, rapidly increases oxygen consumption and consequently increases oxygen supply by 10–15 times, which induces the production of free radicals [7]. Furthermore, oxygen consumption by muscles during exercise is increased by 10–20 times than at rest [8]. Moreover, it activates ROS that attacks cells, which leads to damages to carbohydrates, fats, proteins, and nucleic acids [9]. In particular, hypoxia or local hypoxia causes transferrin to release iron and exacerbates hemolysis. This alters the metabolism, and these responses increase stress or weaken athletic performance [10].

To minimize such adverse physiological responses, many studies have utilized various approaches to examine methods to reduce exercise-induced fatigue and promote recovery [11–15]. In particular, cryotherapy or cold-water immersion (CWI), which involves immersion of a part of the body or the whole body, has been researched in various exercise conditions and treatment durations [11–15]. However, although CWI has more recently been researched in various exercise methods and sports [16,17], past studies on antioxidant activity-CWI involved swimming [18], kayaking [19], and cryotherapy using a chamber; there were no studies investigating the effects of antioxidant-CWI after an actual match involving electronic protective gear, such as a Taekwondo match.

Taekwondo, a combat sport, was introduced as a demonstration sport at the 1988 Summer Olympics at Seoul and the 1992 Summer Olympics at Barcelona. It was confirmed as an official sport at the 2000 Summer Olympics at Sydney. During a Taekwondo match, successful torso punches or kicks and successful head kicks are awarded more points. Thus, a Taekwondo match can result in significant fatigue due to the physical effort involved [20–24].

An appropriate intensity of training is expected to not only reduce the harmful effects of free radicals but also trigger health benefits by stimulating the immune system [25]. However, free radical production and subsequent lipid peroxidation increase proportionate to oxygen consumption, depending on the intensity of exercise, and are known to be positively correlated with skeletal muscle injury [26]. In other words, vigorous exercise at 80–90% of HRmax [27] induces oxidative stress one way or the other, thereby affecting lipid peroxidation and antioxidant enzymes.

Although studies have investigated injuries based on athletic proficiency, sex, body weight, age, mechanism, involving body part, situation, and years or experience [28,29], only a handful of studies were conducted on martial arts athletes. Furthermore, due to the presence of several variables in a Taekwondo competition, including different weight divisions [30], this randomized crossover study aimed to investigate changes in heart rate (HR) during a Taekwondo match and changes in MDA, SOD, and GPX in response to CWI treatment immediately after a match.

Furthermore, although Taekwondo is a well-known sport and an official Olympic sport that is actively researched, antioxidant activity-CWI after a Taekwondo match has never been researched previously. We hypothesized that CWI would have more positive impacts on HR and enzyme activity compared to that only passive resting after a Taekwondo match. Therefore, the aim of this study was to examine the effects of CWI on lipid peroxide and antioxidant enzyme activity in the distal knee after a match in elite male Taekwondo athletes.

2. Materials and Methods

2.1. Participants

Twelve college Taekwondo athletes, with a minimum of 10-year-long careers in the game and who had won a Korean or foreign competition in the past two years, were enrolled. The participants were fully informed about the purpose and method of the study prior to beginning the experiment and signed a written consent form. During the study period, the participants were subjected to an identical experimental condition (exercise, diet, and sleep) at the college dormitory of the place where our study was conducted (Taekwondo Center). In addition, the participants were requested to refrain from the consumption of alcoholic and caffeinated drinks and the use of specific drugs such as anti-inflammatory agents. Moreover, they had to maintain their normal diet until the end of the study. However, the amount of food intake was not controlled. Participant demographics are as follows: (mean age: 20.4 ± 0.8 years; mean height: 181.6 ± 3.2 cm; mean body weight: 71.6 ± 7.9 kg; body mass index: 21.7 ± 2.50 kg/m^2; fat mass: 8.1 ± 2.0 kg; Vo$_{2max}$: 57.7 ± 4.2 mL/kg/min; HR$_{max}$: 201.3 ± 0.8 beats/min).

2.2. Experimental Design

This study was conducted at a college Taekwondo center. The indoor temperature was set to 18–20 °C during the experiment. The participants' Olympic weight classes were evenly distributed (−58 kg to +80 kg), and their body compositions were measured prior to beginning the experiment (Inbody230 Body Composition Analyzer; Inbody Co., Ltd., Seoul, Korea). A graded maximal exercise test to exhaustion using the Bruce protocol was used to measure maximal oxygen consumption (Vo_{2max}), maximum heart rate (HRmax), and time to exhaustion (Quark b2, Cosmed, USA). Prior to testing, we explained rating perceived exertion (RPE) to the participants; they were instructed to provide the RPE every minute during the testing. In addition, their coaches encouraged them to perform maximally. According to the Bruce protocol, the treadmill is started at 2.74 km/h at a gradient of 10%. The incline of the treadmill increases by 2% at 3 min. intervals and the speed increases with each stage. Vo_{2max} was recorded when HR ceased to increase, despite the workload increasing when the RPE reached 17 on the Borg Scale, or when the respiratory exchange ratio was >0.15. The study progression is shown in Figure 1.

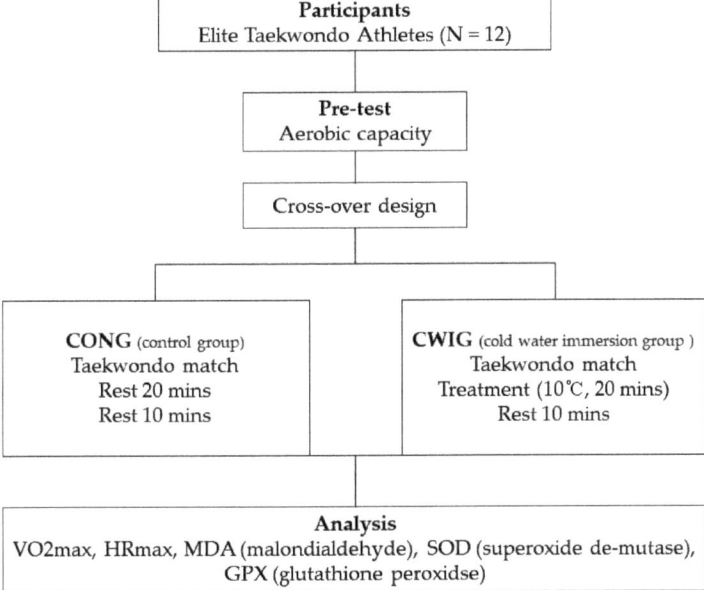

Figure 1. Study progression.

2.3. Taekwondo Competition

The rules of the Taekwondo competition in this study adhered to the 2019 World Taekwondo Federation (WTF) rules. Electronic equipment approved by the WTF and utilized in international competitions was used in this study (electronic body protection, electronic headgear, and electronic socks; KP&P, Seoul, Korea). The duration of each match was 8 min (2 min each for 3 rounds with a 1-min break), similar to that in actual competition. Two coaches cooperated in the study by giving the athletes strategic advice during the match. Further, HR was measured during and after each round (Polar FT1; T31, Polar®, Bethpage, NY, USA).

2.4. Treatment Methods-CWI

A crossover design was used with a control group (CONG) and a cold-water immersion group (CWIG). was measured on visit 1; the second visit was conducted seven days later. A 10-min leisure walk would have had little metabolic impact on elite athletes.

The participants walked from their dorms to the Taekwondo Center on the day of the experiment (10-min walk), and arrived at the center by 8 AM in preparation for the experiment. The participants rested for 30-min before the first blood sampling. After fully preparing for the experiment with the help of research assistants and coaches, the Taekwondo competitions were performed at 10 AM. The second blood sampling was performed immediately after each 2-min match, with 1-min rests between each match. The CONG comfortably sat on the competition mat and rested for 20 min, while the CWIG sat on a chair and underwent CWI of the distal knee area. A research assistant was assigned to each participant to conduct the experiment, and CWIG assisted with supplying ice cubes during CWI to control the temperature of the water (10 °C) (TP-101, Xuzhou Sanhe Automatic Control Equipment Co., Ltd.; Jiangsu, China; RoHS Certification). The duration of treatment (20 min) and water temperature (10 °C) used in this study were determined based on those in previous studies [31–33], as well as our pilot study related to CWI. However, the outcomes varied despite the equal treatment durations [31–33]; hence, the treatment duration used in this study cannot be considered the optimal condition. However, the benefits of this treatment duration and immersion temperature are that they can easily be applied in many sports at a low cost. Both groups underwent a third blood sampling after 20 min of rest and treatment, respectively. Then, both groups comfortably sat on the floor and rested for another 10 min for the final blood sampling. The participants were instructed to limit their water intake to a minimum throughout the experiment, although this was not controlled.

2.5. Blood Analysis

Four blood samples were taken from a vein in the forearm using a disposable syringe after the participants rested. Blood samples were collected in a non-EDTA-treated serum tube and an EDTA-treated plasma tube, centrifuged at 2500 rpm for 15 min, diluted using the assay kit according to the manual, and analyzed for each item using an enzyme-linked immunosorbent assay. Blood analysis was performed at the Green Cross LabCell laboratory in Yong-in, Korea, certified by the Korean Board for Accreditation and Conformity assessment.

2.6. Statistical Analysis

All data were analyzed using SPSS version 24 (SPSS Inc., Chicago, IL, USA) software and presented as mean and standard deviation (SD). Differences in time between groups were analyzed using independent t-tests, and differences in groups, time, and group × time were analyzed using repeated measures analysis of variance (ANOVA). Differences between groups were analyzed with one-way ANOVA followed by Bonferroni correction. Significant differences of p values after testing were presented and explained in the tables using an alphabet. Statistical significance was considered when $p < 0.05$.

3. Results

3.1. Intensity during Taekwondo Competition

HR measured during the Taekwondo match is summarized in Table 1 and Figure 2. The mean pre-Taekwondo match HR was 74.6 ± 6.50 bpm, while mean HR during and post-match were 177.0 ± 13.52 bpm and 183.4 ± 13.52 bpm, respectively. With mean HR_{max} of 201.3 ± 0.75 bpm, intensity during the Taekwondo match represented by mean HR during the match and post-match were 88% and 91% HR_{max}, respectively.

3.2. Change in MDA Concentration

Changes in MDA concentration following CWI are described in Table 2 and Figure 3; they were analyzed using repeated measures ANOVA. Significant differences according to the time of measurement were observed ($F = 8.864$; $p < 0.001$). However, there were no significant differences in MDA concentration between the two groups and no interaction effect. Regarding differences based on time of measurement, the CONG showed a 9%

reduction in MDA concentration after CWI from that immediately after a match, while the CWIG showed a 2% increase in the same period. In addition, the CONG showed a 10% reduction of MDA concentration from immediately after a match until CWI and after rest, while the CWIG showed no changes.

Table 1. Heart rate (HR) during a Taekwondo match.

	t	p
Before	0.370	0.715
Between round 1	1.786	0.088
After round 1	1.108	0.320
Between round 2	0.362	0.720
After round 2	0.502	0.621
Between round 3	0.167	0.869
After round 3	0.413	0.684

Mean ± standard deviation.

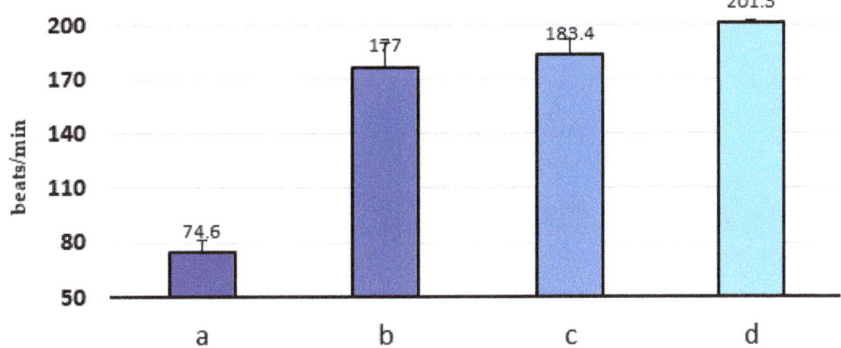

a: Before; b: Average HR between round; c: Average HR after round; d: HRmax

Figure 2. Heart rate during a Taekwondo match.

Table 2. Change in malondialdehyde (MDA) concentration after cold-water immersion (CWI) (unit/μ mol).

Time \ Group	CONG	CWIG	F	
Pre-match	102.5 ± 23.00	119.2 ± 27.61	Group	3.040
Post-match	89.3 ± 17.05	93.9 ± 31.04	Time	8.864 ***
Post-treatment	81.0 ± 16.40	95.3 ± 26.59	Group × Time	0.497
Post-rest	80.7 ± 19.77	93.5 ± 19.88		

Mean ± standard deviation; *** $p < 0.001$; no significant interaction effect was observed for group by time in MDA concentration.

3.3. Change in SOD Concentration

Changes in SOD concentration after CWI are described in Table 3 and Figure 4 and were analyzed using repeated measures ANOVA. Significant differences according to time of measurement were observed ($F = 8.496$; $p < 0.001$). However, there were no significant differences in SOD concentration between the two groups with no interaction effect. Regarding the differences based on time of measurement, the CONG showed a 33% reduction of SOD concentration after CWI from that immediately after a match, while the CWIG showed a 24% reduction in the same period. However, the CONG showed a 10% reduction of SOD from after CWI to after rest, while the CWIG showed a 5% increase in the same period. Furthermore, the CONG showed a 19% increase in SOD concentration after treatment from that before a match compared to the CWIG, but the difference was not statistically significant.

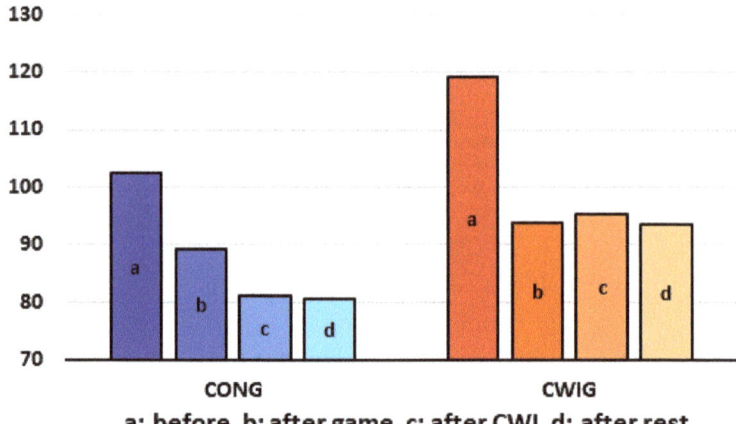

Figure 3. Change in MDA concentration after CWI. (Data are expressed as mean ± standard deviation. A main effect was evident by time $p < 0.001$. CWI: cold-water immersion).

Table 3. Change in SOD concentration after CWI (unit/mL).

Time	Group	CONG	CWIG	F	
Pre-match		1.7 ± 0.90	1.6 ± 1.02	Group	0.158
Post-match		3.0 ± 1.64	2.5 ± 1.52		
Post-treatment		2.0 ± 0.96	1.9 ± 1.08	Time	8.496 ***
Post-rest		1.8 ± 1.04	2.0 ± 1.31	Group × Time	0.945

Mean ± standard deviation; *** $p < 0.001$; no significant interaction effect was observed for group by time in MDA concentration.

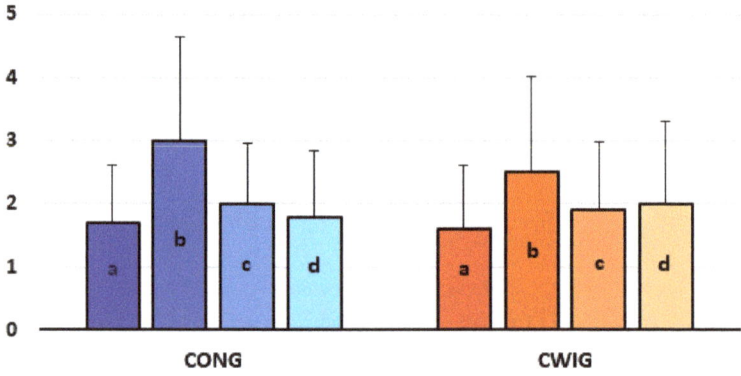

a: Before; b: After game; c: After CWI; d: After rest; CONG: Control group; CWIG: Cold-water immersion group

Figure 4. Change in SOD concentration after CWI. (Data are expressed as mean ± standard deviation. A main effect was evident with respect to time—$p < 0.001$. CWI: cold-water immersion).

3.4. Change in GPX Concentration

Changes in GPX concentration following CWI are described in Table 4 and Figure 5 and were analyzed using repeated measures ANOVA. Significant differences according to the time of measurement were observed ($F = 13.317$; $p < 0.001$). Moreover, there were highly significant differences in interaction ($F = 26.588$; $p < 0.001$). The CONG showed a 2% reduction of GPX concentration after CWI compared to immediately after a match, while the CWIG showed an 8% increase in the same period. Furthermore, the CWIG showed an 89% increase in GPX concentration after rest from the level immediately after a match compared to the CONG ($F = 6.778$; $p < 0.05$).

Table 4. Change in glutathione peroxidase (GPX) concentration after CWI (unit/μ mol).

Time \ Group	CONG	CWIG	F	
[a] Pre-match	112.4 ± 14.37 cd	99.2 ± 37.30 bcd	Group	6.778 *
[b] Post-match	119.1 ± 15.84 cd	65.7 ± 14.35 ad	Time	13.317 ***
[c] Post-treatment	94.3 ± 14.38 ab	70.8 ± 9.78 ad	Group × Time	26.588 ***
[d] Post-rest	93.4 ± 13.74 ab	134.7 ± 24.98 abc		

Mean ± standard deviation, [a]: Pre-match, [b]: Post-match, [c]: Post-treatment, [d]: Post-rest; * $p < 0.05$, *** $p < 0.001$; significant differences in p-values of the Bonferroni post hoc test are indicated with letters.

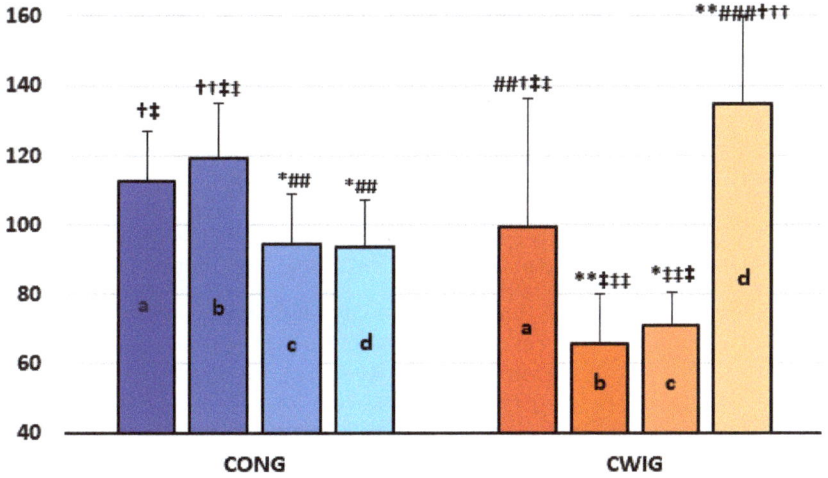

a: Before; b: After game; c: After CWI; d: After rest; CONG: Control group; CWIG: Cold-water immersion group

Figure 5. Change in GPX concentration after CWI. (Data are expressed as mean ± SD; A main effect was evident for time and group × time—$p < 0.001$; differences between each group were statistically significant—$p < 0.05$: difference from before, * $p < 0.5$, ** $p < 0.5$; difference from after game, ## $p < 0.01$, ### $p < 0.001$; difference from before, † $p < 0.05$, †† $p < 0.01$; difference from before, ‡ $p < 0.05$, ‡‡ $p < 0.01$, ‡‡‡ $p < 0.001$. CWI: cold-water immersion.).

4. Discussion

This study was conducted on 12 male elite Taekwondo athletes with the aim to assist with the recovery of the athletes, who need to compete in all their respective matches of a tournament within a single day. To this end, the athletes' HR was measured to investigate the intensity of a Taekwondo match, and CWI was applied to the below-knee area after a match to investigate its effects on the athletes' lipid peroxide and antioxidant enzymes levels. Our study's findings regarding recovery after a match of elite Taekwondo athletes showed that the mean HR after a match was about 91% HR_{max}. CWI treatment after a match neither decreased lipid peroxide concentrations, nor did it confer positive effects on the concentration of SOD. However, it did improve GPX concentrations (Group × Time, $p < 0.001$; Group, $p < 0.05$).

4.1. Athletic Intensity of the Taekwondo Competition

Since being confirmed as an official sport at the 2000 Summer Olympics at Sydney, Taekwondo has been recognized for its values at the Olympics and has advanced as a martial sport [21]. Taekwondo requires players to move quickly and powerfully [34]; thus, the players must have power, muscle strength, muscle endurance, agility, and flexibility [35,36]. In particular, muscle functions, such as muscle strength and endurance of the lower extremities, are important for performing strong and accurate kicks [37,38]. During the three two-min rounds of a Taekwondo competition, athletes employ various techniques and strategies, demanding a substantial amount of energy.

According to a study by Butios (2007) on the intensity of Taekwondo matches in 24 male college Taekwondo athletes, the mean HR of athletes who train for five days per week for an average of 25 h a week was 86% HR_{max} [39]. In seven recreational Taekwondo students, the mean HR was about 80–90% HR_{max} during Taekwondo-combined exercise [27]. Both studies showed a lower HR_{max} than that found in our study, where actual Taekwondo matches were performed.

However, in a study investigating HR responses based on a type and technique combination of Taekwondo in seven elite female Taekwondo athletes, the HR was 186.6 ± 2.5 bpm during a Taekwondo match, with an intensity of 92% HR_{max} [36]. This was consistent with the results of our study, where actual Taekwondo matches were performed with tactical strategies as opposed to previous studies that used Taekwondo as a type of exercise [27,39]. Furthermore, the mean HR of male Taekwondo athletes with an average career of nine years (age: 22 ± 4 years; height 182 ± 0.10 cm; body mass 69.4 ± 3.4 kg) during an international Taekwondo competition was 187 ± 8 bpm after a three-round match at 96% HR_{max} [40]. This shows that HR is higher during a program similar to an actual match than that during Taekwondo performed as an exercise, and that HR is even higher during an actual match, as performed in our study.

4.2. Variation of MDA Concentration after CWI for Taekwondo Athletes

In general, ROS are released from the electron transport chain in the mitochondria, even at rest [3], and they eventually attack the cell membrane and nucleus and form lipid peroxides. Moreover, secondary ROS, produced as a result of ROS activation surpassing the defense system with antioxidant enzymes, stimulate the peroxidation of lipids containing unsaturated fatty acids in cell membranes, thereby elevating the concentration of MDA, the final metabolite of lipid peroxide, and induce injuries [41]. After exercise, ROS concentration can increase so much as to induce acute injuries of muscle fibers and connective tissues, leading to muscle ache, delayed recovery, and diminished exercise performance [42]. Previous studies have examined the effects of types of cryotherapy on such lipid peroxides produced through exercise and antioxidant enzymes [43,44].

Cryotherapies are used for therapeutic purposes in sports, and their effects differ according to the method, duration, treatment site, and the individual's level of physical activity. Among various cryotherapies, crushed ice pack, ice massage, and CWI are the most effective [45]. In a study examining changes of MDA concentration after cold treatment, no change in MDA was found after performing high-intensity jump exercises between the untrained group and the group trained in the exercise; although the levels of lipid peroxidase in muscles, as measured by changes in MDA concentration, varied widely, there were no differences between the two groups [46]. These results seem to be attributable to excellent physical defense regulation in the athletes as a result of prolonged chronic training. These results are consistent with our findings. In this study, MDA concentration immediately after the match was lower than that before the match, but reduced MDA concentration did not differ between after CWI and after rest. However, another study reported that ice-water immersion after 30 min of cycling lowered lipid peroxide concentration [44], which contradicts the results of our study and that of the previously mentioned study [47].

In 2003, Krishnan et al. reported that MDA production is influenced more by exercise intensity or duration, as opposed to the type of exercise performed [47]. Thus, it seems that MDA concentration after jump exercises or a competition that can be performed in a short time [47], and that after a Taekwondo competition, are not markedly influenced by cold treatment or CWI. The reduction of MDA concentration after 30 min of cycling exercise, as reported in a prior study [43], seems to have been a result of the longer duration of the exercise.

There are various study findings regarding long-term chronic training, where some studies report that it bolsters an individual's physical defense mechanisms and decreases MDA even if they engage in exhaustive exercise [48], while other studies report that ROS as well as antioxidant enzymes are produced after exhaustive exercise [49].

This suggests that the gap in the changes of MDA caused by exercise may be attributable to various factors, including study design. Furthermore, the most crucial factor is speculated to be the level of proficiency of participants for the particular type of exercise or perceived exercise intensity; in athletes who underwent prolonged professional training, local CWI seems to have been inadequate to reduce intracellular-intravascular flow to promote recovery from cellular or membrane injuries from free radical production triggered by increased oxygen consumption in the active muscles during a game.

4.3. Variation of Antioxidant Enzyme Concentration According to CWI for Elite Taekwondo Athletes

Taekwondo is a sport in which a player must be nimble enough to exploit the opponent's weak points with explosive kicks; thus, active muscles are utilized alternately at a high intensity. Furthermore, players must compete in at least 5–7 matches in a single day [50,51], during which there is the accumulation of hydrogen ions, phosphorus, ammonia, and lactate. This accumulation has an impact on muscle metabolism, local muscle fatigue, and neuromuscular activities [52,53]. Moreover, high-intensity training, excessive training, and strenuous training without appropriate rest periods also induce fatigue, undermine athletic performance, and can cause sport-related injuries [54]. In addition, they cause muscle contraction and structural damages to cell membranes and muscles, thereby disturbing muscle fiber homeostasis and leading to oxidative stress.

However, lowering ROS levels after exercise can also have the opposite effect [55]. This is attributable to the fact that ROS is needed for appropriate muscle contraction during rest and physical activity [42]. In 1996, Swenson et al. suggested that CWI is a classic method of alleviating muscle injury. Furthermore, they reported that CWI treats muscle injuries by lowering local vascular permeability and edema by inducing vasocontraction while increasing the pain threshold [56]. Another study reported that CWI can regulate the physiological effects of exercise and can be used for treating exercise-induced injuries [57]. Regarding prior research on cold treatment, one study reported that a single session using ice increased antioxidant enzyme activity in untrained volunteers [19]. However, our findings showed that a single CWI session partially increased antioxidant enzyme activity. That is, there were no significant differences in SOD levels between groups, but there was an interaction effect. Moreover, CWI treatment increased GPX concentration, and there were interactions between groups. Thus, a single CWI session can be applied in different ways according to the study methodology. In another similar study, low-temperature stimulation once per day increased SOD activity [58], showing that the outcomes varied, even with the same cold treatment.

However, ice-cold water treatment did not increase antioxidant enzyme activation [43], which is in line with our findings, but inconsistent with the findings of other studies [44,58].

Elevated antioxidant enzyme activity attests to increased ROS concentration. However, such ROS production could be beneficial, as it may cause stimulating changes, and does not damage the body [18,59]. Therefore, as an oxidant, ice-water immersion stimulates and enhances antioxidant capacity [43]. In another study utilizing cold treatment, a whole-body cryotherapy (WBC) session used as a pre-training stimulation in a multiday training camp had adverse effects on elite athletes by diminishing both lipid peroxide level and antioxidant enzyme activities [60,61]. Nevertheless, WBC and CWI are increasingly used in professional sports to facilitate rehabilitation following an injury, as they lower oxidative stress, inflammatory reactions, and pain from vigorous exercise [19,57,60,61]. In particular, CWI continues to be researched using various study designs, which help support the claim that it is an effective method to delay or prevent physical fatigue, muscle fatigue, and diminished athletic performance suffered by athletes who undergo high-intensity training or compete in multiple games.

Therefore, the inconsistent effects of CWI on the oxidant/antioxidant balance in the human body would probably be helpful in maintaining an ROS concentration that is the most appropriate for both rest and exercise [43].

Inconsistent results pertaining to the effects of CWI on lipid peroxide and antioxidant enzymes were shown in previous studies [43,44,60,61]. Our study clarifies the tasks to be addressed by researchers in the future using new methodologies for the type of participant, duration of exercise, method of exercise, and CWI treatment duration and site. Furthermore, the exact mechanism of the antioxidant system and cold treatment must be researched.

4.4. Limitations of the Study

We acknowledge the following limitations of this study. First, we only enrolled adult men and analyzed three blood samples. Second, while all athletes were in the same Taekwondo weight category and were trained in the same training program prior to the study, we could not control for the amount of continuous training. Therefore, it may be difficult to draw definitive conclusions due to individual athletes' physical responses to continuous training, including free radical production, cell injury, and antioxidant enzymatic system. However, the significance of this study is that we tackled a novel area of research involving antioxidant activity-CWI after an actual Taekwondo game.

Therefore, our findings highlight the need to restrict continued physical training, amount of food intake, and drug use for a certain period and to expand the scope of study parameters.

5. Conclusions

Regarding the exercise intensity of a Taekwondo match, the mean HR during the match was 88% HR_{max} and post-match was 91% of HR_{max}. CWI treatment after the Taekwondo match had no effect on the reduction of MDA concentration in elite Taekwondo athletes. SOD concentration in the CWIG was 19% higher than that in the CONG, suggesting that CWI effectively increases SOD concentration. Further CWI after the Taekwondo match effectively increased GPX concentration.

In conclusion, although CWI at 10 °C for 20 min after a Taekwondo match did not alter lipid peroxide levels, it may promote antioxidant enzyme activation in elite Taekwondo players. However, the theoretical grounds for the effects of CWI on antioxidant enzymes have not yet been established. Additional studies employing diverse methods are needed to examine post-match treatment for sports that use protective devices on the head, trunk, hands, and feet, such as Taekwondo.

We found that CWI, which can be readily applied after a high-intensity Taekwondo match, may promote the more rapid recovery of Taekwondo athletes who are required to play multiple matches in one day from their qualifications to the finals.

Author Contributions: E.-H.P. was the main researcher and writer, contributed to the study design, collected data, and took part in manuscript preparation. S.-W.C. and Y.-K.Y. helped conceptualize the study, participated in its design and statistical analysis. All authors have read and agreed to the published version of the manuscript.

Funding: This research received no external funding.

Institutional Review Board Statement: Not applicable.

Informed Consent Statement: Not applicable.

Data Availability Statement: Not applicable.

Acknowledgments: The authors would like to express their gratitude to the people who supported this study and the participants who joined the program voluntarily.

Conflicts of Interest: The authors declare no conflict of interest.

References

1. Niess, A.M.; Sommer, M.; Schneider, M.; Angres, C.; Tschositsch, K.; Golly, I.C.; Fehrenbach, E. Physical exercise-induced expression of inducible nitric oxide synthase and heme oxygenase-1 in human leukocytes: Effects of RRR-α-tocopherol supplementation. *Antioxid. Redox Signal.* **2000**, *2*, 113–126. [CrossRef]
2. Fernández-Lázaro, D.; Mielgo-Ayuso, J.; Seco Calvo, J.; Córdova Martínez, A.; Caballero García, A.; Fernandez-Lazaro, C.I. Modulation of exercise-induced muscle damage, inflammation, and oxidative markers by curcumin supplementation in a physically active population: A systematic review. *Nutrients* **2020**, *12*, 501. [CrossRef]
3. Halliwell, B. Free radicals, antioxidants, and human diseases: Curiosity, cause, or consequence? *Lancet* **1994**, *344*, 721–724. [CrossRef]
4. Jones, J.I.; Clemmons, D.R. Insulin-like growth factors and their binding proteins: Biological actions. *Endocr. Rev.* **1995**, *16*, 3–34. [PubMed]
5. Ji, L.L. Antioxidant enzyme response to exercise and aging. *Med. Sci. Sports Exerc.* **1993**, *25*, 225–231. [CrossRef] [PubMed]
6. Jenkins, R.R.; Goldfarb, A. Introduction: Oxidant stress, aging and exercise. *Med. Sci. Sports Exerc.* **1993**, *25*, 210–212. [CrossRef] [PubMed]
7. Reznick, A.Z.; Steinhagan-Thiessen, E.; Gershon, D. The effect of exercise on enzymes activities in cardiac muscle of mice of various ages. *Biochem. Med.* **1992**, *28*, 347–352. [CrossRef]
8. Holloszy, J.O.; Booth, F.W. Biochemical adaptations to endurance exercise in muscle. *Ann. Rev. Physiol.* **1976**, *38*, 273–291. [CrossRef]
9. Slattery, K.; Bentley, D.; Coutts, A.J. The role of oxidative, inflammatory and neuroendocrinological systems during exercise stress in athletes: Implications of antioxidant supplementation on physiological adaptation during intensified physical training. *Sports Med.* **2015**, *45*, 453–471. [CrossRef]
10. Andriichuk, A.; Tkachenko, H.; Tkachova, I. Oxidative stress biomarkers and erythrocytes hemolysis in well-trained equine athletes before and after exercise. *J. Equine Vet. Sci.* **2016**, *36*, 32–43. [CrossRef]
11. Bailey, D.M.; Erith, S.J.; Griffin, P.J.; Dowson, A.; Brewer, D.S.; Gant, N.; Williams, C. Influence of cold-water immersion on indices of muscle damage following prolonged intermittent shuttle running. *J. Sport Sci.* **2007**, *25*, 1163–1170. [CrossRef]
12. Vaile, J.; Halson, S.; Gill, N.; Dawson, B. Effect of cold water immersion on repeat cycling performance and thermoregulation in the heat. *J. Sport Sci.* **2008**, *26*, 431–440. [CrossRef] [PubMed]
13. Delextrat, A.; Calleja-González, J.; Hippocrate, A.; Clarke, N.D. Effects of sports massage and intermittent cold-water immersion on recovery from matches by basketball players. *J. Sport Sci.* **2013**, *31*, 11–19. [CrossRef]
14. Rowsell, G.J.; Coutts, A.J.; Reaburn, P.; Hill-Haas, S. Effects of cold-water immersion on physical performance between successive matches in high-performance junior male soccer players. *J. Sport Sci.* **2009**, *27*, 565–573. [CrossRef]
15. Ascensão, A.; Leite, M.; Rebelo, A.N.; Magalhães, S.; Magalhães, J. Effects of cold water immersion on the recovery of physical performance and muscle damage following a one-off soccer match. *J. Sport Sci.* **2011**, *29*, 217–225. [CrossRef] [PubMed]
16. Racinais, S.; Oksa, J. Temperature and neuromuscular function. *Scand. J. Med. Sci. Sports* **2010**, *20*, 1–18. [CrossRef] [PubMed]
17. Stocks, J.M.; Taylor, N.A.S.; Tipton, M.J.; Greenleaf, J.E. Human physiological responses to cold exposure. *Sport Aviat. Space Environ. Med.* **2004**, *75*, 444–457.
18. Siems, W.G.; Brenke, R.; Sommerburg, O.; Grune, T. Improved antioxidative protection in winter swimmers. *QJM* **1999**, *92*, 193–198. [CrossRef] [PubMed]
19. Wozniak, A.; Mila-Kierzenkowska, C.; Szpinda, M.; Chwalbinska-Moneta, J.; Augustynska, B.; Jurecka, A. Whole-body cryostimulation and oxidative stress in rowers: The preliminary results. *Arch. Med. Sci.* **2013**, *9*, 303. [CrossRef] [PubMed]
20. Lee Kyung, K.T.; Choi, Y.S.; Lee, Y.K.; Lee, J.P.; Young, K.W.; Park, S.Y. Extensor hallucis longus tendon Injury in Taekwondo Athletes. *Phys. Ther. Sport* **2009**, *10*, 101–104.
21. Kim, Y.J.; Cha, E.J.; Kim, S.M.; Kang, K.D.; Han, D.H. The effects of Taekwondo training on brain connectivity and body intelligence. *Psychiatry Investig.* **2015**, *12*, 335–340. [CrossRef] [PubMed]
22. Pieter, W.; Zemper, E.D. Incidence of reported cerebral concussion in adult Taekwondo athletes. *Perspect. Public Health* **1998**, *118*, 272–279. [CrossRef] [PubMed]

23. Pieter, W.; Zemper. E.D. Head and neck injuries in young Taekwondo athletes. *J. Sport Med. Phys. Fit.* **1999**, *38*, 147–153.
24. Kasemi, M.; Pieter, W. Injuries at a Canadian national Taekwondo championships: A prospective study. *BMC Musculoskel. Disord.* **2004**, *5*, 22. [CrossRef] [PubMed]
25. Bøyum, A.; Wiik, P.; Gustavsson, E.; Veiby, O.P.; Reseland, J.; Haugen, A.H.; Opstad, P.K. The effect of strenuous exercise, calorie deficiency and sleep deprivation on white blood cells, plasma immunoglobulins and cytokines. *Scand. J. Immunol.* **1996**, *43*, 228–235. [CrossRef] [PubMed]
26. Kanter, M.M.; Nolte, L.A.; Hollosszy, J.O. Effects of an antioxidant vitamin mixture on lipid peroxidation at rest and postexercise. *J. Appl. Physiol.* **1993**, *74*, 965–969. [CrossRef]
27. Beis, K.; Pieter, W.; Abatzides, G. Taekwondo techniques and competition characteristics involved time-loss injuries. *J. Sport Sci. Med.* **2007**, *6*, 45–51.
28. Pieter, W.; Paul, G.F.; Michael, D.O. Competition injuries in Taekwondo: A literature review and suggestions for prevention and surveillance. *Br. J. Sport Med.* **2012**, *46*, 485–491. [CrossRef]
29. Kazemi, M.; Judith, W.; Morgan, C.; White, A.R. A profile of Olympic Taekwondo competitors. *J. Sport Sci. Med.* **2006**, *5*, 114–121.
30. De Pauw, K.; De Geus, B.; Roelands, B.; Lauwens, F.; Verschueren, J.; Heyman, E.; Meeusen, R.R. Effect of five different recovery methods on repeated cycle performance. *Med. Sci. Sport Exerc.* **2011**, *43*, 890–897. [CrossRef]
31. Schniepp, J.; Campbell, T.S.; Powell, K.L.; Pincivero, D.M. The effects of cold-water immersion on power output and heart rate in elite cyclists. *J. Strength Cond. Res.* **2002**, *16*, 561–566.
32. Crowe, M.J.; O'Connor, D.; Rudd, D. Cold water recovery reduces anaerobic performance. *Int. J. Sport Med.* **2007**, *28*, 994–998. [CrossRef] [PubMed]
33. Pieter, W.; Bercades, L.T.; Kim, G.D. Relative total body fat and skinfold patterning in Filipino national combat sport athletes. *J. Sport Sci. Med.* **2006**, *5*, 35–41.
34. Bouhlel, E.; Jouini, A.; Gmada, N.; Nefzi, A.; Ben Abdallah, K.; Tabka, Z. Heart rate and blood lactate responses during Taekwondo training and competition. *Braz. J. Biomotricity* **2006**, *21*, 285–290. [CrossRef]
35. Markovic, G.; Vucetic, V.; Cardinale, M. Heart rate and lactate responses to Taekwondo fight in elite women performers. *Bio Sport* **2008**, *25*, 135–146.
36. Cools, A.M.; Geerooms, E.; Dorien, F.M.; Berghe, V.D.; Cambier, D.C.; Witvrouw, E. Isokinetic scapular muscle performance in young elite gymnasts. *J. Athl. Train.* **2007**, *42*, 458–563. [PubMed]
37. Fritzsche, J.; Raschka, C. Body composition and somatotype of German top Taekwondo practitioners. *Paper Anthropol.* **2008**, *17*, 58.
38. Butios, S.; Tasika, N. Changes in heart rate and blood lactate concentration as intensity parameters during simulated Taekwondo competition. *J. Sport Med. Phys. Fit.* **2007**, *47*, 179–185.
39. Pieter, W.; Taaffe, D.; Heijmans, J. Heart rate response to Taekwondo forms and technique combinations. A pilot study. *J. Sport Med. Phys. Fit.* **1990**, *30*, 97–102.
40. Bride, C.A.; Jones, M.A.; Drust, B. Physiological responses and perceived exertion during international Taekwondo competition. *Int. J. Sport Physiol. Perform.* **2009**, *4*, 485–493. [CrossRef]
41. Quash, G.; Ripoll, H.; Gazzolo, L.; Doutheau, A.; Saba, A.; Gore, J. Malondialdehyde production from spermine by homog-enates of nomal and transformed cells. *Biochimie* **1987**, *69*, 101–108. [CrossRef]
42. Clanton, T.L.; Zuo, L.; Klawitter, P. Oxidants and skeletal muscle function: Physiologic and pathophysiologic implications. *Proc. Soc. Exp. Biol. Med.* **1999**, *222*, 253–262. [CrossRef] [PubMed]
43. Sutkowy, P.; Woźniak, A.; Boraczyński, T.; Mila-Kierzenkowska, C.; Boraczyński, M. Postexercise impact of ice-cold water bath on the oxidant-antioxidant balance in healthy men. *BioMed. Res. Int.* **2015**, *2015*, 706141. [CrossRef] [PubMed]
44. Lubkowska, A.; Dołęgowska, B.; Szyguła, Z.; Bryczkowska, I.; Stańczyk-Dunaj, M.; Sałata, D.; Budkowska, M. Win-ter-swimming as a building-up body resistance factor inducing adaptive changes in the oxidant/antioxidant status. *Scand. J. Clin. Lab. Investig.* **2013**, *38*, 315–325. [CrossRef] [PubMed]
45. Merrick, M.A.; Jutte, L.S.; Smith, M.E. Cold modalities with different thermodynamic properties produce different surface and intramuscular temperatures. *J. Athl. Train.* **2003**, *38*, 28–33.
46. Krishnan, R.K.; Evans, W.J.; Kirwan, J.P. Impaired substrate oxidation in healthy elderly men after eccentric exercise. *J. App. Physiol.* **2003**, *94*, 716–723. [CrossRef]
47. Ortenblad, N.; Madsen, K.; Djurhuus, M.S. Antioxidant status and lipid peroxidation after short-term maximal exercise in trained and untrained humans. *Am. J. Physiol. Regul.* **1997**, *272*, 1258–1263. [CrossRef]
48. Ji, L.L. Exercise-induced modulation of antioxidant defense. *Ann. N. Y. Acad. Sci.* **2002**, *959*, 82–92. [CrossRef]
49. Child, R.B.; Wilkinson, D.M.; Fallowfield, J.L. Effects of a training taper on tissue damage indices, serum antioxidant capacity and half-marathon running performance. *Int. J. Sports Med.* **2000**, *21*, 325–331. [CrossRef]
50. Chiodo, S.; Tessitore, A.; Cortis, C.; Cibelli, G.; Lupo, C.; Ammendolia, A.; De Rosas, M.; Capranica, L. Stress-related hormonal and psychological changes to official youth Taekwondo competition. *Scand. J. Med. Sci. Sports* **2011**, *21*, 111–119. [CrossRef]
51. Tsai, M.L.; Chou, K.M.; Chang, C.K.; Fang, S.H. Changes of mucosal immunity and antioxidation activity in Elite Male Taiwanese taekwondo athletes associated with intensive training and rapid weight loss. *Br. J. Sport Med.* **2011**, *45*, 729–734. [CrossRef] [PubMed]
52. Iaia, F.M.; Perez-Gomez, J.; Nordsborg, N.; Bangsbo, J. Effect of previous exhaustive exercise on metabolism and fatigue development during intense exercise in humans. *Scand. J. Med. Sci. Sports* **2010**, *20*, 619–629. [CrossRef]

53. Ravier, G.; Dugué, B.; Grappe, F.; Rouillon, J.D. Maximal accumulated oxygen deficit and blood responses of ammonia, lactate and PH after anaerobic test: A comparison between international and national elite karate athletes. *Int. J. Sport Med.* **2006**, *27*, 810–817. [CrossRef] [PubMed]
54. Halson, S.L.; Jeukendrup, A.E. Does overtraining exist? *Sport Med.* **2004**, *34*, 967–981. [CrossRef] [PubMed]
55. Peternelj, T.-T.; Coombes, J.S. Antioxidant supplementation during exercise training. *Sport Med.* **2011**, *41*, 1043–1069. [CrossRef] [PubMed]
56. Swenson, C.; Swärd, L.; Karlsson, J. Cryotherapy in sports medicine. *Scand. J. Med. Sci. Sports* **1996**, *6*, 193–200. [CrossRef]
57. Bleakley, C.M.; Bieuzen, F.; Davison, G.W.; Costello, J.T. Whole-body cryotherapy: Empirical evidence and theoretical perspectives. *Open Access J. Sports Med.* **2014**, *5*, 25. [CrossRef]
58. Miller, E.; Markiewicz, Ł.; Saluk, J.; Majsterek, I. Effect of short-term cryostimulation on antioxidative status and its clinical applications in humans. *Eur. J. Appl. Physiol.* **2012**, *112*, 1645–1652. [CrossRef] [PubMed]
59. Siems, W.G.; van Kuijk, F.J.; Maass, R.; Brenke, R. Uric acid and glutathione levels during short-term whole body cold exposure. *Free Radic. Biol. Med.* **1994**, *16*, 299–305. [CrossRef]
60. Wozniak, A.; Wozniak, B.; Drewa, G.; Mila-kierzenkowska, C. The effect of whole-body cryostimulation on the prooxidant–antioxidant balance in blood of elite kayakers after training. *Eur. J. Appl. Physiol.* **2007**, *101*, 533–537. [CrossRef]
61. Rakowski, A.; Jurecka, A.; Rajewski, R. Whole-body cryostimulation in kayaker women: A study of the effect of cryogenic temperatures on oxidative stress after the exercise. *J. Sport Med. Phys. Fit.* **2009**, *49*, 201–207.

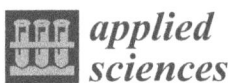

Article

Achieve Personalized Exercise Intensity through an Intelligent System and Cycling Equipment: A Machine Learning Approach

Yichen Wu [1,2,3], Zuchang Ma [1], Huanhuan Zhao [1,2,4], Yibing Li [1,2,5] and Yining Sun [1,*]

[1] Anhui Province Key Laboratory of Medical Physics and Technology, Institute of Intelligent Machines, Hefei Institutes of Physical Science, Chinese Academy of Sciences, Hefei 230031, China; wuyichen@mail.ustc.edu.cn (Y.W.); zcma@iim.ac.cn (Z.M.); zhh174@mail.ustc.edu.cn (H.Z.); liyibing@mail.ustc.edu.cn (Y.L.)
[2] Science Island Branch of Graduate School, University of Science and Technology of China, Hefei 230031, China
[3] School of Electronic and Information Engineering, Anhui Jianzhu University, Hefei 230601, China
[4] School of Computer and Information Engineering, Chuzhou University, Chuzhou 239000, China
[5] School of Computer Science and Technology, HeFei Normal University, Hefei 230601, China
* Correspondence: health-promotion@iim.ac.cn

Received: 12 October 2020; Accepted: 28 October 2020; Published: 30 October 2020

Featured Application: With the development of artificial intelligence, Internet technology, smart exercise equipment, and smart wearable devices, more and more people are becoming willing to use these technologies for exercise, whether out of curiosity or because they want to use them for scientific fitness. At the same time, many non-invasive static human data acquisition devices have become commonplace, and many hospitals and communities are already using them. The smart health system that we designed can easily process the in-exercise and non-exercise data collected by the above two ways. The system, which includes a mobile application, website, cloud server, smart wearable device, and other platforms, generates personalized prescriptions for users by learning the data. The system also includes many functions for public health, and exercise prescription is just one module of it.

Abstract: Using absolute intensity methods (metabolic equivalent of energy (METs), etc.) to determine exercise intensity in exercise prescriptions is straightforward and convenient. Using relative intensity methods (heart rate reserve (%HRR), maximal heart rate (%HR_{max}), etc.) is more recommended because it is more personalized. Taking target heart rate (THR) given by the relative method as an example, compared with just presenting the THR value, intuitively providing the setting parameters for achieving the THR with specific sport equipment is more user-friendly. The objective of this study was to find a method which combines the advantages (convenient and personalized) of the absolute and relative methods and relatively avoids their disadvantages, helping individuals to meet the target intensity by simply setting equipment parameters. For this purpose, we recruited 32 males and 29 females to undergo incremental cardiopulmonary exercise testing with cycling equipment. The linear regression model of heart rate and exercise wattage (the setting parameter of the equipment) was constructed for each one ($R^2 = 0.933$, $p < 0.001$), and the slopes of the graph of these models were obtained. Next, we used an iterative algorithm to obtain a multiple regression model (adjusted $R^2 = 0.8336$, $p < 0.001$) of selected static body data and the slopes of participants. The regression model can accurately predict the slope of the general population through their static body data. Moreover, other populations can guarantee comparable accuracy by using questionnaire data for calibration. Then, the predicted slope can be utilized to calculate the equipment's settings for achieving a personalized THR through our equation. All of these steps can be assigned to the intelligent system.

Keywords: exercise prescriptions; sports equipment; exercise intensity; intelligent system; machine learning

1. Introduction

Exercise intensity refers to the amount of force exerted during an action and the degree of tension in the body. It is one of the main factors that determines exercise load and has a great stimulating effect on the human body. There are positive dose–response health/fitness benefits that result from increasing exercise intensity [1]. Appropriate exercise intensity can effectively promote bodily functions, thereby enhancing physical fitness. If the intensity of exercise is too high, it will reduce bodily functions and even cause sports injuries. Determining the exercise intensity is key to obtaining exercise benefits (improvement of cardiorespiratory fitness (CRF), muscular strength and endurance, flexibility, body composition, neuromotor fitness, etc.) and is one of the core steps in generating personalized exercise prescriptions [2].

There are many effective exercise intensity calculation methods that can be used to formulate personalized exercise prescriptions [1]. Absolute methods (oxygen uptake (VO_2), metabolic equivalent of energy (METs), etc.), relative methods (heart rate reserve (%HRR), maximal heart rate (%HR_{max}), maximal oxygen uptake (%VO_{2max}), etc.), and actual energy expenditure (EE) are commonly used. Although the absolute method can easily provide the exercise items necessary for achieving the target intensity (such as a comparison table of physical activity intensity [3,4]), it does not consider an individual's CRF level, age, physiology differences, health status, living habits, or other personal factors. Thus, when estimating exercise intensity, the result may be too high or too low [5,6], leading to misclassification of exercise intensity [7–9], and the recommended exercise is unreasonable. Therefore, it is more often recommended to use relative methods to formulate exercise prescriptions under the guidelines issued by the American College of Sports Medicine [9,10], but the relative methods also have shortcomings. Relative methods do not directly give the specific exercise to achieve the target intensity but indirectly express the exercise intensity through other indicators. Among them, the commonly used %HRR method, the oxygen uptake reserve (VO_2R) method, the %HR_{max} method, and the %VO_{2max} method obtain exercise intensity in terms of target heart rate (THR) and target VO_2R, but the exercise wattage (amount of exercise) required by different individuals to reach a specific THR or target VO_2R is different, which is affected by multiple factors such as gender, height, and weight.

Exercise prescriptions are used to guide the public to exercise. For most ordinary exercisers who perform exercise prescriptions, their exercise knowledge is relatively limited, or they do not have with smart wearable devices. Prescriptions for these types of persons that define intensity only in terms of THR or target VO_2R for exercise often result in the exerciser having difficulty understanding the meaning of the prescription and then performing it with an inappropriate intensity. Users will still encounter these problems when using exercise prescriptions for the first time, even if they have the knowledge and devices. In the current Chinese society, sports equipment has become popular, especially indoor electronic sports equipment. Not only do many communities provide free sports equipment for residents to use, but also, each family spends more on purchasing such equipment. Compared to traditional sports such as running and dancing, the use of sports equipment is more controllable because of the fewer external factors (such as running road conditions and dancing types). Therefore, the manner in which to combine sports equipment to accurately achieve target exercise intensity has become more important.

This study used a linear regression model to find the relationship between heart rate and exercise wattage (because we changed the exercise load by adjusting the setting parameters (wattage) of the equipment) and describes the relationship with the slope S of the model's graph. Afterward, we used statistics and machine learning methods to predict the slope S through static human body data. Then, when generating a prescription, we used the predicted slope S and the THR obtained by the relative intensity method, combined with the resting heart rate (RHR) and HR_{max} (Fox-HR_{max}, Tanaka-HR_{max}, etc.), to determine the wattage of the bicycle equipment (spinning). This was calculated using Equation (1) as follows:

$$\text{Wattage of bicycle} = \frac{\text{THR} - \text{RHR}}{\text{slope}} \quad (1)$$

We collected data such as anthropometric data, cardiac and vascular function indicators, body composition, and bone density. These are universal human indicators that can reflect cardiovascular health, heart and lung capacity, skeletal muscle system, etc. We tried many commonly used multiple regression models (e.g., random forest and elastic net), and then selected the best one.

Using absolute methods is convenient and fast, but it is not personalized enough, while using relative methods is personalized but relatively complex and risky to operate. The method proposed by us combines the advantages of the two methods and relatively avoids their disadvantages. Based on the personalized THR obtained by using the relative method, our method can predict the input parameters of specific equipment (wattage for the smart cycling equipment) required to reach THR through static body data that can be used by exercisers conveniently. However, training and optimization of the model proposed in our method will remain ongoing through the interconnection of the data of the modules, such as electronic fitness equipment, intelligent systems, and smart wearable devices. Therefore, a closed loop of data acquisition, data learning, model optimization, and results presentation was formed.

2. Materials and Methods

2.1. Participants

This study was carried out at the Institute of Intelligent Machines, Chinese Academy of Sciences, Hefei, China. This study was approved by the Ethics Committee of the Hefei Institutes of Physical Science, Chinese Academy of Sciences (No. Y-2018-29). Participants were recruited through social media, advertisements in public places, and word of mouth. Sixty-one participants (aged 24–58 years) volunteered to participate in the study (32 males and 29 females), comprised of college students, scientific researchers, young and middle-aged white-collar workers, retired people, etc. All participants were informed about the study and signed a written informed consent form prior to participation. They had no contraindications for long-term or strenuous exercise, and none of them had experience in executing exercise prescriptions given by professionals or intelligent systems for a long time before the experiment. Their weekly exercise time and intensity was irregular.

2.2. Experimental Protocol

The experiment was scheduled to take place at least two hours after a meal (10:00 to 12:00 in the morning or 2:30 to 4:30 in the afternoon), maintaining the same ambient temperature (25 °C) and avoiding any sports 24 h before the test and try to maintain a static rest state between a meal and the start of the test. Using the maximum load (W-max) formula proposed by Wasserman et al. [11], we set the grading load experiment according to 20%, 40%, 50%, 70%, 85%, 100% of the W-max, and the load power of the bicycle ergometer (manufacturer: Lode BV Medical Technology, the Netherlands. IEC 60601-1. REF no. 960912) was intermittently adjusted from low to high until the participant was exhausted. This kind of experimental equipment, like many types of civilian cycling fitness equipment, uses wattage to adjust the exercise load, except that it is more expensive and more complicated. Exercise duration of each level was 3 min, as was the interval between each level, specifically measuring exercise heart rate. If a participant was unable to complete the 3-min test, the data could not be used until the heart rate had stabilized, and data which could not reach this stabilization were discarded. Each participant's RHR (wattage is 0, 0% of W-max) was used with the heart rate and power data of each level to construct a linear regression model of heart rate and wattage and to obtain the slope S of the graph of the linear model.

2.3. Measured Features and Statistical Analysis

We chose to use static human body data (non-exercise (Non-Ex) data) to predict the slope S, which is much more convenient than obtaining the slope S directly from a cardiopulmonary exercise test. Before the experiment, the static human body data were collected for each participant. Then, the relevant questionnaires were carried out, including lifestyle, medical history, family history, and others. Pearson correlation analysis on the slope S was performed for all quantifiable features (all data in Table 1) except for the questionnaire data. The features were arranged from high to low in the Pearson correlation to form a feature matrix. The data of the 61 participants were divided into a training set (50 participants) and a test set (11 participants), and it was ensured that there was no significant difference in the main features of the two sets, such as gender and age.

2.4. Algorithm Design

The algorithm (for the training set) can automatically select the best feature set from the feature matrix mentioned in Section 2.3 and can then analyze the related performance through multiple iterations. The specific steps are as follows:

1. Select the *i*-th feature in the feature matrix as the *j*-th feature of the regression model for machine learning (i and j both start at 1).
2. Perform multiple regression models to predict the slope S.
3. Use the leave-one-out method to verify and save the adjusted R^2 value of the model.
4. Select another feature (i + 1) from the feature matrix and then perform steps 1–3 until all of the features in the feature matrix have been traversed.
5. Select the feature with the best predictive effect, and then delete the selected features from the feature matrix. Add another feature (j + 1) of the regression model and repeat steps 1–4.
6. Continue to add new features until the adjusted R^2 value of the model drops for two consecutive time; then, the iteration is terminated.

We performed this algorithm separately for the linear regression, random forest, elastic net, polynomial regression, ridge regression, and lasso regression. Depending on the data in the iterations, we analyzed the performance of each model, selected the model with the best prediction effect, and determined the final feature set.

Table 1. Static human body data for the participants according to sex. Values refer to mean ± standard deviation (SD).

Data Type	Feature	Females (n = 29)	Males (n = 32)	Data Type	Feature	Females (n = 29)	Males (n = 32)
Anthropometric	Height, cm	161.1 ± 4.68	172.4 ± 7.07	Demographic	Age, years	37.2 ± 11.85	35.6 ± 10.75
	Weight, kg	57.3 ± 10.67	69.5 ± 9.74	Heart and blood vessels	EF, %	0.404 ± 0.034	0.389 ± 0.032
	BMI	22.0 ± 3.75	23.3 ± 2.54		SBP, mmHg	108.0 ± 12.91	115.8 ± 8.35
	WHR	0.83 ± 0.081	0.86 ± 0.031		DBP, mmHg	67.6 ± 8.04	73.0 ± 6.33
Physical fitness	Grip strength, kg	25.3 ± 4.77	41.0 ± 6.82		PP, mmHg	40.4 ± 6.67	42.8 ± 6.94
	Vital capacity, ml	2496.9 ± 545.89	3851.1 ± 857.63		AI, %	0.68 ± 0.150	0.55 ± 0.146
	Reaction time, sec	0.56 ± 0.128	0.49 ± 0.106		Cap, mmHg	95.3 ± 15.34	96.1 ± 10.74
	Sit-and-reach, cm	11.7 ± 8.94	9.7 ± 9.18		Left BAPWV, m/s	11.98 ± 1.41	12.11 ± 1.13
	Balance ability, s	48.5 ± 54.77	35.4 ± 29.81		Right BAPWV, m/s	12.84 ± 1.72	12.83 ± 1.29
Body composition	Body fat, %	0.227 ± 0.065	0.17 ± 0.045		Left lower limb ABI	1.19 ± 0.066	1.18 ± 0.065
	Moisture, %	0.517 ± 0.044	0.581 ± 0.034		Right lower limb ABI	1.17 ± 0.058	1.19 ± 0.070
	Protein, %	0.176 ± 0.019	0.204 ± 0.011		SEVR	1.21 ± 0.17	1.30 ± 0.18
	Inorganic salt, %	0.041 ± 0.0033	0.042 ± 0.0026		STI	96 ± 15.42	105 ± 17.47
	Left lower limb muscle, kg	6.45 ± 0.81	9.67 ± 1.67	Bone density	BUA	45.98 ± 4.42	48.69 ± 6.03
	Right lower limb muscle, kg	6.53 ± 0.74	9.85 ± 1.69		SOS	1582 ± 27.14	1595 ± 30.10
	Left upper limb muscle, kg	1.65 ± 0.32	2.41 ± 0.61		T-value	−0.5 ± 0.83	−0.04 ± 0.91
	Right upper limb muscle, kg	1.76 ± 0.34	2.55 ± 0.64		Z-value	−0.02 ± 0.99	0.38 ± 1.18
	Trunk muscle, kg	22.25 ± 1.89	29.47 ± 2.94		STI/expected value of peers	0.99 ± 0.156	1.04 ± 0.184

BMI, body mass index; WHR, waist-to-hip ratio; reaction time, the time measured by the human eye from seeing different signal lights to triggering the button by hand, which can express human agility; sit-and-reach, used to measure human flexibility; balance ability, time to stand on one foot with eyes closed; EF, ejection fraction; SBP, systolic blood pressure; DBP, diastolic blood pressure; PP, pulse pressure; AI, augmentation index; Cap, central arterial pressure; BAPWV, brachial-ankle pulse wave velocity; ABI, ankle/brachial index; SEVR, radial artery subendocardial viability ratio; STI, bone strength index; BUA, the slope of the relationship between ultrasonic attenuation and frequency after passing through the medium in a certain frequency band; SOS, the propagation speed of ultrasound in the medium; T-value, the degree of deviation of the tester's bone strength in terms of being higher or lower than the reference mean of young adults; Z-value, the degree of deviation of the tester's bone strength in terms of being higher or lower than the expected average of their peers. Number of participants in each age group: aged 20–29 years, n = 23 (11 females and 12 males); aged 30–39 years, n = 15 (6 females and 9 males); aged 40–49 years, n = 13 (5 females and 8 males); aged 50–59 years, n = 9 (7 females and 2 males); aged 60–69 years, n = 1 (1 male). Body composition data were measured by the bioelectrical impedance analysis method using a body composition analyzer. The bone density data were measured by the ultrasonic transmission method using an ultrasonic bone density meter. Grip strength was measured by a grip dynamometer. Participants used their dominant hand to hold the grip dynamometer as hard as they could while measuring.

3. Results

Twenty-eight percent of the participants completed all six levels, 52% completed five levels, and the rest completed less than five levels. Half of the participants who achieved less than five levels were middle-aged, with an average age of 38.9 years. Therefore, they may have been affected by the degree of subjective coordination or other unknown subjective and objective factors that could lead to a lower level of completion.

3.1. Linear Regression Model of Heart Rate and Wattage

The data of different load levels and RHR were used one-by-one to construct a linear regression model for each participant. For each individual's data, one single level of data was randomly selected as the test set, and the rest of the levels were used as the training set for the model. The average R^2 value of all of the individuals' models was 0.979, the standard deviation was 0.019, and the average p-value was 5.64×10^{-4}. This shows that the linear regression model has high prediction accuracy, so the use of the univariate slope S can describe the graphic characteristic of the model well and can determine the required exercise load wattage. Then, we included all levels of data (regardless of training or test set) to reconstruct the model for each person. The slope S of the model's graph was obtained from each participant (mean value = 0.684, standard deviation = 0.139, median = 0.678, maximum = 0.95, minimum = 0.441). The slope S was used as a dependent variable for training and validation by the model described later.

3.2. Feature Matrix and Regression Algorithm Analysis

3.2.1. Model Selection and Feature Analysis

In the process of using the iterative method to filter the features for predicting the slope S, the p-value obtained by each iteration of each model was much less than 0.001. The features finally selected by each model are shown in Figure 1. The adjusted R^2 value and the selected feature of each model in the iteration are shown in Figure 2 and Table 2. Compared to several other models, the ridge regression achieved the largest adjusted R^2 value and the smallest prediction error at the end of the iteration, so it was selected as the prediction model. Figure 2 shows that the adjusted R^2 value reached the highest when the ridge regression model was iterated to four features. Based on the above situation, a final feature set of four features was selected to predict the slope S: the waist-to-hip ratio (WHR), grip strength (GS), left lower limb muscle (LLLM), and bone strength index (STI). However, we can easily find that the final set of four features is not the combination that achieves the highest correlation with the slope, which seems unreasonable. This is actually because the algorithm that we propose is result-oriented. The algorithm tried a huge number of feature combinations to select the one with the highest predictive accuracy, regardless of whether the combination of features made sense. For example, the algorithm selects LLLM but not RLLM, which is easy to cause doubts. However, such a result is just because we can obtain better prediction results through LLLM by the existing experimental data. This does not mean that LLLM be more important than RLLM. The accuracy of using RLLM is only slightly lower than that of using LLLM. This difference may be due to differences in population or dominant feet. Thus, the choice of LLLM and RLLM mainly depends on the equipment that the individual already owns. Of course, we can also put forward a new feature (lower limb muscle) to remove people's doubts and make the result easier to figure out. The lower limb muscle (LLM) is the mean of LLLM and RLLM, which makes a lot more sense since, in cycling, the average power is generated by the average power of the two legs. The method of integrating features is also applicable to other pairs of body data that distinguish between right and left.

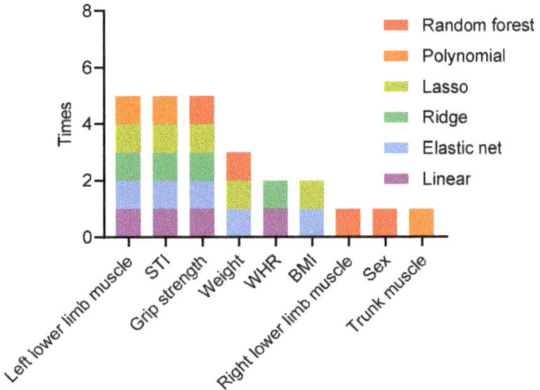

Figure 1. Features used when each model was iterated to the optimal.

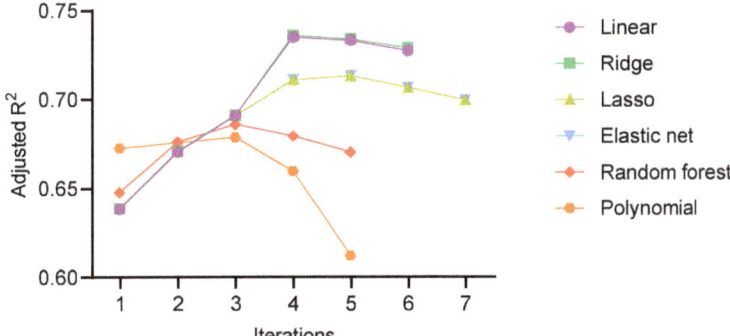

Figure 2. In each iteration, all of the remaining features in the matrix were traversed to obtain the best prediction result. The plot shows how the adjusted R^2 of the various models changed as features were iteratively added.

Table 2. Feature selected by each model in each iteration.

Number of Iterations	Machine Learning Model				
	Linear	Ridge	Lasso	Elastic Net	Polynomial
1st	Left lower limb muscle	Left lower limb muscle	Left lower limb muscle	Left lower limb muscle	Left lower limb muscle
2nd	Bone strength index	Bone strength index	Bone strength index	Bone strength index	Bone strength index
3rd	Grip strength	Grip strength	Grip strength	Grip strength	Grip strength
4th	Waist-to-hip ratio	Waist-to-hip ratio	BMI	BMI	BUA
5th	AI	AI	Weight	Weight	Right upper limb muscle
6th	BUA	BUA	Right lower limb muscle	Right lower limb muscle	-
7th	-	-	Left upper limb muscle	STI/Expected value for Peers	-

Random forest is a model that uses decision trees, whose training results are random each time. Therefore, the features selected by the random forest model in the training are not listed in the table. The adjusted R^2 in Figure 2 is also the average value obtained from the multiple training results.

3.2.2. Ridge Regression Model Analysis

The adjusted R^2 was 0.7363, the root-mean-square error (RMSE) was 0.068, the *p*-value was 2.089×10^{-16}, which was obtained by the leave-one-out method when the final feature set and regression model were determined, and the mean absolute error of each individual was 0.054 ± 0.041 (since the slope S is a ratio, we used the absolute error instead of the relative error). Eight of them had an absolute error greater than 0.1 and an average of 0.126.

We used the questionnaires filled out by participants and exercise experimental data to find the key factors that cause large errors (see Table 3). In the experimental data of these eight individuals, some individuals had an exhaustive heart rate that was more than 15 bpm lower than the HR_{max} calculated by the formula but had completed at least five levels of load. This shows that their cardiopulmonary exercise ability is stronger than that of the same type of people, and that the highest experimental level can no longer make them reach the HR_{max}. However, this situation may not be reflected through the collected static human body data, and it was not covered in the questionnaire either. There were also individuals whose exhausted heart rate was 15 bpm or more than 15 bpm lower than the maximum HR_{max} calculated by the formula and their completed load level was less than five. The load level they accomplished was lower and their exhausted heart rate was far from the theoretical HR_{max}, indicating that there may be other influencing factors in the experiment, such as poor subjective cooperation of the participants or errors in the experimental data collected. These are problems with exercise experimental data, indicating that the slope S obtained by linear regression of those individuals may deviate from the true value. Using an inaccurate slope S as the dependent variable to train the multiple regression model would undoubtedly cause a large error. In other individuals, some had fatty livers (which has a certain impact on exercise ability [12]), and some never exercised. The information obtained from the questionnaire shows that the static body data in the feature matrix used are not comprehensive enough and are only applicable to normal people, which may cause large errors. After excluding individuals with large errors, the model was re-trained, and the adjusted R^2 was 0.8336, the RMSE was 0.049, the *p*-value was 4.43×10^{-18}, and the average prediction absolute error was 0.041 ± 0.028.

Table 3. Features of the samples with high prediction errors mined from existing questionnaires and exercise data.

Number of Individuals	Feature	Predicted Result
2	Exhausted HR is more than 15 bpm lower than the formula HR_{max} (the load level is 5 or more)	Higher
2	Exhausted HR is more than 15 bpm lower than the formula HR_{max} (the load level is less than 5)	Uncertain
2	Fatty liver	Lower
1	Never exercise	Lower
1	Unknown	

Exhausted HR was the participant's real-time heart rate when he was no longer able to continue the experiment. HR_{max} is the maximum heart rate calculated by the formula.

Finally, the following regression equation was obtained:

$$Slope = 1.7015 - 2.676 \times 10^{-2} \times LLLM - 1.654 \times 10^{-3} \times STI \\ -6.143 \times 10^{-3} \times GS - 0.5188 \times WHR \quad (2)$$

We substituted the test set data into the equation and achieved an adjusted R^2 of 0.7068 and a *p*-value of 6.92×10^{-5}. Then, relying on the information reflected in the lifestyle questionnaire and the experimental data, we eliminated two cases of large error data. The adjusted R^2 value after correction was 0.8247, the *p*-value was 4.046×10^{-5}, and the predicted value was significantly correlated with the measured value, which shows that the above formula can predict the slope S of the general population. The scatter plots of the training and test sets are shown in Figure 3.

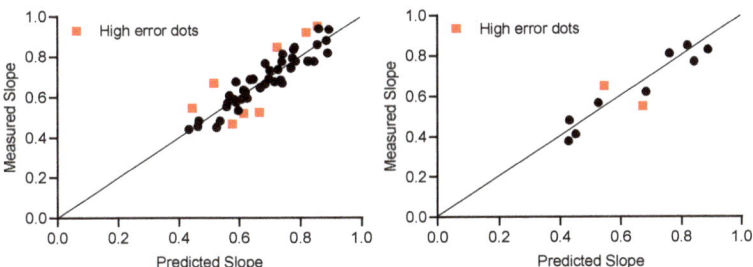

Figure 3. The slope obtained by the prediction and the slope measured in the experiment. Training set on the left, test set on the right.

4. Discussion

This research proposed a new idea that uses static human body data (input of the model) to predict the slope (output of the model) through the machine learning model. Then, we can use the Equation (1) to easily figure out the parameters of the cycling equipment required to reach the THR. We use wattage here only because most smart cycling equipment uses it as the input parameter (although there are other examples, such as the speed of treadmills and rowing machine). If MPH is going to be an input parameter for most smart cycling equipment in the future, then the slope we need might be in terms of heart rate and MPH.

For wattage prediction, we focused on verifying our ideas and the model's concepts. The purpose of this was not only to determine the final specific regression Equation (2), because in our main scenario (intelligent health system), a high-performance computer coupled with network technology can efficiently use and optimize the model, without the need of specific regression formulas. Our study showed that the slope could be accurately predicted through the static data we had, and that the predicted results could be further optimized through the key information obtained from the questionnaire, so as to expand the applicable scope of the model. After the model training is completed, using slope can help exercisers reach the target intensity accurately without the need for smart wearable devices. In daily use, the exerciser only needs to enter the predicted wattage into the smart cycling equipment to reach the target intensity. Of course, we certainly encourage people who are able to utilize wearable devices to use them because, in this way, we can obtain more in-exercise data. These data also do not require exercisers to observe and record. The device automatically uploads data when it is connected to the network. These data can be utilized to continuously optimize our models to provide better services.

Our method is relatively complex. It requires specific static body data monitoring equipment, rather than directly and continuously monitoring heart rate to reach exercise intensity. However, our method has specific usage scenarios because, among Chinese exercisers who use cycling equipment, only some people use exercise prescriptions. They obtained their prescriptions from professional departments, so they could easily obtain the static body data when they visit. Then, they can use our method without buying this equipment (body composition analyzer, an ultrasonic bone density meter, and other equipment). Other exercisers who did not utilize exercise prescriptions exercised more casually, lacked exercise knowledge, or even did not know what THR is. Even if they have a smart watch, they may be unable to accurately and scientifically use it to reach the THR. For those exercisers who have the ability to use a wearable device to reach the intensity without our method, they are more likely to suffer sports injuries during exercise, especially when they implement prescriptions for the first time because exercisers need to continue to pay attention to the changes in the heart rate data of the wearable device and whether the data remains stable throughout the exercise. When exercisers engage in exercises of moderate intensity or above, a lack of concentration can easily to cause sport injuries. On the other hand, many exercisers are not even sure if they can maintain their THR heart rate and complete the recommended exercise time. In this case, the exerciser may feel palpitation, chest tightness, cramps, and so on during the exercise, which also may cause sport injuries.

When the training set was initially set to 35 samples, the adjusted R^2 was 0.63, while the adjusted R^2 was 0.71 after excluding high error samples from the questionnaires or experimental data. In the process of continuous iteration, it was found that with an increase in the number of training samples, the adjusted R^2 gradually increased and the model improved. At the same time, the regression equation obtained by the iteration constantly changed. The equation parameters obtained in this study were the optimal choices under the existing data volume. Although the selected features changed, they were mainly concentrated in the data such as body composition, bone density, and anthropometrics (see Figure 1). The features in the figure are strongly related to the slope S, and the slope S can be predicted accurately.

Cardiopulmonary fitness (aerobic capacity) is of great significance in basic medicine, clinical medicine, and sports medicine research. The body composition index is related to exercise ability, exercise habits, cardiopulmonary fitness, etc. [13–15]. On the other hand, there are some studies that show that bone density has similar characteristics [16–18]. Improving exercise habits through scientific exercise can improve exercise ability and cardiorespiratory health, which is accompanied by improvements in body composition and bone density. Moreover, the relationship between body composition and bone density to exercise ability and cardiorespiratory health can also be reflected in some people with diseases [19–21]. The above results are consistent with our research: the slope S reflected the exercise ability at a specific heart rate, which was capable of evaluating a person's cardiorespiratory fitness (aerobic capacity). Thus, the slope S it is also closely related to body composition, bone density, and anthropometric data.

We constructed a dynamic machine learning closed loop consisting of smart wearable devices, human body data measurement devices, and Internet-based intelligent systems, which eventually became an important module in the entire smart health system (see Figure 4). This closed loop was gradually put into operation, continuously collecting data. Since the system had only just been put into operation, we only obtained a small amount of data; however, the data we did collect confirmed our ideas. With an increase in the number of users and daily usage, relevant static human body data, questionnaire data, and exercise data will be continuously input into the machine learning model that we built. In this way, not only the accuracy of the model will be continuously improved, but also the key factors that cause large prediction errors will be continuously found from the questionnaire. Among the above factors, definite positive or negative ones can be used to roughly calibrate the predicted results, resulting in a wider range of users for the model. However, on the one hand, the existing questionnaire types are relatively insufficient. This is because it is not completely clear which type of data obtained from the questionnaires will affect the results of the prediction. The impact factor of one of the eight large error samples could not be found from the sport experimental data and the existing questionnaire data. The reason for this may be the inherent prediction error of the model itself, but it is more likely that the positive and negative impact factors that cause the large error have not been discovered. On the other hand, a lot of information in the questionnaire is therefore difficult to quantify. This type of information is often described by adjectives such as yes/no, high/medium/low, and mild/moderate/severe. Since such data cannot be input into the machine learning model, they can only be used for a rough calibration of results. A positive factor means an increase in the predicted value, while a negative one reflects a reduction (the fourth and fifth rows of Table 3), but the amount that needs to be calibrated cannot be accurately determined. This requires us to continue to optimize the questionnaire and to find a suitable quantitative method in follow-up work. For some positive and negative factors, we found that there are some offsetting phenomena. For example, one participant in our exercise test had received systematic physical training before. Although he has fatty liver now, the prediction error was still within a reasonable range. With the increasing amount of data, it will be proven whether this offset phenomenon really exists and the specific factors that can be offset will become clearer.

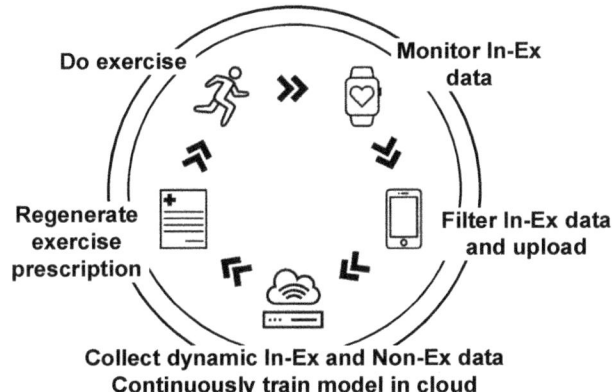

Figure 4. The various parts of the closed loop containing the prediction model.

Moreover, our participants were all from Hefei, a city in Central China. For the global population, the final results may vary. We will build more models based on different exercise equipment in the next stage of our research. With the gradual improvement of our designed prescriptions, the threshold of the end users will be significantly reduced. Ultimately, the smart health system will solve the problem of shortage of sports science professionals and the high learning cost of exercise intensity execution, and it will also allow people to establish the habit of using exercise prescriptions for scientific fitness, which was the purpose of our research. We will try to join in-exercise (In-Ex) impact factor data (such as exercise pulse wave signal (photoplethysmography—PPG), exercise oxygen consumption, road conditions, weather, and wind speed) to study its effects. On the other hand, we also want to see if slope S can be used as a measure of the human body in the same way as HR_{max} and VO_{2max}.

5. Conclusions

The slope S obtained by the linear regression model can determine the parameters of electronic sports equipment (cycling equipment) to achieve the target exercise intensity. The multiple regression model obtained by machine learning using body static data can achieve an accurate prediction of the slope S for the general population, and we can make the model applicable to more people by using our questionnaire to calibrate the results. Combined with the intelligent system, the model can be continuously trained, optimized, and will expand through cloud technology in the future.

Author Contributions: Conceptualization, Y.W., Z.M., and Y.S.; data curation, H.Z.; funding acquisition, Z.M. and Y.S.; investigation, H.Z.; methodology, Y.W.; project administration, Z.M. and Y.S.; software, Y.W. and Y.L.; supervision, Z.M.; validation, Y.L.; writing—original draft, Y.W.; writing—review and editing, Y.W. and Z.M. All authors read and agreed to the published version of the manuscript.

Funding: This research was funded by the major special project of the Anhui Science and Technology Department (grant number 18030801133), the Science and Technology Service Network Initiative (grant number KFJ-STS-ZDTP-079), and the key projects of the National Natural Science Foundation of universities in Anhui Province (grant number KJ2020A0112).

Acknowledgments: The authors would like to thank the participants and support personnel that took part in the study.

Conflicts of Interest: The authors declare no conflict of interest.

References

1. Garber, C.E.; Blissmer, B.; Deschenes, M.R.; Franklin, B.A.; Lamonte, M.J.; Lee, I.M.; Nieman, D.C.; Swain, D.P. Amer Coll Sports M: Quantity and Quality of Exercise for Developing and Maintaining Cardiorespiratory, Musculoskeletal, and Neuromotor Fitness in Apparently Healthy Adults: Guidance for Prescribing Exercise. *Med. Sci. Sports Exerc.* **2011**, *43*, 1334–1359. [CrossRef] [PubMed]
2. Thompson, P.D.; Arena, R.; Riebe, D.; Pescatello, L.S. ACSM's New Preparticipation Health Screening Recommendations from ACSM's Guidelines for Exercise Testing and Prescription, Ninth Edition. *Curr. Sports Med. Rep.* **2013**, *12*, 215–217. [CrossRef] [PubMed]
3. Butte, N.F.; Watson, K.B.; Ridley, K.; Zakeri, I.F.; McMurray, R.G.; Pfeiffer, K.A.; Crouter, S.E.; Herrmann, S.D.; Bassett, D.R.; Long, A.; et al. A Youth Compendium of Physical Activities. *Med. Sci. Sports Exerc.* **2018**, *50*, 246–256. [CrossRef] [PubMed]
4. Ainsworth, B.E.; Haskell, W.L.; Herrmann, S.D.; Meckes, N.; Bassett, D.R.; Tudor-Locke, C.; Greer, J.L.; Vezina, J.; Whitt-Glover, M.C.; Leon, A.S. 2011 Compendium of Physical Activities. *Med. Sci. Sports Exerc.* **2011**, *43*, 1575–1581. [CrossRef] [PubMed]
5. Mezzani, A.; Hamm, L.F.; Jones, A.M.; E McBride, P.; Moholdt, T.; A Stone, J.; Urhausen, A.; A Williams, M. Aerobic exercise intensity assessment and prescription in cardiac rehabilitation: A joint position statement of the European Association for Cardiovascular Prevention and Rehabilitation, the American Association of Cardiovascular and Pulmonary Rehabilitation and the Canadian Association of Cardiac Rehabilitation. *Eur. J. Prev. Cardiol.* **2012**, *20*, 442–467. [PubMed]
6. Swain, D.P. Energy cost calculations for exercise prescription: An update. *Sports Med.* **2000**, *30*, 17–22. [CrossRef] [PubMed]
7. Ainsworth, B.E.; Haskell, W.L.; Leon, A.S.; Jacobs, D.R.; Montoye, H.J.; Sallis, J.F.; Paffenbarger, R.S. Compendium of physical activities–classification of energy costs of human physical activities. *Med. Sci. Sports Exerc.* **1993**, *25*, 71–80. [CrossRef] [PubMed]
8. Ainsworth, B.E.; Haskell, W.L.; Whitt, M.C.; Irwin, M.L.; Swartz, A.M.; Strath, S.J.; O'Brien, W.L.; Bassett, D.R.; Schmitz, K.H.; O Emplaincourt, P.; et al. Compendium of Physical Activities: An update of activity codes and MET intensities. *Med. Sci. Sports Exerc.* **2000**, *32*, S498–S516. [CrossRef] [PubMed]
9. Howley, E.T. Type of activity: Resistance, aerobic and leisure versus occupational physical activity. *Med. Sci. Sports Exerc.* **2001**, *33*, S364–S369. [CrossRef]
10. Nelson, M.E.; Rejeski, W.J.; Blair, S.N.; Duncan, P.W.; Judge, J.O.; King, A.C.; Macera, C.A.; Castaneda-Sceppa, C. Physical Activity and Public Health in Older Adults: Recommendation from the American College of Sports Medicine and the American Heart Association. *Med. Sci. Sports Exerc.* **2007**, *39*, 1435–1445. [CrossRef]
11. Wasserman, K.; Hansen, J.; Sue, D.Y.; Stringer, W.; Sietsema, K.; Sun, X.G.; Whipp, B.J. *Principles of Exercise Testing and Interpretation: Including Pathophysiology and Clinical Applications*, 10th ed.; Wolters Kluwer Health: Philadelphia, PA, USA, 2018.
12. Duarte, S.M.; Rezende, R.E.; Stefano, J.T.; Perandini, L.A.; Dassouki, T.; Sa-Pinto, A.L.; Roschel, H.; Gualano, B.; Carrilho, F.J.; Oliveira, C.P. Impaired aerobic capacity and cardiac autonomic control in sedentary postmenopausal women with nonalcoholic fatty liver disease (NAFLD). *J. Hepatol.* **2015**, *62*, S733. [CrossRef]
13. Chin, E.C.; Yu, A.P.; Lai, W.K.C.; Fong, D.Y.; Chan, D.K.; Wong, S.H.; Sun, F.-H.; Ngai, H.H.; Yung, P.S.H.; Siu, P.M. Low-Frequency HIIT Improves Body Composition and Aerobic Capacity in Overweight Men. *Med. Sci. Sports Exerc.* **2020**, *52*, 56–66. [CrossRef] [PubMed]
14. McDaniel, B.B.; Naquin, M.R.; Sirikul, B.; Kraemer, R.R. Five Weeks of Aquatic-Calisthenic High Intensity Interval Training Improves Cardiorespiratory Fitness and Body Composition in Sedentary Young Adults. *J. Sci. Med. Sport* **2020**, *19*, 187–194.
15. Wang, T.Y. Effects of High Intensity Circuit Training on Body Composition, Cardiopulmonary fitness and Metabolic Syndrome Markers in Middle Aged Male. *Med. Sci. Sports Exerc.* **2016**, *48*, 988–989. [CrossRef]
16. Schwarz, P.; Jørgensen, N.R.; Nielsen, B.; Laursen, A.S.D.; Linneberg, A.; Aadahl, M. Muscle strength, power and cardiorespiratory fitness are associated with bone mineral density in men aged 31–60 years. *Scand. J. Public Heal.* **2014**, *42*, 773–779. [CrossRef]

17. Scott, M.; Johannsen, N.M.; Welsch, M.A.; Credeur, D.P.; Church, T.S.; Ravussin, E.; Allen, J.D. Changes in Body Composition, Bone Mineral Density, Muscle Strength and Functional Ability following Exercise Training in Old Adults. *Med. Sci. Sports Exerc.* **2013**, *45*, 274.
18. Ravnholt, T.; Tybirk, J.; Jorgensen, N.R.; Bangsbo, J. High-intensity intermittent "5-10-15" running reduces body fat, and increases lean body mass, bone mineral density, and performance in untrained subjects. *Eur. J. Appl. Physiol.* **2018**, *118*, 1221–1230. [CrossRef]
19. Grabenbauer, A.; Grabenbauer, A.J.; Lengenfelder, R.; Grabenbauer, M.G.G.; Distel, L.V. Feasibility of a 12-month-exercise intervention during and after radiation and chemotherapy in cancer patients: Impact on quality of life, peak oxygen consumption, and body composition. *Radiat. Oncol.* **2016**, *11*, 42. [CrossRef]
20. Hayashi, F.; Kaibori, M.; Sakaguchi, T.; Matsui, K.; Ishizaki, M.; Kwon, A.; Iwasaka, J.; Kimura, Y.; Habu, D. Loss of skeletal muscle mass in patients with chronic liver disease is related to decrease in bone mineral density and exercise tolerance. *Hepatol. Res.* **2017**, *48*, 345–354. [CrossRef] [PubMed]
21. Youn, J.C.; Lee, S.J.; Lee, H.S.; Oh, J.; Hong, N.; Park, S.; Choi, D.; Rhee, Y.; Kang, S.-M.; Lee, S.-H. Exercise capacity independently predicts bone mineral density and proximal femoral geometry in patients with acute decompensated heart failure. *Osteoporos. Int.* **2015**, *26*, 2121–2129. [CrossRef]

Publisher's Note: MDPI stays neutral with regard to jurisdictional claims in published maps and institutional affiliations.

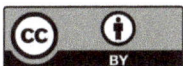

© 2020 by the authors. Licensee MDPI, Basel, Switzerland. This article is an open access article distributed under the terms and conditions of the Creative Commons Attribution (CC BY) license (http://creativecommons.org/licenses/by/4.0/).

Article

Introduction of Open-Source Engineering Tools for the Structural Modeling of a Multilayer Mountaineering Ski under Operation

Lorenzo Fraccaroli and Franco Concli *

Faculty of Science and Technology, Free University of Bolzano/Bozen, Piazza Università 1, 39100 Bolzano, Italy; lorenzo.fraccaroli@unibz.it
* Correspondence: franco.concli@unibz.it; Tel.: +39-0471-017748

Received: 29 June 2020; Accepted: 28 July 2020; Published: 31 July 2020

Abstract: Winter sports have significantly developed in the last century. Among others, skiing is a winter-sport branch in which the equipment makes the difference in the performances. While in the beginning of the last century skis were simply made of wood, nowadays the increasing demand of performances and weight reduction has promoted the adoption of composite materials. However, no significant progress has been made in the engineering approach to design such equipment which are very often still designed on the basis of several physical prototypes and trials. This is particularly true in the niche sector of ski mountaineering, where the production batches are significantly smaller with respect to those of alpine skis and at the same time the weight reduction plays a determinant role. In this context, finite elements analysis (FEA) could represent an important tool to shorten the development times and costs leading to a more effective design process. The aim of this research is the development of an accurate virtual model of an existing mountaineering ski, capable of reproducing the behavior of the real component under operation. A preliminary characterization of all the materials used for the different layers of the ski was performed via tensile tests on flat dog-bone-shaped samples in combination with digital image correlation (DIC) techniques. Samples were laser cut from sheets. The tensile tests were performed in the two principal directions for each material. In combination with DIC, these tests allowed us to estimate the four in-plane (XY) elastic properties, namely, the two elastic modules, the shear module, and the Poisson ratio (Ex, Ey, Gxy, νxy). The DIC acquisitions were elaborated with the free software GOM-Correlate. The digital model of the ski was created and simulated in an open-source environment: Code_Aster/Salome-Meca. The reason for using an open-source software is the possibility to parallelize the calculation without restrictions due to licenses and to customize the code according to the specific problem of interest. These aspects underline the potential of open-source software to improve the design process. The results of the simulations were compared with the response of the real ski in a three-point bending and a torsion-bending tests. Differences of 2.5–10% with respect to the real ski were observed for the different modeling techniques. Moreover, the validated virtual model of the ski was used to study the behavior of the ski when interacting with the snow for different roll angles and loads.

Keywords: ski mountaineering; FEM; Code_Aster; DIC; composite materials; Salome-Meca; snow

1. Introduction

Ski mountaineering is a niche sector of winter sports in which the equipment, namely the skis, is determinant for the performances of the athletes. Most of the races foresee the climbing of a hill; in this condition having a light ski is fundamental. Moreover, during the downhills, the lightweight is not as important as the stiffness of the ski. Finding the best compromise between these 2 main properties means designing a good ski. However, the optimization process requires several attempts and, considering that the current design approaches of ski-mountaineering (skimo or skialp) are characterized by a relevant testing activity, the whole development of a new model could be very expensive and time consuming. A preliminary screening of the multifarious designs is made by simplified laboratory tests, such as three-point-bending or torsional tests. Only the most promising prototypes are tested by skilled professional skiers, like mountain guides, or athletes that can give a more accurate evaluation of the properties of the ski in real conditions which characterize their practical use. This trial and error approach has significant economical disadvantages and requires long times for assembling and testing all the ski variants. Having the possibility to reduce the number of physical prototypes with a virtual preliminary screening could represent a significant improvement of the whole design and manufacturing process.

Finite element analysis (FEA) is already used for the development and design phases of alpine downhill skis [1–4]. In literature, several works in which the mechanical behavior of alpine or carving skis is analyzed are present [5–7]. However, the adoption of these modeling techniques for the development of mountaineering skis seem to be not yet widespread. It must be highlighted that for ski-mountaineering the necessity to find a balance between performances and lightweight design represents an additional issue which complicates the design [8]. The aim of the present study is to develop a reliable numerical model of an existing mountaineering ski. The model is based on the geometrical data of the ski and the results of material characterization tests of the different layers of the ski obtained combining tensile tests on flat dog-bone-shaped samples with digital image correlation (DIC) measurements. The dog-bone-shaped specimens were produced by laser cutting. Each material was tested in two different directions. For the materials for which it was possible, the tensile test was repeated twice. Digital image correlation [9–16] combined with the Campbell [17] hypothesis allowed the estimation of the four in-plane elastic properties.

Moreover, a real prototype (ski available on the market) was also tested in three-point-bending and bending-torsional tests. Simulations of these two conditions were performed with different levels of simplifications. The numerical results were compared with those obtained from three-point bending and torsion-bending tests on the real ski [18].

Once the numerical model of the ski was validated, its behavior in different working conditions was studied. In particular, the ski–snow interaction was simulated. The snow was modeled according to Lintzèn [19]. Different roll angles and loads were simulated to better understand the behavior of the ski under operation.

2. Materials and Methods

2.1. Ski Overview

Modern skis are composed of a multilayer composite structure, with a wood or honeycomb softcore that guarantees good flexibility and low weight. This core is wrapped with different layers. These are typically carbon-, basalt- and glass-fiber-reinforced materials. Resistance and stiffness of the ski are mainly determined by the material of these wrapping layers. The upper and the bottom layers do not have structural purposes. The first one is just required for a better appearance of the ski while the latter is chosen in order to reduce the friction between ski and snow. To obtain a high-performing ski, it is important to find a good balance between weight, resistance, and stiffness. Solutions with an increased number of layers ensure the most performing designs. However, increasing the number of layers and materials also implies the need for producing and testing many more prototypes. Without FE simulations, this is very difficult and time consuming, and the experience of the manufacturer represents the only available tool for speeding up the development.

2.2. Methods

To give a general validity to the adopted approach, the mechanical properties of the different materials were obtained with dedicated tensile tests combined with DIC techniques. These allow the characterization of the 4 in-plane elastic properties of each material used in the ski successively tested. The materials used in the ski manufacturing are composited themselves. They have two major constituents, fibers and matrix. Fibers ensure the resistance and stiffness, while matrix plays the role of keeping the fibers together and protecting them from external agents. The theory of orthotropic laminas and laminated structures could be used for describing these materials. The assumption of having (for each material) just one principal direction was made. Orthotropic materials can be described in the space with 9 independent elastic parameters (for a completely non-isotropic material the constants are 21). For a lamina of small thickness and with longitudinal continuous fibers, the elastic behavior can be described with 4 elastic constants only: The 2 in-plane elastic modules, the in-plane shear module, and one of the two in-plane Poisson ratios. The 2 elastic modules can be obtained directly from unidirectional tensile tests while the Poisson's ratio can be extrapolated from digital image correlation (DIC) measurements. The shear module was evaluated by means of the approximated Campbell formula [17].

The tested materials are identified with a code number. Specifically, 9, 24, 139, 207, 290, 135, 31, 86, and 217.

Tensile tests were performed on the STEPLab UD04 (Figure 1) testing machine available in the labs of the Free University of Bolzano/Bozen. It is capable to apply static forces up to 4.5 kN. Each test was performed with a crosshead speed 0.1 mm/min.

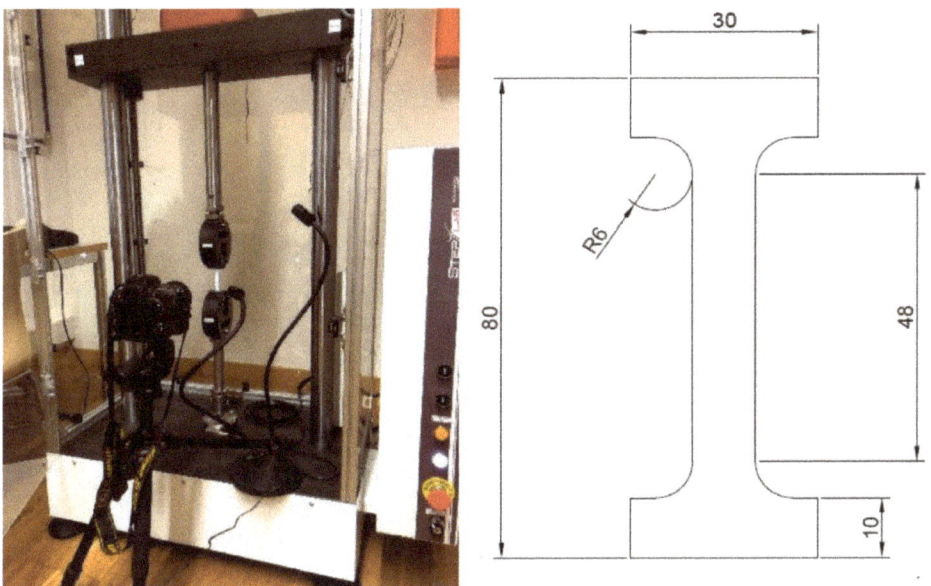

Figure 1. STEPLab UD04 tensile machine and testing setup; (right) dog-bone sample geometry and dimensions.

While the Young's modules can be directly derived from the monoaxial tests, the estimation of the Poisson's ratio requires the calculation of the strains in 2 perpendicular directions (Equation (1)).

$$\nu_{xy} = -\frac{\varepsilon_y}{\varepsilon_x}; \quad \nu_{yx} = -\frac{\varepsilon_x}{\varepsilon_y} \qquad (1)$$

Digital image correlation (DIC) was used for this purpose. A reflex Nikon D750 camera with a 24–85 zoom, 32 MPixel resolution, and a stabilizer was placed perpendicularly to the specimen surfaces.

It acquired pictures of the sample at each 0.5 s. External light sources were used for a better illumination of the specimen's surface.

Two-dimensional digital image correlation is an advanced optical measurement technique allowing displacement and strain fields on a planar surface to be reconstructed.

Firstly, a characteristic black and white "speckle" pattern was created on the specimen surface. Pictures were acquired at a fixed rate for the entire tensile test. The first picture acquired (undeformed sample) was used as reference. Cross correlation operations allowed the recognition of facets (subsets of the specimen's surface) across all the time steps (corresponding to different images and deformations) (Figure 2). Once all subsets were recognized for each timestep, the displacement field and successively the strain field of the tested component could be reconstructed. The software used was GOM-Correlate [20].

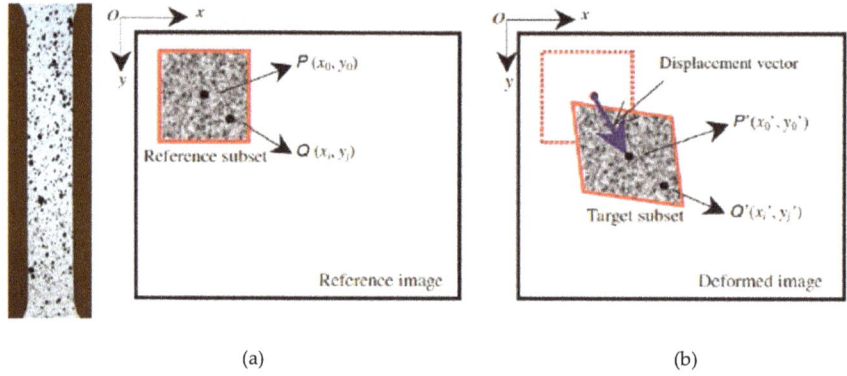

(a)   (b)

Figure 2. Digital image correlation (DIC); (**a**) surface pattern; (**b**) cross correlation.

Knowing the strains in 2 independent directions allowed the calculation of the Poisson's ratio according to Equation (1). The shear module could be finally obtained using the Campbell equation (Equation (2)).

$$\frac{1}{G_{xy}} = \frac{(1+v_{xy})}{E_x} + \frac{(1+v_{yx})}{E_y} \qquad (2)$$

2.3. SKI

In this research the open-source software Code_Aster/Salome-Meca was used. Three-point-bending and bending-torsional tests were numerically reproduced. Figure 3 shows the schematic representation of the loaded ski.

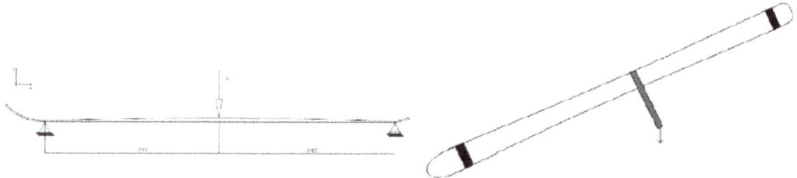

Figure 3. Schematic representation of the three-point bending and torsion-bending tests—reference case for the FE simulations.

2.3.1. Shell Model

Figure 3 shows the schematic layout of the three-point-bending test. In the virtual model, just half of the structure was simulated, taking advantage of the symmetry. Moreover, the tail and the tip of the ski were not modeled to simulate only the part of the component that falls within supports. Due to their very low-resistant contribution and their very small section, the steel edges were considered negligible and were not modeled as well. A multilayered shell approach was used. The ski was divided into 145 sectors to achieve a good approximation of the curvature of the ski—this ensured a good reproduction of the effective thicknesses along the whole ski. The final grid consisted of about 22 k quadrangular elements. Figure 4 shows the 2D model of the ski.

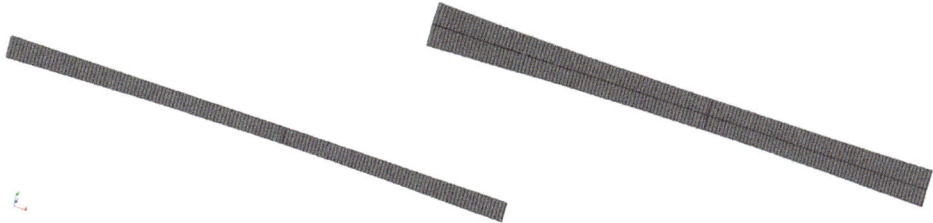

Figure 4. Shell models used for the three-point-bending (left) and torsion-bending (right) simulations.

The torsion-bending test was simulated numerically in a similar way, without exploiting the z–x plane-symmetry.

2.3.2. Solid Model

The same geometrical simplifications of the shell model were also used for the 3D simulations (symmetry for the three-point-bending model and cutting of tail and tip for both models). Moreover, additional assumptions have been made in order to obtain all the 9 constants necessary for the proper description of the materials in the space. According to [21], materials with unidirectional long fibers have the same elastic module in each radial direction (perpendicular to the reinforcing fibers). The characterization tests were performed on thin laminates and it was not possible to characterize the remaining out of plane properties. The shear module G and the Poisson's ratio ν founded in the xy plane were used also for the other 2 directions (zx and yz). While in the 3D modeling approach some additional hypothesis were introduced for the material properties, from a geometrical point of view the 3D model (Figures 5 and 6) better reproduced the real shape of the ski, as it also included the lateral protective layer that was neglected in the shell approach.

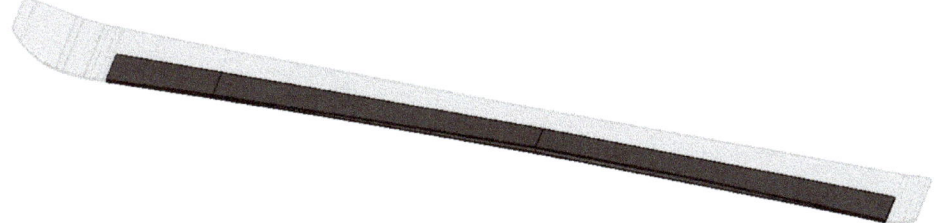

Figure 5. Isometric view of the solid model used for the three-point-bending test.

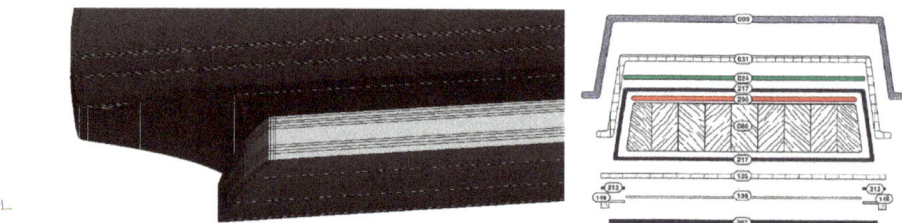

Figure 6. Different layers of the solid model.

The mesh was made of quadratic hexahedrons only. A total number of about 500 k cells was used for the symmetric model reproducing the three-point-bending configuration. The bending-torsional model was made of about 1 M cells.

3. Experimental Results and Validation of the Virtual Model of the Ski

The results of the monoaxial tests are presented in Figures 7–13.

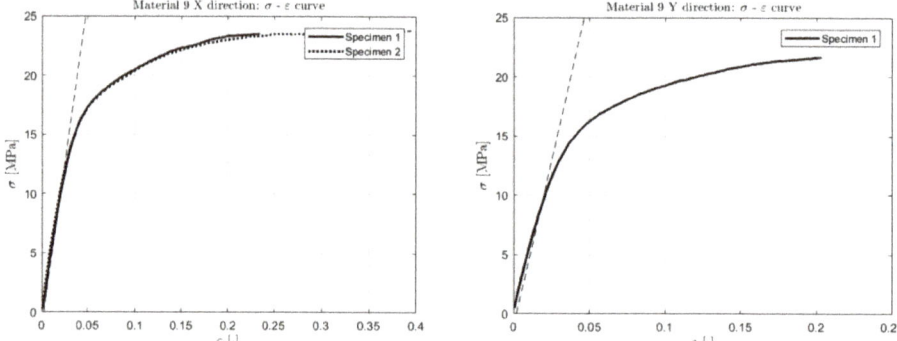

Figure 7. Material 9 tensile tests.

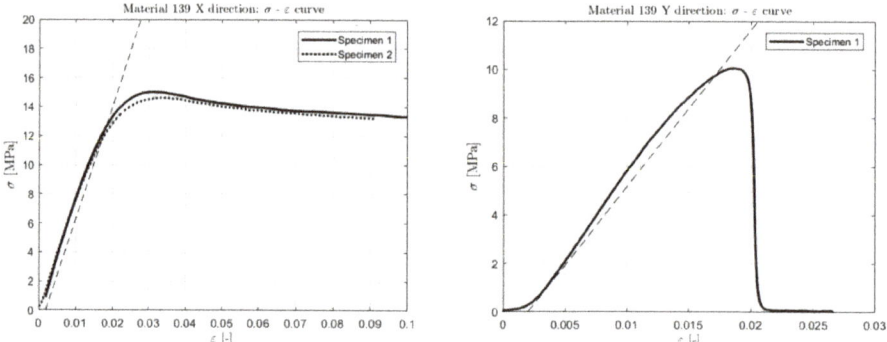

Figure 8. Material 139 tensile tests.

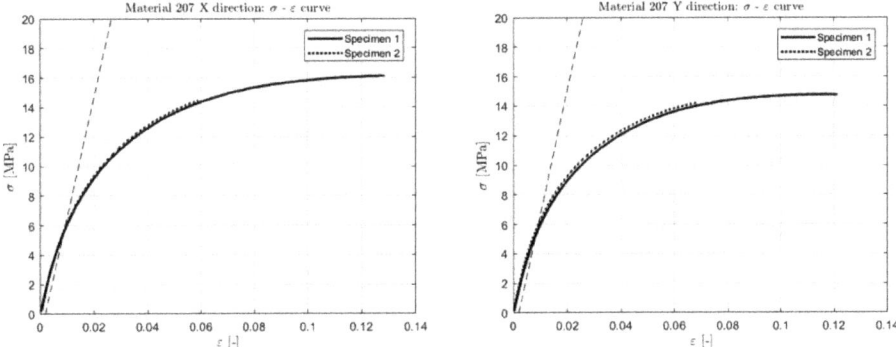

Figure 9. Material 207 tensile tests.

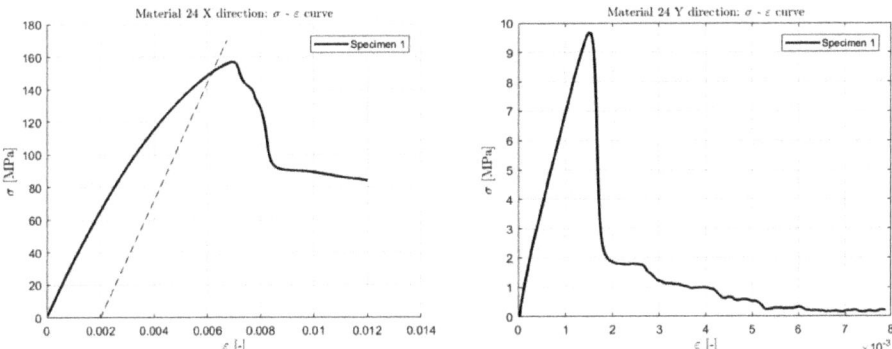

Figure 10. Material 24 tensile tests.

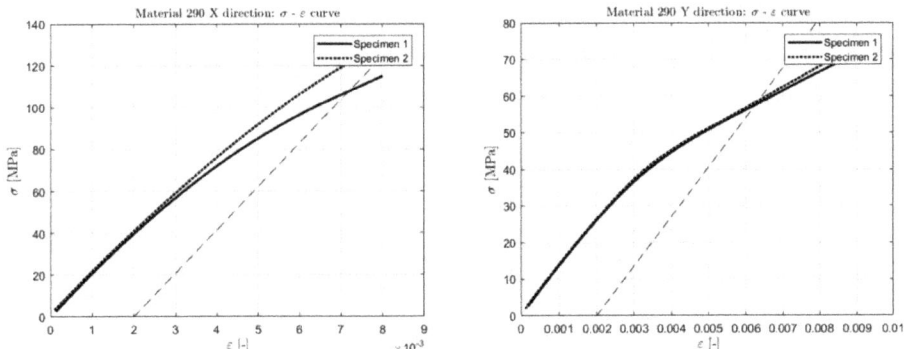

Figure 11. Material 290 tensile tests.

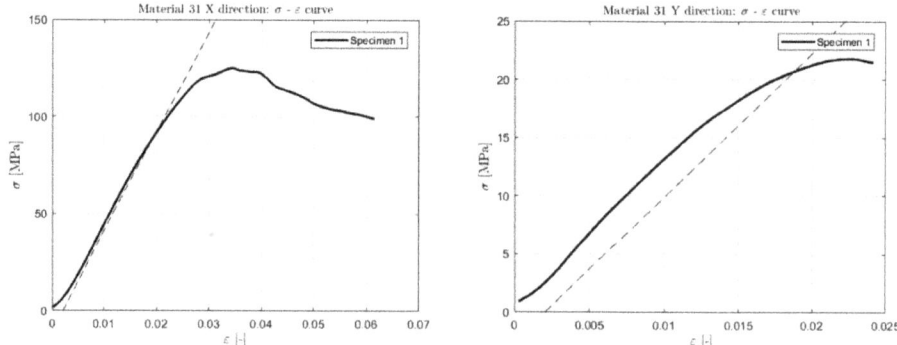

Figure 12. Material 31 tensile tests.

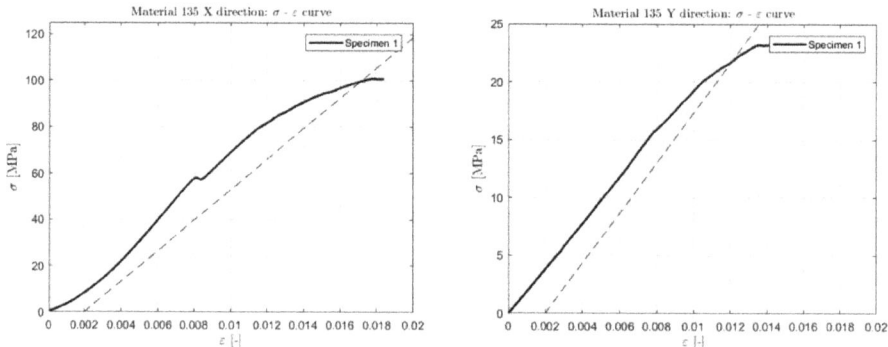

Figure 13. Material 135 tensile tests.

Table 1 reports the in-plane parameters for each material.

Table 1. Material elastic properties.

	Material								
	9	24	139	207	290	135	31	86	217
E_x [MPa]	550	35,000	800	850	20,000	4000	2000	13,700	35,000
E_y [MPa]	567	8700	750	897	13,700	569	127	420	12,436
ν_{xy} [-]	0.45	0.23	0.45	0.42	0.18	0.39	0.39	0.40	0.56
ν_{yx} [-]	0.43	0.35	0.38	0.30	0.12	0.39	0.39	0.40	0.48
G_{xy} [MPa]	776	35,010	1097	1291	29,125	3009	1184	10,086	25,327
σ_x [MPa]	11	152	10	6	110	98	87	-	-
σ_y [MPa]	10	9	13	6	57	22	21	-	-
Thickness [mm]	0.35	0.35	0.50	1.10	1.20	0.55	0.55	0–5.45	0.5

* The sub-indexes x and y refer to the longitudinal and axial ski direction, respectively.

Table 2 reports the maximum displacement in the midpoint of the ski when bended under a load of 120 N in the three-point-bending tests. Measured values were compared with those obtained from the two different FEM analyses (with shell and solid elements).

Table 2. Comparison of the maximum deflection of the ski in the three-point bending test: Finite element analysis (FEM) vs. experiments.

Model	Displacement [mm]	Simulation Time * [min]	Error [%]
Experimental	40		
Shell	41	35	2.5%
Solid	44	60	10.0%

* on a 9.6 GFLOPS workstation.

Table 3 reports the results of the torsion-bending tests (40N @ 0.45m) and the related numerical predictions.

Table 3. Comparison of the maximum deflection of the ski in the torsion-bending test: FEM vs. experiments.

Model	Rotation Angle [°]	Simulation Time * [min]	Error [%]
Experimental	4.44		
Shell	4.61	35	3.0%
Solid	4.86	60	9.5%

* on a 9.6 GFLOPS workstation.

Figure 14 shows the normal stresses in the thickness of the ski (on the symmetry plane and the position where the load was applied—0 corresponds to the bottom part) during the three-point-bending test. Figure 15 refers to the bending-torsion test.

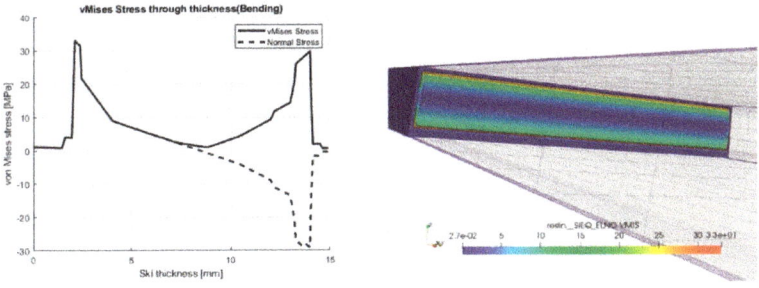

Figure 14. Solid model results—three-point-bending test (normal and Von Mises stresses in the section).

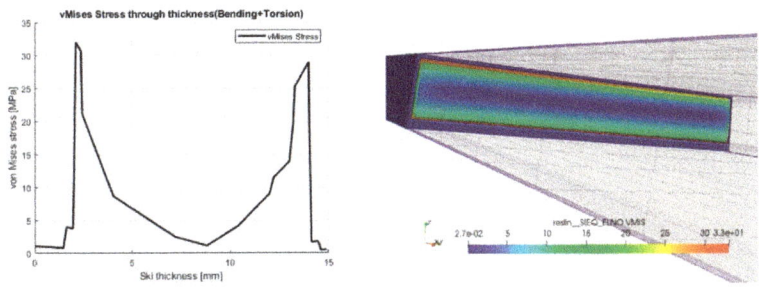

Figure 15. Solid model results—torsion-bending test (normal and Von Mises stresses in the section).

Both tests were repeated increasing the load up from the first yielding. The most loaded layer was the n. 217, in which the stress reached a value of about 32 MPa both in the three-point-bending and in the bending-torsion test.

Nevertheless, even if the first yielding took place for a relative low force, these specific loading conditions (very useful to validate the model because easily reproducible with lab tests) were not representative of the real loading condition of a ski during operation. The contact with the snow, in fact, promoted a more uniform load transfer from the ski to the ground and, therefore, a significantly less critical stress state for the same applied loads. For this reason, the numerical model was improved including the interaction with the snow to study the behavior of the ski during operation. Friction was neglected.

4. Behavior of the Ski during a Carving Turn

To study the behavior of the ski during a downhill turn, the ski–snow interaction had to be modeled. For doing this, the Lintzèn [19] model of snow was used. It is based on experimental compression tests on big frozen snow cylindrical samples. Lintzèn came up with a relation that described the snow as a piece-wise linear function as shown in Figure 16. The snow was characterized by an initial linear behavior in which the elastic constant assumed a value that varied between E_{tan} = 115 (old snow) and E_{tan} = 160 MPa (artificial snow). For higher strains, the behavior could be still described with a linear relation in which elastic module assumed a value between E_{res} = 9 and E_{res} = 35 MPa.

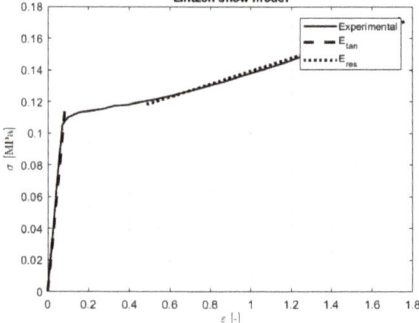

Figure 16. Snow model according to Lintzèn—adapted from [19].

The previously developed and validated solid model of the ski was improved by adding the interaction with the snow. The ski was tested for different roll angles and loads. The roll angle describes the rotation of the ski along its longitudinal axis with respect to the ground. Table 4 shows the studied combinations.

Table 4. Roll angles and forces applied.

Roll Angle [°]	Force Applied [kg]	Maximum Deflection [mm]	Maximum Snow Penetration [mm]
10	50	2.85	8.26
10	100	2.88	8.29
10	200	2.94	8.35
30	50	9.00	12.82
30	100	9.07	12.89
30	200	9.15	12.97
45	50	15.01	17.01
45	100	15.15	17.17
45	200	15.30	17.32
60	50	29.02	22.59
60	100	29.31	22.88
60	200	29.61	22.18

* The roll angle is defined as the angle at which an object must be rotated about its longitudinal axis to bring its sagittal- into a horizontal-plane.

Simulations were performed with a non-linear solver using a large strain formulation. The snow was modeled using a von Mises elastoplastic law with linear isotropic hardening. The contact was modeled as discrete. The models of contact and friction were drawn up from already discretized quantities, i.e., displacements and nodal forces. The problem of contact/friction was solved by uncoupling it from the problem of the equilibrium of structure.

Figure 17 shows the deformed ski under load. Figures 18 and 19 show the deformed shape of the ski along the symmetry plane for several levels of load and different roll angles. These results were fundamental to understand the downhill behavior of the ski: The combination of its carving, roll angle, and load applied determined the turning angle (assuming a conductive turn was done, i.e., without sliding between the ski and the snow). The actual stiffness of the ski was fundamental in this regard: A stiffer ski would require a much higher load to ensure the same turning angle (at equal carving and roll angle). Therefore, skis having the same geometry should have different stiffnesses according to the weight of the athlete. Numerical simulations could be an effective tool for designing the perfect ski.

Figure 20 shows the relation between the roll angle and the turning radius. The relation is well described by a decreasing power function.

$$r_{turn} = 1529.5 \cdot \vartheta_{roll}^{-1.129} \tag{3}$$

The applied load seemed to have a moderate effect on the ski deflection compared to the roll angle. With a roll angle of 45°, in the hypothesis of the conduction turn, the ski showed a turning radius of about 22 m. The geometrical rounding radius of the ski was 40 m. For lower roll angles (30° and 10°), the rounding radius results equaled to 34 and 111 m, respectively. At a roll angle of 60°, the turning radius decreased to 14 m.

Figure 21 shows the von Mises stress in the cross-section of the ski for different roll angles and loads. Differently from what was observed during the three-point-bending and torsion-bending tests, the interaction with the snow prevented big deformations and the maximum stress level results were far below the yielding for each layer.

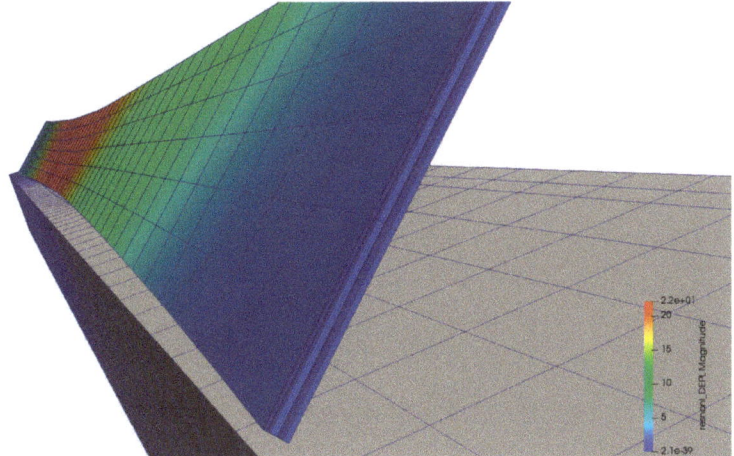

Figure 17. Ski in contact with the snow: Roll angle 45°, load 200 kg.

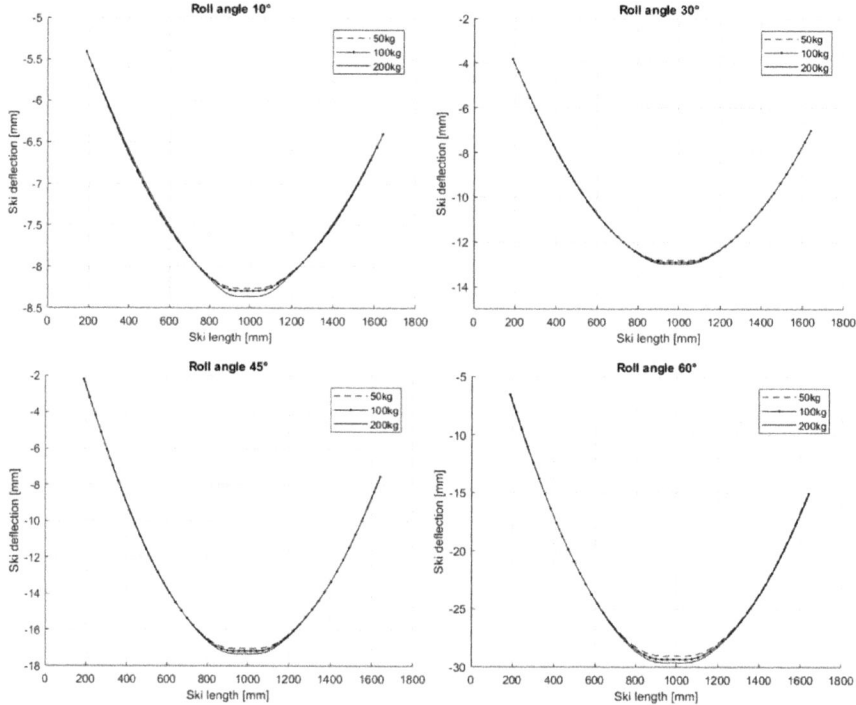

Figure 18. Deflection of the ski for different roll angles and loads.

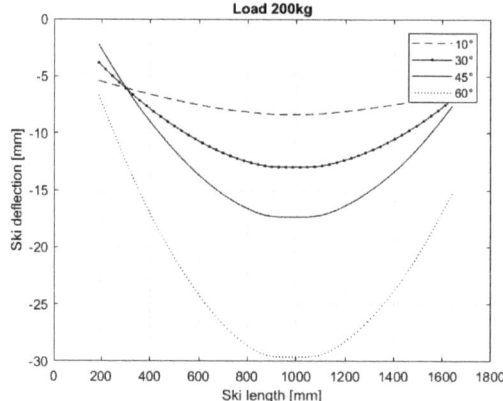

Figure 19. Deflection of the ski for different roll angles and 200 kg.

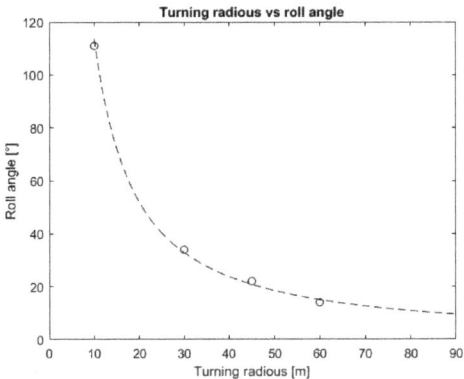

Figure 20. Turning radius vs. roll angle.

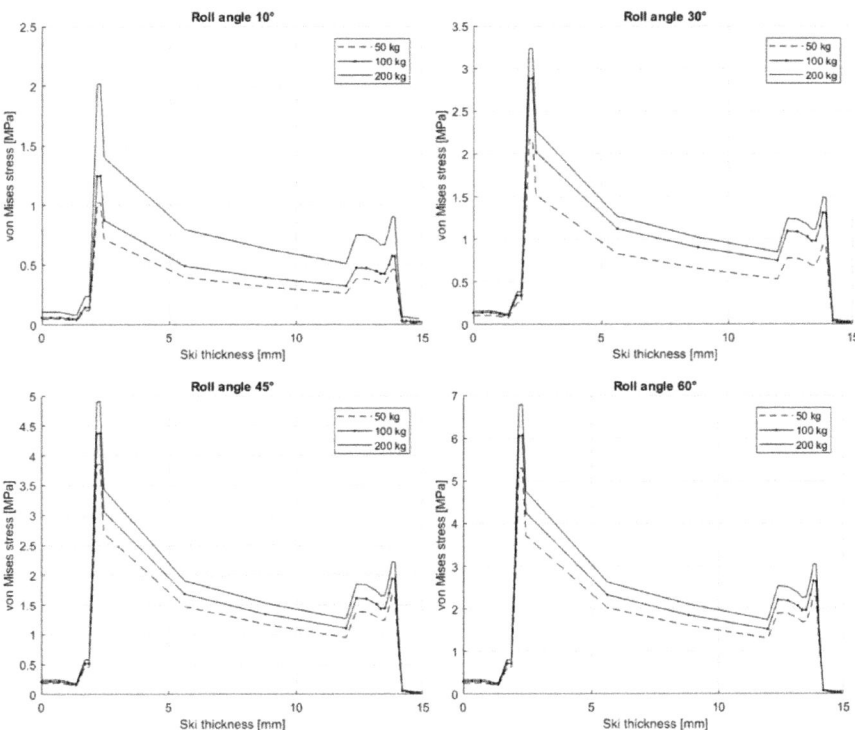

Figure 21. Von Mises stress in the cross-section of the ski for different roll angles and loads.

5. Discussion

For its nature, the ski works in the elastic field only. Plastic deformations should be avoided. Therefore, during the experimental measurements, the constitutive law was characterized up to the yielding only. Most of the tested materials showed a good repeatability in the results. In some cases, due to low availability of materials, only one specimen was tested. Repetitions were possible for material 207 (both directions), 290 (both directions), 139 (X direction), and 9 (X direction). The discrepancies between repetition were very small, confirming the correct configuration of the testing setup and adequacy of the measuring devices. Materials #207 and #9 showed the same behavior in both directions. The tests performed on material #135 and #31, in which the single fibers were easily visible, were performed with a special sample with a rectangular geometry instead of a dog-bone-shaped one. After measuring the thickness and width of a single fiber, the resistant area was computed by multiplying the area of a single fiber by the total number of fibers of each specimen.

FEM results were fully validated by the experimental data for both modeling approaches (shell and solid). The 2D analysis presented a maximum displacement (in the three-point-bending) of 41 mm, showing a 2.5% difference with respect to the experimental data, while the 3D model predicted a maximum displacement of 44 mm (10% difference vs experiments). In the torsion-bending analysis, the 2D model predicted a rotation of 4.60°, and the 3D model a rotation of 4.86°. The difference with respect to the experimental data result was 3% and 9.5%, respectively.

For the shell model, discrepancies in the predicted displacement/rotation with respect to the measured one could be attributed to the following reasons:

- The ski was modeled with multiple sections having different heights; thus, the perfect curved shape of the ski was not correctly replicated;
- The steel edges and the lateral layers (cage) were not modeled.

On the other side, the simplification in the 3D models are:

- The longitudinal curvature of the ski was not considered;
- The assumption on the material properties taken during material characterization affected results.

Both the 2D and the 3D models had the same maximum width, but the lateral layers were modeled in the 3D model only. The second order (area) moment of these vertical layers was lower with respect to the horizontal ones; therefore, it is reasonable that the 2D models resulted in a stiffer quality compared to the 3D one. From Figure 7 to Figure 13, it can be observed that not all layers had structural purposes. The lower and the upper layers were not significantly loaded despite the maximum strain. This was due to their low elastic modulus. The material of the bottom layer, for example, was aimed to reduce friction with snow and to insulate the ski from humidity. FEA allowed for an accurate evaluation on how each layer contributed to the total stiffness of the ski.

The discrepancies observed in the torsion-bending analysis can be explained with the geometrical and material simplifications already explained, but also considering that the shear module G plays a fundamental role. The fact that it was approximated with the Campbell simplification may affects results.

The simulations of the real behavior of the ski in contact with the snow showed that the rolling angle played a much more significant role with respect to the applied load in terms of turning radius. This was equal to about 22 m for a roll angle equal to 45°, 34 m for a roll angle equal to 30°, and 111 m for a roll angle of 10°. The geometrical rounding radius of the ski was 40 m. The turning radius decreased to 14 m when the roll angle was increased to 60°.

6. Conclusions

An accurate physical model of a real ski is a hard engineering challenge. In this paper, only a 2.5–10% error with respect to experimental data was obtained. The difficulty to properly describe the materials that composed the sandwich structure hugely influenced the model replication. The material sheets had small sizes and did not permit us to follow standards for testing their mechanical properties. The elastic module was extracted directly from the tensile tests on each material (apart from textile and the wood core, of which the properties were available in literature). DIC was used to obtain a complete material characterization. The comparison between the experimental measurements and numerical results of three-point bending and torsion-bending tests showed a satisfactory agreement. Better results were obtained with the 2D approach. The 3D model showed a higher error due to material parameter simplifications. However, theoretical predictions of the stress state and the behavior of the ski when subjected under bending were confirmed by an experimental test. For the torsion-bending shell model, a maximum error of 3% was found, while for the solid one a 9.5% discrepancy was recorded. As for the bending case, the plane model presented more reliable results. This fact was due to the lower level of approximation used in the 2D problem.

The model was validated with experimental observations. It is now possible to easily change material properties and layer dimensions and compare different solutions in the early stages of the design phase. This can lead to a reduction of the time needed for ski development. Moreover, the need to produce several physical prototypes may no longer be necessary. As a consequence, the R&D costs could be reduced thanks to the implemented models.

Once the model was validated, a real operating condition (interaction with the snow) was modeled. The simulation's results allowed us to quantify the stress levels in the ski together with its turning radius under different loads and roll angles. This was fundamental to optimize the equipment for a specific athlete/specific race, avoiding the massive need of expensive prototypes and experimental tests.

Author Contributions: All authors contributed actively in every part of the work. All authors have read and agreed to the published version of the manuscript.

Funding: This research received no external funding.

Acknowledgments: We would like to thank the Free University of Bolzano/Bozen for giving us the access to laboratories and for the support during the work.

Conflicts of Interest: The authors declare that they have no competing interests.

References

1. Wolfsperger, F.; Szabo, D.; Rhyner, H. Development of Alpine Skis Using FE Simulations. *Proced. Eng.* **2016**, *147*, 366–371. [CrossRef]
2. Federolf, P.; Roos, M.; Lüthi, A.; Dual, J. Finite element simulation of the ski-snow interaction of an alpine ski in a carved turn. *Sports Eng.* **2010**, *12*, 123–133. [CrossRef]
3. Zboncak, R. Experimental Verification of Ski Model for Finite Element Analysis. In Proceedings of the 56th International Conference on Experimental Stress Analysis, Harrachov, Czech Republic, 5–7 June 2018; pp. 450–456.
4. Mössner, M.; Innerhofer, G.; Schindelwig, K.; Kaps, P.; Schretter, H.; Nachbauer, W. Measurement of mechanical properties of snow for simulation of skiing. *J. Glaciol.* **2013**, *59*, 1170–1178. [CrossRef]
5. Nordt, A.A.; Springer, G.S.; Kollar, L.P. Computing the mechanical properties of alpine skis. *Sports Eng.* **1999**, *2*, 65. [CrossRef]
6. Hirano, Y.; Tada, N. Mechanics of a turning snow ski. *Int. J. Mech. Sci.* **1994**, *36*, 421–429. [CrossRef]
7. Cresseri, S.; Jommi, C. Snow as an elastic viscoplastic bonded continuum: A modelling approach. *Ital. Geotech.* **2005**, *4*, 43–58.
8. Braghin, F.; Cheli, F.; Maldifassi, S.; Melzi, S.; Sabbioni, E. *The Engineering Approach to Winter Sports*; Springer: New York, NY, USA, 2016.
9. Musotto, Z. Digital Image Correlation: Applicazione Di Tecniche Convenzionali E Sviluppo Di Soluzioni La Stima E L'Incremento Dell'Accuratezza. Master's Thesis, ING IV-Scuola di Ingegneria Industriale, Monteluco di Roio, Italia, 2012.
10. Crammond, G.; Boyd, S.W.; Dulieu-Barton, J.M. Speckle pattern quality assessment for digital image correlation. *Opt. Lasers Eng.* **2013**, *51*, 1368–1378. [CrossRef]
11. Makeev, A.; He, Y.; Carpentier, P.; Shonkwiler, B. A method for measurement of multiple constitutive properties for composite materials. *Compos. Part A. Appl. Sci. Manuf.* **2012**, *43*, 2199–2210. [CrossRef]
12. Kowalczyk, P. Identification of mechanical parameters of composites in tensile tests using mixed numerical-experimental method. *Meas. J. Int. Meas. Confed.* **2019**, *135*, 131–137. [CrossRef]
13. Schreier, H.W.; Sutton, M.A. Systematic Errors in Digital Image Correlation Due to Undermatched Subset Shape Functions. *Exp. Mech.* **2002**, *42*, 303–310. [CrossRef]
14. Wattrisse, B.; Chrysochoos, A.; Muracciole, J. Analysis of Strain Localization during Tensile Tests by Digital Image Correlation. *Exp. Mech.* **2000**, *41*, 29–39. [CrossRef]

15. Peters, W. Digital image techniques in experimental stress analysis. *Opt. Eng.* **1982**, *21*, 427–431. [CrossRef]
16. Górszczyk, J.; Malicki, K.; Zych, T. Application of Digital Image Correlation (DIC) Method for Road Material Testing. *Materials* **2019**, *12*, 2349. [CrossRef] [PubMed]
17. Yokoyama, T.; Nakai, K. Evaluation of in-plane orthotopic elastic constants of paper and paperboard. *Proc. SEM Ann. Conf. Expo. Exp. Appl. Mech.* **2007**, *3*, 1505–1511.
18. Fraccaroli, L. Structural Modelling of Multilayer Skis. M.Sc. Thesis, Free University of Bozen-Bolzano, Bolzano, Italy, 2019.
19. Lintzén, N.; Edeskär, T. Uniaxial strength and deformation properties of machine-made snow. *J. Cold Reg. Eng.* **2015**, *29*, 04014020. [CrossRef]
20. GOM. Available online: www.gom.com (accessed on 1 May 2020).
21. Tecnologie E Materiali Aerospaziali. CAPITOLO 32-Materiali Compositi: La Legge Costitutiva Ortotropa. Available online: Https://www.andreadd.it/appunti/polimi/ingegneria/corsi/en_mec_aes/ing_aerospaziale/anno3/TecnologieMaterialiAerospaziali/viewer.html?file=appunti/Teoria_Riassunto.pdf (accessed on 1 May 2020).

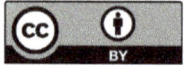

© 2020 by the authors. Licensee MDPI, Basel, Switzerland. This article is an open access article distributed under the terms and conditions of the Creative Commons Attribution (CC BY) license (http://creativecommons.org/licenses/by/4.0/).

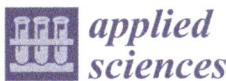

Article

A Predictive Model on the Intention to Accept Taekwondo Electronic Protection Devices

Sung-Un Park [1], Dong-Kyu Kim [2,*,†] and Hyunkyun Ahn [3,*,†]

1. Department of Sport & Leisure Studies, College of Arts & Physical Education, Shingyeong University, Hwaseong-si 18274, Korea; psu@sgu.ac.kr
2. Department of Sport Management, Graduate School of Technology Management, Kyung Hee University, Yongin-si 17104, Korea
3. Department of Sport & Leisure Studies, Division of Arts & Health, Myongji College, Seoul 03656, Korea
* Correspondence: khudk04@khu.ac.kr (D.-K.K.); ahnhk@mjc.ac.kr (H.A.); Tel.: +82-31-201-2130 (D.-K.K.); +82-2-300-3877 (H.A.)
† These authors contributed equally to this work.

Abstract: This study's purpose was to establish a predictive model of the intention to accept Taekwondo electronic protector devices through the application of the technology acceptance model. Two hundred and twenty collegiate Taekwondo practitioners affiliated with the Korea Taekwondo Association participated in a survey that included 28 questions (4 relating to demographic characteristics, 12 to precursor variables, and 12 to the technology acceptance model). Correlation and structural equation modeling analyses were applied and a significance level of 0.05 was used. The results were as follows. Perceived quality had a significant influence on perceived ease of use ($\beta = 0.380$, $t = 3.481$, $p < 0.001$) and perceived usefulness ($\beta = 0.544$, $t = 5.098$, $p < 0.001$). Visual attractiveness had no significant influence on either perceived ease of use ($\beta = 0.159$, $t = 1.798$, $p = 0.072$) or perceived usefulness ($\beta = -0.010$, $t = -0.131$, $p = 0.896$). Wearability had a significant influence on perceived ease of use ($\beta = 0.234$, $t = 2.867$, $p < 0.01$), but a significantly negative influence on perceived usefulness ($\beta = -0.218$, $t = -2.932$, $p < 0.01$). Functionality had no significant influence on either perceived ease of use ($\beta = 0.116$, $t = 1.031$, $p = 0.302$) or perceived usefulness ($\beta = 0.107$, $t = 1.093$, $p = 0.274$). Perceived ease of use had a significant influence on perceived usefulness ($\beta = 0.418$, $t = 4.361$, $p < 0.001$) and acceptance intention ($\beta = 0.361$, $t = 4.031$, $p < 0.001$). Perceived usefulness had a significant influence on acceptance intention ($\beta = 0.525$, $t = 5.758$, $p < 0.001$). These results suggest that improving the perceived quality and wearability of the devices will enhance their acceptance. We believe that this study provides an appropriate verification model for the intention to accept Taekwondo electronic protection devices.

Keywords: Taekwondo; Taekwondo electronic protection devices; technology acceptance model

1. Introduction

Taekwondo is a traditional Korean martial art and has been an official Olympic combat sport since the 2000 Sydney Olympic Games [1]. More than 200 countries are affiliated with the World Taekwondo Federation (WT) and a growing number of individuals are participating in Taekwondo competitions globally [2]. However, a critical issue related to the scoring system used during competitions arose, interrupting the further development of Taekwondo competitions [3]. To ensure the fairness and smooth operation of Taekwondo competitions, an electronic body protector and scoring system were introduced in the 2012 London Olympic Games and have been used in all subsequent Olympic Games [4,5]. These systems not only protect Taekwondo players against injury but also result in more reliable and accurate scoring [6]. In other words, Taekwondo electronic protection devices (TEPDs) (such as headgear, body protectors and hand–foot protectors) have a technical feature that automatically recognizes the effective attack power by means of a sensor equipped with an

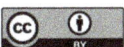

advanced electronic chip attached to the protector, which automatically transmits it to the score monitor through a wireless transmission device. Thus, the WT endorses TEPDs as official equipment at the World Taekwondo Championships, Olympic Games, and other Taekwondo megaevents.

The use of wearable protective devices for the head, body, hands, and feet that measure striking power through sensors and electronic chips has changed the paradigm of Taekwondo from a game to an objective, qualitative, and scientific sport [7]. Despite these scientific advancements, no study has been published that provides details about the safety performance of the current equipment, except for head and body protectors [8–11]. During the match, sometimes the score is overestimated or underestimated because sensors and devices do not operate accurately while recognizing the TEPDs' score [12]. Additionally, Moon and Jung [13] have observed that the electronic scoring system was undesirably activated, suggesting the need for future improvements.

Thus, at this point, it is relevant to study the precursor variables that affect the intention to accept TEPDs by applying the technology acceptance model (TAM). In fact, research has been conducted on the acceptance of other devices for other purposes using surveys [14–16]. Therefore, this study examines the factors that influence TEPD acceptance and then suggests a predictive model for the intention to accept TEPDs. We believe that this study provides important academic data about TEPDs for developing Taekwondo competitions.

2. Literature Review

Davis [17] developed the theory of TAM to predict and explain the behavior of information technology (IT) users. In other words, TAM is a significant information systems theory that is relevant to the acceptance and use of IT [18–20]. TAM is based on the theory of reasoned action (TRA) [21] and the theory of planned behavior (TPB) [22]. These theories are representative behavioral intention models that predict behavior through attitude. TAM is an adaptation of the TRA by Fishbein and Ajzen [21]. It was designed for modeling user acceptance of IT [23]. Furthermore, TPB expands TRA by adding subjective norms and perceived behavior control variables; however, these were excluded from TAM [24]. Assessing changing attitudes and behavioral intentions is common among TAM, TRA, and TPB. Nevertheless, TAM differs from the other two theories as it examines perceived usefulness and perceived ease as factors that explain the difference in the degree of acceptance of technology and innovation. It is believed that these factors influence attitudes.

TAM can predict users' behavioral intention and actual behavior by examining the relationship between perceived ease of use (PEU), perceived usefulness (PU), attitude toward using, and behavioral intention to use (BI) [17]. This model hypothesizes that system use is directly determined by BI, which in turn is influenced by users' AT, the system, and the system's PU [25]. It is important to emphasize that while TPB is a general theory, designed to explain almost any human behavior [26], TAM exclusively focuses on the use of technological innovations and is appropriate for analyzing this type of behavior [17,27]. This theory states that PEU and PU significantly influence the acceptance to use a technology [28]. Davis et al. [23] have stated that various external variables, other than the abovementioned, can also influence the acceptance of a technology. Consequently, this study extends the TAM by including perceived quality, visual attractiveness, wearability, and functionality as factors that influence the use of a technology.

In an attempt to expand TAM, a recent study applied structural equation modeling (SEM) to improve the understanding of the use of wearable technology [29]. Therefore, the hypotheses and research model (Figure 1) established in this study are as follows.

Hypothesis 1. *The perceived quality of Taekwondo electronic protector devices significantly influences perceived ease of use and perceived usefulness.*

Hypothesis 2. *The visual attractiveness of Taekwondo electronic protector devices significantly influences perceived ease of use and perceived usefulness.*

Hypothesis 3. *The wearability of Taekwondo electronic protector devices significantly influences perceived ease of use and perceived usefulness.*

Hypothesis 4. *The functionality of Taekwondo electronic protector devices significantly influences perceived ease of use and perceived usefulness.*

Hypothesis 5. *The perceived ease of use of Taekwondo electronic protector devices significantly influences perceived usefulness and acceptance intention.*

Hypothesis 6. *The perceived usefulness of Taekwondo electronic protector devices significantly influences acceptance intention.*

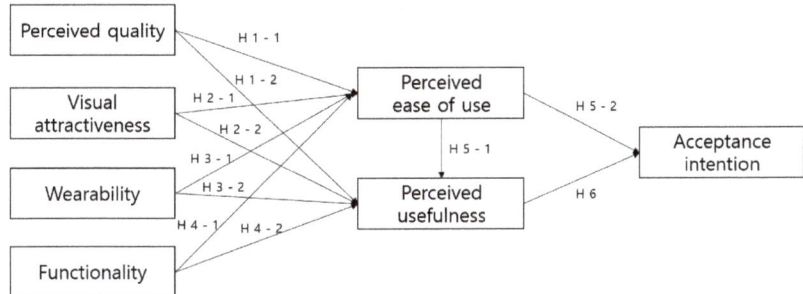

Figure 1. Research model.

3. Materials and Methods
3.1. Data Collection

In January 2019, we conducted a survey of college Taekwondo athletes who were registered with the Korea Taekwondo Association (KTA). The KTA is an official member of the Korean Olympic Committee and is the representative organization that manages the Korean Taekwondo system. We ruled out four responses because of lack of sincerity, analyzed the remaining 220 responses, and compiled the general characteristics of the study participants, as shown in Table 1.

Table 1. Demographics of the participants (N = 220).

Variables	Category	Numbers	Ratio (%)
Gender	Male	160	72.7
	Female	60	27.3
Grade	Freshmen	73	33.2
	Sophomore	71	32.3
	Junior	56	25.5
	Senior	20	9.1
Period of wearing	Less than 1 year	11	5.0
	1–3 years	14	6.4
	3–5 years	40	18.2
	Greater than 5 years	155	70.5
Preferred brand	Daedo (Daedo International, Barcelona, Spain) (http://daedo.com)	37	16.8
	KPNP (KPNP Co., Ltd., Seoul, Korea) (http://kpnp.net)	183	83.2

3.2. Survey Instrument

A survey questionnaire, comprising 28 questions (out of which four were related to demographic factors: gender, school grade, period of using TEPD, and preference for a TEPD brand) was used to collect data. Kim and Choi's [30] questionnaire was modified to obtain the items for perceived quality, and Lee's [31] questionnaire was modified to obtain the items for visual attractiveness, wearability, and functionality. The modified questionnaire used in Park [32], which was based on Davis's [17] TAM, was applied to obtain the items for PU, PEU, and BI. With the exception of the demographic questions, the answers to the questions related to the TAM were based on a 5-point Likert scale ranging from 1 (strongly disagree) to 5 (strongly agree).

3.3. Statistical Analysis

This study utilized IBM PASW 23.0 and AMOS 23.0 (IBM Corp., Armonk, NY, USA) for data analysis. Frequency analysis was conducted to check the demographic characteristics of the research participants, while confirmatory factor and reliability analyses were used to check the validity and reliability of the research tools. Technical statistics analysis was employed to verify the normality of the data. Correlation analysis and structural equation modeling were performed to investigate the relationship between the predetermined variables. The statistical significance was set at 0.05.

4. Results

4.1. Validity and Reliability of Research Tools

This study conducted confirmatory factor analysis to verify the convergent and discriminant validity of the survey. The validity of the measurement model is shown in Table 2.

Table 2. Validity and reliability of research tools.

	Measurement Items	Estimate	SE	C.R	CR	AVE	α
Perceived quality	TEPDs are reliable.	0.776	0.067	12.529	0.842	0.641	0.848
	TEPD manufacturing skill levels are high.	0.672	0.057	15.431			
	The quality of TEPDs is excellent.	0.748	-	-			
Visual attractiveness	The exterior design of TEPDs is excellent.	0.728	0.079	11.511	0.887	0.729	0.854
	The overall look of TEPDs is visually attractive.	0.906	0.081	14.248			
	TEPDs give a visually sophisticated feel.	0.813	-	-			
Wearability	TEPDs can be worn for long periods of time.	0.802	0.090	12.178	0.850	0.655	0.863
	TEPDs are not restricted in their movement.	0.905	0.091	13.307			
	There is no inconvenience in wearing TEPDs.	0.770	-	-			
Functionality	TEPDs have various functions.	0.776	0.103	10.138	0.837	0.632	0.775
	TEPDs are easily mixed with other devices.	0.672	0.115	8.995			
	TEPDs provide a variety of information.	0.748	-	-			
Perceived ease of use	The function of the TEPD is convenient.	0.786	0.106	10.967	0.868	0.622	0.842
	Adaptation of the TEPD is easy.	0.740	0.112	10.350			
	TEPDs are easy to use.	0.754	0.107	10.535			
	TEPD functioning is easy to understand.	0.733	-	-			
Perceived usefulness	TEPDs are useful for practice.	0.768	0.074	13.098	0.908	0.713	0.888
	TEPDs are useful for games.	0.831	0.072	14.718			
	TEPDs are useful for improving performance.	0.825	0.074	14.552			
	TEPDs are generally useful.	0.841	-	-			

Table 2. Cont.

	Measurement Items	Estimate	SE	C.R	CR	AVE	α
Acceptance intention	I am willing to use the TEPD again.	0.827	0.092	12.800	0.895	0.681	0.879
	I am willing to continue to use TEPDs	0.835	0.093	12.946			
	I will recommend TEPDs to other people.	0.776	0.093	11.892			
	I will talk positively about TEPDs to others.	0.772	-	-			
	X^2 = 432.365, DF = 231, Q = 1.872, CFI = 0.939, IFI = 0.940, TLI = 0.927, RMSEA = 0.063						

Note: TEPD = Taekwondo electronic protection device, SE = standard error; C.R = critical ratio, AVE = average variance extracted; CR = construct reliability; x^2 = chi square, DF = degrees of freedom, Q = x^2/DF, CFI = comparative fit index, IFI = incremental fit index, TLI = Tucker–Lewis index, RESEA = root mean square error of approximation.

Table 2 shows that the results—comparative fit index (CFI) > 0.90, incremental fit index (IFI) > 0.90, Tucker–Lewis index (TLI) > 0.90, root mean square error of approximation (RMSEA) < 0.10—meet the validity standard suggested by Kline [33], which indicates that they can be generally accepted. To analyze the convergent validity of each variable used during the study, construct reliability (CR) and the average variance extracted (AVE) were calculated. The results ensured convergent probability based on the criteria presented by Hair et al. [34], as the CR for all observed variables was between 0.837 and 0.908, while the AVE was between 0.622 and 0.729. In addition, if the squared value of the correlation coefficient between the construct conceptions is higher than the AVE of the related concept in the verification of the validity of each concept, the AVE of all factors is greater, and is thereby judged to have secured valid judgment among the concepts [35]. Finally, the reliability of the research tools was tested by referring to the Cronbach's α values: perceived quality (0.848), visual attractiveness (0.854), wearability (0.863), functionality (0.775), PEU (0.842), PU (0.888), and acceptance intention (0.879), thereby ensuring overall confidence [36].

4.2. Verification of Technical Statistical Analysis, Correlation, and Normality

The normality of the data was verified based on the technical statistics of the variables. According to West et al.'s [37] criteria for obtaining normality when verifying univariate normal distribution, the data are normalized when displaying values within the range of ±2 for skewness and ±7 for kurtosis. Additionally, the results of the correlation analysis presented in Table 3 show that there are no multicollinearity problems as the correlation between variables was less than 0.85 in all cases [33].

Table 3. Correlation analysis and normality of data.

	1	2	3	4	5	6	7
Perceived quality	1						
Visual attractiveness	0.529 **	1					
Wearability	0.499 **	0.491 **	1				
Functionality	0.578 **	0.478 **	0.484 **	1			
Perceived ease of use	0.581 **	0.508 **	0.479 **	0.482 **	1		
Perceived usefulness	0.675 **	0.445 **	0.301 **	0.485 **	0.616 **	1	
Acceptance intention	0.655 **	0.458 **	0.444 **	0.460 **	0.618 **	0.673 **	1
Mean	3.471	3.457	2.948	3.497	3.601	3.855	3.656
Standard deviation	0.826	0.776	0.951	0.679	0.736	0.778	0.791
Skewness	−0.176	0.209	0.026	0.257	−0.127	−0.568	−0.449
Kurtosis	0.093	−0.294	−0.491	0.294	−0.048	0.748	0.721

** $p < 0.01$.

4.3. Structural Equation Modeling

Maximum likelihood (ML) was used as an SEM parameter estimation method; as Table 4 shows, the goodness-of-fit indices indicate that the structural model is an acceptable fit to the data (χ^2 = 445.814, DF = 235, CFI = 0.936, IFI = 0.937, TLI = 0.925, RMSEA = 0.064).

Table 4. Result for structural equation modeling.

Items	Path	β	SE	C.R	p
1–1	Perceived quality -> Perceived ease of use	0.380	0.078	3.481	0.000
1–2	Perceived quality -> Perceived usefulness	0.544	0.088	5.089	0.000
2–1	Visual attractiveness -> Perceived ease of use	0.159	0.076	1.798	0.072
2–2	Visual attractiveness -> Perceived usefulness	−0.010	0.076	−0.131	0.896
3–1	Wearability -> Perceived ease of use	0.234	0.061	2.867	0.004
3–2	Wearability -> Perceived usefulness	−0.218	0.064	−2.932	0.003
4–1	Functionality -> Perceived ease of use	0.116	0.117	1.031	0.302
4–2	Functionality -> Perceived usefulness	0.107	0.117	1.093	0.274
5–1	Perceived ease of use -> Perceived usefulness	0.418	0.109	4.361	0.000
5–2	Perceived ease of use -> Acceptance intention	0.361	0.116	4.031	0.000
6	Perceived usefulness -> Acceptance intention	0.525	0.104	5.758	0.000

X^2 = 445.814, DF = 235, Q = 1.897, CFI = 0.936, IFI = 0.937, TLI = 0.925, RMSEA = 0.064

β = standard coefficient, SE = standard error; C.R = critical ratio, x^2 = chi square, DF = degrees of freedom, Q = x^2/DF, CFI = comparative fit index, IFI = incremental fit index, TLI = Tucker–Lewis index, RESEA = root mean square error of approximation.

A closer look at the results of the structural model analysis confirms the following (Figure 2). First, perceived quality positively (+) affects PEU (β = 0.380, t = 3.481) and PU (β = 0.544, t = 5.089). Second, visual attractiveness does not significantly affect either PEU (β = 0.159, t = 1.798) or PU (β = −0.100, t = −0.131). Third, wearability had a positive (+) effect on PEU (β = 0.234, t = 2.867), but a negative (−) effect on PU (β = −0.218 and t = −2.932). Fourth, functionality did not significantly affect either PEU (β = 0.116, t = 1.031) or PU (β = 0.107, t = 1.093). Fifth, PEU had a positive (+) effect on PU (β = 0.418, t = 4.361) and acceptance intention (β = 0.361, t = 4.031). Sixth, PU had a positive (+) effect on acceptance intention (β = 0.525, t = 5.758).

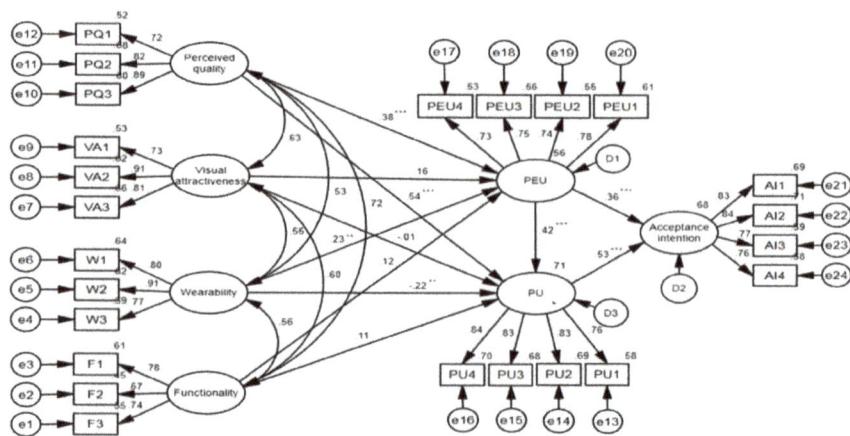

Figure 2. Acceptance intention prediction model for Taekwondo electronic protection devices. Note: *** p < 0.001, ** p < 0.01, PQ = perceived quality, VA = visual attractiveness, W = wearability, F = functionality, PEU = perceived ease of use, PU = perceived usefulness, AI = acceptance intention.

5. Discussion

First, perceived quality has a significant influence on PEU and PU. In particular, in this study, perceived quality was found to be the most significant factor affecting PEU and PU—the quality of the TEPD has a direct effect on the competition. Considering that TEPDs are used to ensure fairness in the Taekwondo competition, efforts to enhance their perceived quality are critical. In the past, for example, Taekwondo athletes observed that a purportedly strong kick did not register a point, while weak force did [38]. These problems were raised as technical issues with TEPDs, among not only Taekwondo athletes but also spectators, as they expressed doubts about PEU and PU. Therefore, efforts should be made to maintain a consistent standard of TEPD quality and to enhance athletes and spectators' perception of the device's quality through continuous technical development.

Second, visual attractiveness does not have a significant influence on the PEU and PU. Falcó et al.'s study [39] supports these results, as their research shows that there is no significant relationship between the appearance and performance of TEPDs. The appearance of various TEPD brands is similar; moreover, their design is similar to that of a typical product without the electronic components. Therefore, this study confirms that the visual attractiveness that Taekwondo athletes perceive does not have a significant effect on their PEU and PU.

Third, wearability has a significant positive influence on PEU, while it has a significantly negative (−) effect on PU. Taekwondo competition scoring happens quickly over a short period. Taekwondo athletes are very sensitive to this movement and therefore, the higher the TEPD wearing sensibility, the greater the PEU. Conversely, wearability has been shown to have a negative effect on PU. This indicates that Taekwondo athletes tend to recognize highly wearable TEPDs as good products and believe that the latest updated TEPDs will easily record the score of opponent strikes on themselves. Therefore, it seems that the higher the wearing sensation, the less useful it will be. More importantly, Sevinc and Colak [40] indicate that TEPD wearability is a leading factor that significantly affects Taekwondo performance. Therefore, manufacturing companies must maintain the product condition and continue to make efforts to improve its material and technical ability to improve product durability.

Fourth, functionality does not have a significant influence on the PEU and PU. Considering that the function of TEPDs is to ensure fairness in competitions [41], this study confirms that PEU and PU are not recognized for functions other than this purpose. Given that some individuals did not trust the functioning of the earlier versions of the TEPD because of their technical issues [42], TEPD manufacturers need to focus more on the development of products that enhance fairness in their functionality.

Fifth, PEU has a significant influence on PU and acceptance intention. There were many technical problems with the initial model of the device, including errors with the sensor recognition process during use. However, recent improvements in material development and technical skills have improved athletes' competency and provided them with motivation and objective feedback. Electronic systems help analyze the performance, strength, and functional capacity of athletes, and assist in improving their skills and monitoring these improvements. Additionally, these systems help develop strategies, motivate athletes, and provide objective feedback [43]. PEU of TEPDs, athletes' PU, and acceptance intention are also judged to have increased.

Sixth, PU has a significant influence on acceptance intention. As TEPDs have been used in all recent international competitions, one can expect that the higher the PU of the TEPD, the more the acceptance intention increases. Notably, the rules have been gradually amended to increase athletes' acceptance of the TEPD since its introduction [44]. However, as Taekwondo is a spectator sport, it is necessary to address technical problems so that spectators can also recognize the use of TEPDs and their usefulness.

6. Conclusions

The TAM provides a critical theoretical model for predicting the acceptance of TEPDs. The importance of PEU and PU as leading variables in predicting TEPD acceptability means that continuous improvement in perceived quality and wearability are required to develop athletes' TEPD skills and improve the performance and fairness of Taekwondo competitions. As such, this study presents factors that enhance the effectiveness of the TAM and provides a predictive model appropriate for measuring athletes' intention to accept TEPDs.

Author Contributions: Study design, S.-U.P. and D.-K.K.; study conduct, S.-U.P., D.-K.K., and H.A.; data collection, D.-K.K.; data analysis, S.-U.P. and D.-K.K.; data interpretation, S.-U.P. and D.-K.K.; drafting manuscript, S.-U.P., D.-K.K. and H.A.; revising the manuscript content, S.-U.P., D.-K.K. and H.A. All authors have read and agreed to the published version of the manuscript.

Funding: This research received no external funding.

Acknowledgments: This study supplemented the contents announced at the 2019 International Conference on Biotechnology and Sports Engineering.

Conflicts of Interest: The authors declare no conflict of interest.

References

1. International Olympic Committee. Taekwondo. Available online: https://www.olympic.org/taekwondo/ (accessed on 28 January 2021).
2. World Taekwondo Federation. ABOUT WT. Available online: http://www.worldtaekwondo.org/about-wt/about.html (accessed on 28 January 2021).
3. Korea Institute of Sport Science. Taekwondo Olympic Games Status Maintenance Plan. Available online: https://www.sports.re.kr/pyxis-api/1/digital-files/bea28d12-5830-45d2-ae24-65c7bd4776b6/ (accessed on 28 January 2021).
4. Kim, J. Electronic Hogu, 'OK' for London Olympic Games. Available online: http://www.mookas.us/media_view.asp?news_no=1655/ (accessed on 5 April 2011).
5. Ko, Y.J.; Cattani, K.; Chang, Y.; Hur, Y. Do spectators and competitors accept the use of scoring technology in Taekwondo competitions? *Int. J. Sport Manag. Mark.* **2011**, *9*, 238–253. [CrossRef]
6. Del Vecchio, F.B.; Franchini, E.; Del Vecchio, A.H.M.; Pieter, W. Energy absorbed by electronic body protectors from kicks in a taekwondo competition. *Biol. Sport* **2011**, *28*, 75–78. [CrossRef]
7. Song, Y.; Jeon, Y.; Park, G.; An, H.; Hwang, T.; Lee, H.; Lee, S. Development of taekwondo trainer system for training on electronic protector with hitting target indicator. *Int. J. Comput. Sci. Netw. Secur.* **2010**, *10*, 51–56.
8. Bae, Y.S. Relationship between the impact value of electronic body protector and the impact force of force platform in the Taekwondo. *Korean J. Sport Biomech.* **2013**, *23*, 125–130. [CrossRef]
9. Jeong, H.S.; O'sullivan, D.M.; Lee, S.C.; Lee, S.Y. Safety evaluation of protective equipment for the forearm, shin, hand and foot in taekwondo. *J. Sports Sci. Med.* **2019**, *18*, 376–383.
10. O'Sullivan, D.M.; Fife, G.P. Impact attenuation of protective boxing and taekwondo headgear. *Eur. J. Sports Sci.* **2016**, *16*, 1219–1225. [CrossRef]
11. O'Sullivan, D.M.; Fife, G.P.; Pieter, W.; Shin, I. Safety performance evaluation of taekwondo headgear. *Br. J. Sports Med.* **2013**, *47*, 447–451. [CrossRef]
12. Cho, E.H. Regional Perception in Searching for the 'Recognized Electronic Protectors Problems'. *Korean J. Meas. Eval. Phys. Educ. Sport Sci* **2015**, *17*, 47–56.
13. Moon, W.J.; Jung, K.C. The Technical Analysis Based in the Types of Olympic Taekwondo Game. *Sports Sci.* **2014**, *31*, 85–92.
14. David, M.L.; Zoe Co, L.P.; Newmark, A.R.; Groisser, A.; Jay, H.; Jennifer, S.H.; David, W.B. Design and testing of a mobile health application rating tool. *NPJ Digit. Med.* **2020**, *3*, 1–7.
15. Peter, B.; Relish, C.; Yaoqi, Z. Large expert-curated database for benchmarking document similarity detection in biomedical literature search. *Database* **2019**, 1–66.
16. Shih-Cheng, H.; Tanay, K.; Imon, B.; Chris, C.; Robyn, L.B.; Norah, B.; Andrew, H.; Bhavik, N.P.; Pranav, R.; Jeremy, I.; et al. PENet—a scalable deep-learning model for automated diagnosis of pulmonary embolism using volumetric CT imaging. *NPJ Digit. Med.* **2020**, *3*, 1–9.
17. Davis, F.D. Perceived usefulness, perceived ease of use, and user acceptance of information technology. *Mis Q.* **1989**, *13*, 319–340. [CrossRef]
18. Lee, Y.; Kozar, K.A.; Larsen, K.R. The technology acceptance model: Past, present, and future. *Commun. Assoc. Inf. Syst.* **2003**, *12*, 50. [CrossRef]
19. Lucas, H.C.; Spitler, V.K. Implementation in a world of workstations and networks. *Inf. Manag.* **2000**, *38*, 119–128. [CrossRef]

20. Venkatesh, V.; Davis, F.D. A theoretical extension of the technology acceptance model: Four longitudinal field studies. *Manag. Sci.* **2000**, *46*, 186–204. [CrossRef]
21. Fishbein, M.; Ajzen, I. *Belief, Attitude, Intention, and Behavior: An Introduction to Theory and Research*; Addison-Wesley: Reading, MA, USA, 1975.
22. Ajzen, I. From Intentions to Actions: A Theory of Planned Behavior. In *Action Control*; Springer: Berlin/Heidelberg, Germany, 1985; pp. 11–39.
23. Davis, F.D.; Bagozzi, R.P.; Warshaw, P.R. User acceptance of computer technology: A comparison of two theoretical models. *Manag. Sci.* **1989**, *35*, 982–1003. [CrossRef]
24. Ajzen, I. The theory of planned behavior. *Organ. Behav. Hum. Decis. Process.* **1991**, *50*, 179–211. [CrossRef]
25. Lee, M.C. Factors influencing the adoption of internet banking: An integration of TAM and TPB with perceived risk and perceived benefit. *Electron. Commer. Res. Appl.* **2009**, *8*, 130–141. [CrossRef]
26. Herrera, S.I.; Fénnema, M.C. Tecnologías móviles aplicadas a la educación superior. In *XVII Congreso Argentino de Ciencias de la Computación*; SEDICI: Buenos Aires, Argentina, 2011; pp. 620–630.
27. Gómez-Ramirez, I.; Valencia-Arias, A.; Duque, L. Approach to M-learning acceptance among university students: An integrated model of TPB and TAM. *Int. Rev. Res. Open Distrib. Learn.* **2019**, *20*, 141–164. [CrossRef]
28. Sung, H.J.; Jeon, H.M. Untact: Customer's Acceptance Intention toward Robot Barista in Coffee Shop. *Sustainability* **2020**, *12*, 8598. [CrossRef]
29. Lunney, A.; Cunningham, N.R.; Eastin, M.S. Wearable fitness technology: A structural investigation into acceptance and perceived fitness outcomes. *Comput. Hum. Behav.* **2016**, *65*, 114–120. [CrossRef]
30. Kim, B.G.; Choi, Y.H. Effects of perceived quality on brand attitudes and purchase intention by the Taekwondo electronic hogu experience. *Korean J. Sport* **2017**, *15*, 513–522.
31. Lee, S.I. A Study of the Influence of Technical and Indivisual Characteristics on the Acceptance Intention and Performance Expectation of Healthcare Werable Devices. Ph.D. Thesis, Konkuk University, Seoul, Korea, 2017.
32. Park, S.U. Prediction of intention to use internet Taekwondo media using extended technology acceptance model. *Taekwondo J. Kukkiwon* **2020**, *11*, 47–59.
33. Kline, R.B. *Principle and Practice of Structural Equation Modeling*; Guilford Press: New York, NY, USA, 1998.
34. Hair, J.F.; Black, W.C.; Babin, B.J.; Anderson, R.E.; Tatham, R.L. *Multivariate Data Analysis*, 6th ed.; Pearson Prentice Hall: Upper Saddle River, NJ, USA, 2006.
35. Fornell, C.; Larcker, D.F. Evaluating structural equation models with unobservable variables and measurement error. *J. Mark. Res.* **1981**, *18*, 39–50. [CrossRef]
36. Nunnally, J.C.; Bernstein, I.H. The assessment of reliability. *Psychom. Theory* **1994**, *3*, 248–292.
37. West, S.G.; Finch, J.F.; Curran, P.J. Structural Equation Models with Nonnormal Variables: Problems and Remedies. In *Structural Equation Modeling: Concepts, Issues, and Applications*; Hoyle, R.H., Ed.; Sage: Thousand Oaks, CA, USA, 1995; pp. 56–75.
38. Leveaux, R. 2012 Olympic Games Decision Making Technologies for Taekwondo Competition. *Commun. IBIMA* **2012**, 1–8. [CrossRef]
39. Falcó, C.; Conchado, A.; Estevan, I. The effect of color on the use of electronic body protectors in taekwondo matches. *Percept. Mot. Ski.* **2016**, *122*, 812–824. [CrossRef]
40. Sevinç, D.; Çolak, M. The effect of electronic body protector and gamification on the performance of taekwondo athletes. *Int. J. Perform. Anal. Sport* **2019**, *19*, 110–120. [CrossRef]
41. Tasika, N. Reliability & linearity of an electronic body protector employed in taekwondo games: A preliminary study. *J. Hum. Sport Exerc.* **2013**, *8*, S622–S632.
42. Kailian, G.S. *Sport Taekwondo Referee Primer*; Word Association Publishers: Tarentum, PA, USA, 2010.
43. Ball, N.; Nolan, E.; Wheeler, K. Anthropometrical, physiological, and tracked power profiles of elite taekwondo athletes 9 weeks before the Olympic competition phase. *J. Strength Cond. Res.* **2011**, *25*, 2752–2763. [CrossRef]
44. Moenig, U. Rule and equipment modification issues in World Taekwondo Federation (WTF) competition. Ido Movement for Culture. *J. Martial Arts Anthropol.* **2015**, *15*, 3–12.

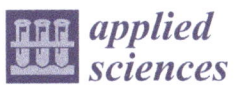

Article

Relative Weights of Physical Strength Factors in Sports Events: Focused on Similarity Sports Events Group According to the Sports Physiological View

Kyoung-Hyun Lee [1], Jin-Seok Lee [2], Byung-Chan Lee [3] and Eun-Hyung Cho [2,*]

1. Center for Sport Science in Gwangju, 278, Geumhwa-ro, Seo-gu, Gwangju 62048, Korea; brion118@skku.edu
2. Department of Sports Science, Korea Institute of Sport Science, 727, Hwarang-ro, Nowon-gu, Seoul 01794, Korea; js0420@kspo.or.kr
3. Department of Physical Education, Sichuan Agricultural University, Ya'an 625014, China; wongkei@korea.ac.kr
* Correspondence: ehcho@kspo.or.kr; Tel.: +82-970-9564

Received: 31 October 2020; Accepted: 11 December 2020; Published: 21 December 2020

Abstract: The purpose of this study was to investigate the relative weights of physical strength factors in sports events. We selected 16,645 people as a sample group who participated in physical fitness measurements through eight sports science centers across the country from 2016 until August of 2018, and divided into four sports types depending on the sports physiological view: type A: short-term muscular power and short-term muscular endurance, type B: mid-term muscular power, type C: long-term cardiorespiratory endurance, type D: coordination capability (CC), agility, flexibility, and balance. Categorized the performance level into excellent athletes and non-excellent athletes, and standardized (T-score) the measured value after considering sex, age and sports type group. Used logistic regression analysis for the method of analysis, and calculated the relative weights of physical strength factor with different sports by using Wald value which was calculated from logistic regression analysis. As a result, the relative weights of physical factor in type A were power 30%, muscular power (MP) 18%, CC 16%, agility 11%, flexibility 10%, cardiorespiratory endurance (CE) 1%, and balance 0%. The relative weights of physical factor in type B were muscular endurance (ME) 43%, MP 25%, power 20%, balance 9%, CE 2%, flexibility 1%, agility 0%, and CC 0%. The relative weights of physical factor in type C were ME 41%, CE 37%, power 10%, agility 8%, flexibility 2%, CC 2%, ME 0%, and balance 0%. Need more specific classification standard for type D sports. Hope the results of this study were used to measure physical fitness level and used as baseline data for recruiting future talents.

Keywords: sports events; physiological view; physical strength factor; relative weight

1. Introduction

It's a proven fact through many studies that physical strength is a vital factor to improve performance in sports. However, the importance of physical strength differs by sport event. It is necessary to find out the physical factors that affect the performance of each sport.

If one examines the studies about finding out the physical factors that are related with the performance, you can see that they are sorted by two big categories which are theoretical studies about the literature, or content validity with collections of expert opinions [1] and studies based on measurement of physical fitness data [2,3].

The first category has strength in internal validity and contents as it applies literature and the opinions of experts, while the other category has strength in objectivity as it applies physical fitness data. However, both methods can verify the priorities of important physical factors of each sport, and has limitations in finding out the magnitude of the importance. For example, for a judo athlete one can verify that power is a more important factor than muscular endurance, but we cannot verify how more important it is. In other words, it has weakness in assigning relative weights to each factor.

Verifying relative weights of physical factors can quantify the physical factors that individuals have and can be used as important baseline data when recruiting future talent [4]. If you look at the selection process of future talent within countries, they apply different importances of performance, physique, and physical factors to each sport, and also apply different importances of physical factors to each sport according to detailed measurement items [5]. However, even though verifying relative weights of physical factors is a very crucial data which can be used for recruiting, precedent research is not enough and inadequate. One of the reasons why verifying relative weights of physical factors in each sport is not enough and inadequate, is the problem of the amount of data. To secure the validity of the verified weights, we need data analysis based on big data and collecting enough physical data of elite athletes is just too difficult unless it happens to be available at a national level.

Meanwhile, the Korean Ministry of Culture is operating a pilot project to provide sports science support to local elite athletes which is provided by the Korea Institute of Sports Science which is applying it to national team athletes to improve the performance of the local athletes since 2015. Year 2018 as it is now, there are eight local sports science centers operating across the country and their goal is to provide sports science support to 1400 athletes at each center annually. Therefore, if we use accumulated measurement data from the local sports centers, we can estimate the validity of verified relative weights of physical factors in each sport. Thus, the purpose of this study is to verify the relative weights of physical factors in each sport using accumulated big data measured at the local sports science centers.

2. Subjects and Statistical Analysis

2.1. Data Collection

To achieve the purpose of this study, selected 16,645 athletes as a population who participated in physical fitness measurement from eight sports science centers across the country from 2016 until August of 2018. Table 1 shows the sex and number of the populations by age groups.

Table 1. Sex and number of populations by age groups.

Sex	Elementary School (Age: 8–13)	Middle School (Age: 14–16)	High School (Age: 17–19)	Adults (Age: 20–30)	Total
Male	1627	3721	3289	2430	11,067
Female	897	1519	1705	1457	5578
Overall	2524	5240	4994	3887	16,645

2.2. Classification Criteria of Similar Sports Types

Based on the 'Research task report on local sports science 2017' and the development of physical training in each sport [6], they are categorized into five types depending on the sports physiological viewpoint. Concretely, the five types are sports events focused on short-term muscular power and short-term muscular endurance (Type A, 24 sports), mid-term muscular endurance (Type B, 19 sports), long-term cardiorespiratory endurance (Type C, 10 sports), agility, coordination capability, balance (Type D, 25 sports), and speed endurance (Type E, 11 sports). On the basis of this, in this research, through the discussion of experts, we excluded sports events focused on speed endurance (Type E) to fit the character of research materials and recategorized as four events (A, B, C, D). Table 2 shows the classification standard of similar sports events depending on the sports physiological viewpoint.

Table 2. Classification criteria of similar sports type grouped according to the sports physiological viewpoint.

Type	Classification Criteria	Detailed Sports Type
A	Physical factors that decide performance: short-term muscular power, short-term muscular endurance Short-term muscular power and anaerobic endurance training sports Anaerobic 40~100%, aerobic 0~60% sports Super Short time (less than 10 s), shot-term performance (10~180 s) sports	Track & field (100~800 m), athletics (jumping), athletics (throwing), cycle (200~1000 m), short-track (500~1500 m), diving, gymnastics, judo, wrestling, ssireum, golf, fencing, kendo, weightlifting, bodybuilding, sports climbing, snowboarding (cross), alpine skiing, freestyle skiing (cross)
B	Physical factors that decide performance: mid-term muscular endurance Mid-term muscular endurance and aerobic training sports Anaerobic 10~40%, aerobic 60~90% sports Short time (3~20 min), mid time performance (21~60 min) sports	Track & field (1000~10,000 m), cycling (4000 m), short-track (3000 m), speed skating, boxing, taekwondo, synchronized swimming, canoe, water polo, kayak, rowing, kickboxing, wushu, aerobics, race walking, inline skating, swimming, fin swimming
C	Physical factors that decide performance: long-term cardiorespiratory endurance Long-term muscular endurance and long-term cardiorespiratory endurance training sports anaerobic 0~10%, aerobic 90~100% sports Long-time (1~4 h) performance sports	Modern pentathlon, marathon, cycling (MTB), cycling (road), yachting, biathlon, triathlon, cross country skiing, Nordic skiing, ice hockey, cycling (long distance)
D	Physical factors that decide performance: agility, coordination capabilities, flexibility and balance Agility, coordination capabilities training sports ATP-PCr 60~90%, glycolysis 0~20% sports	Basketball, baseball, volleyball, table tennis, handball, tennis, badminton, cricket, shooting, archery, curling, cycling (BMX), field hockey, figure skating, snowboarding (half pipe), rugby, soccer, sepaktakraw, softball, archery, squash, tennis, billiards

A: short-term muscular power and short-term muscular endurance, B: mid-term muscular endurance. C: long-term cardiorespiratory endurance, D: agility, coordination capability, balance. Reference: Research task report on local sports science 2017 from the development of physical training in each sports event [6].

2.3. Assessment Tools to Physical Fitness

Physical factors chosen to achieve the purpose of this study are strength, muscle endurance, power, cardiorespiratory function, agility, flexibility, balance and coordination, and each method of measurement is shown in Table 3.

2.4. Categorized the Performance Level

The performance level is categorized into excellent athletes and non-excellent athletes. Categorization criteria were first selected as domestic and international standing status and second, they were classified according to close support status. Close support is a program that provides sports science support from the local sports centers to those with high performance and with high chance of winning the medals. Table 4 shows the sports events and sample sizes in athletes.

2.5. Data Standardized and Sampling

The age of the sample group for this research is from elementary through high school students and adults, sex is both. Therefore, the use of raw data means age and sex could be variables. For example, an excellent elementary athlete could have better physical ability than a non-excellent adult athlete or an excellent female athlete could have better physical ability than a non-excellent male athlete. To solve this problem, I considered sex, age, sport events, and calculated the personalized T-score which is standardized to each group. Calculation formula of T-score is as follows.

$$T = \left(\frac{X - M_i}{S_i}\right) \times 10 + 50 \tag{1}$$

In Equation (1), X means individuals' original score, and M_i means the average of sex, age, and sport type group. S_i means the standard deviation between sex, age and sport type group. After calculating the T-score of individuals, if it scores over than 90 and less than 10, I regarded them as churn values and deleted them. For the physical score, used average of each measurement items to calculate.

Table 3. Assessment tools according to physical fitness.

Sex	Assessment Tools
Strength	Grip Strength (kg) Back Strength (kg)
Muscle endurance	Sit-Up (count/60 s) Push-Up (count/60 s)
Power	Sargent Jump (cm) Standing Long Jump (cm)
Cardiorespiratory function	FEV_1 (%) 20-m Shuttle Run Test (count)
Agility	Reaction Time (1/1000 s) Side-Step Test (count/20 s)
Flexibility	Trunk Flexion (cm) Trunk Extension (cm)
Balance	One Leg Balance with Eyes Closed (s) Dynamic Balance (s/min.)
Coordination	Eye-Hand Coordination (s)

FEV: forced expiratory volume.

Table 4. Sports events and sample sizes in athletes.

Sex	A	B	C	D	Overall
Excellent	530	378	77	888	1873
Non-excellent	3421	3138	642	7571	14,772
Overall	3951	3516	719	8459	16,645

A: short-term muscular power and short-term muscular endurance, B: mid-term muscular endurance. C: long-term cardiorespiratory endurance, D: agility, coordination capability, balance.

In Table 4, as suggested earlier, the number of sports events group excellent athletes and non-excellent ones differs. Among a total number of 16,645 athletes, excellent athletes are 1873, which represents 11.3%. When a logistic regression model is applied, if there is a big difference in the sample sizes of a dependent variables, so the fidelity of the model could be low. Concretely, the non-excellent athletes sample size is larger, so there is a possibility of the model that might focus on classification prediction of the non-excellent athletes. While this makes more classification of non-excellent athletes more accurate, it lowers however the accuracy of the classification of excellent athletes. To solve this problem, we implemented stratified randomization random sampling which considers sex and age [7]. Table 5 shows the characteristics of the finally selected sample groups.

Table 5. Sports events and sample sizes in athletes.

Sex	A	B	C	D	Total
Excellent	231	156	46	304	737
Non-excellent	231	156	46	304	737
Total	462	312	92	608	1474

A: short-term muscular power and short-term muscular endurance, B: mid-term muscular endurance. C: long-term cardiorespiratory endurance, D: agility, coordination capability, balance.

2.6. Statistical Analysis

We used Excel 2014 (Microsoft, Redmond, WA, USA) to organize the data and calculate T-scores. We implemented logistic regression analysis to explore the physical factors of performance determinants. For calculation of relative weigh values, we used logistic regression analysis Wald values so the sum of each physical factor become 100% through the proportions. We used SPSS version 25.0 (SPSS Inc., Chicago, IL, USA) for statistical processing, and set the statistical significance level at 0.05.

3. Results

3.1. Results of Logistic Regression Goodness of Fit Model

Table 6 presents the results of the goodness of fit of our logistic regression analysis by sport events. The constants of the type A, B and C models appear to have a X^2 significance probability value that is statistically reasonable—between 2LL and the theoretical model that the researchers set (intercept model-theory model), on the other hand, type D appear to have no significance probability. Nagelkerke R^2 generally appeared low in all sport type groups, but in case of logistic regression analysis, the sums of the coefficient of determinations differ depending on the value of a dependent variable, but still that value is generally low as well. If one looks at the classification precision, it shows that type A is 58.9%, B is 65.4%, C is 69.6%, and D is 55.4%.

Table 6. The goodness of fit of the logistic regression analysis by sport events.

Validation Method		A	B	C	D
-2LL		616.3	383.7	109.0	828.7
X^2		24.1	48.9	18.5	14.1
df		8	8	8	8
p		0.002	0.001	0.018	0.079
Nagelkerke R^2		0.068	0.193	0.243	0.031
Classification precision	Excellent	57.1%	65.4%	67.4%	53.6%
	Non-excellent	60.6%	65.4%	71.7%	57.2%
	overall	58.9%	65.4%	69.6%	55.4%

A: short-term muscular power and short-term muscular endurance, B: mid-term muscular endurance. C: long-term cardiorespiratory endurance, D: agility, coordination capability, balance.

3.2. Results of Relative Weight of Physical Fitness

To calculate the relative weighs of physical factors by sport event group, we used Wald values from the logistic regression analysis. Concretely, these were calculated through a proportional expression so that the sum of Wald values is 100% for each physical factor. The relative weighs resulting from this are shown in Table 7.

For A type, the values are power 30%, strength 18%, coordination 16%, agility 11%, flexibility 10%, cardiorespiratory function 1%, balance 0%. For B type they are muscle endurance 43%, strength 25%, power 20%, balance 9%, cardiorespiratory function 2%, flexibility 1%, agility 0%, coordination 0%. For C type, they appear to be muscle endurance 41%, cardiorespiratory function 37%, power 10%, agility 8%, flexibility 2%, coordination 2%, strength 0%, balance 0%. For D type, they are coordination

29%, flexibility 24%, strength 21%, balance 16%, muscle endurance 7%, power 2%, cardiorespiratory function 1%, agility 0%.

Table 7. The relative weights of physical fitness factors.

Physical Fitness Factor	Sport Type Group			
	A	B	C	D
Strength	18%	25%	0%	21%
Muscle endurance	14%	43%	41%	7%
Power	30%	20%	10%	2%
Cardiorespiratory function	1%	2%	37%	1%
Agility	11%	0%	8%	0%
Flexibility	10%	1%	2%	24%
Balance	0%	9%	0%	16%
Coordination	16%	0%	2%	29%

A: short-term muscular power and short-term muscular endurance, B: mid-term muscular endurance, C: long-term cardiorespiratory endurance, D: agility, coordination capability, balance.

3.3. Results of Logistic Regression Analysis

As a result, a statistical significance about physical factors of performance by sport event group is obtained. For type A, only the factor of power (Wald = 6.153, $p = 0.013$) appeared to have statistical significance, for type B, the factors of strength (Wald = 6.533, $p = 0.011$), muscular endurance (Wald = 11.298, $p = 0.001$, and power (Wald = 5.215, $p = 0.022$) appeared to have statistical significance. For type C, the factors of muscular endurance (Wald = 4.901, $p = 0.027$) and cardiorespiratory function (Wald = 4.462, $p = 0.035$) appeared to have statistical significance, whereas for type D none of the physical factors appeared to have statistical significance (Table 8).

Table 8. Results of physical fitness factors on performance by sport type (logistic regression analysis).

Type	Variables	B	SE	Wald	df	p	Exp(B)
A	Strength	0.021	0.011	3.711	1	0.054	1.021
	Muscle endurance	0.020	0.012	2.837	1	0.092	1.020
	Power	0.032	0.013	6.153	1	0.013	1.032
	Cardiorespiratory function	−0.005	0.012	0.184	1	0.668	0.995
	Agility	0.002	0.015	2.145	1	0.143	1.022
	Flexibility	−0.018	0.012	2.000	1	0.157	0.982
	Balance	0.003	0.010	0.094	1	0.759	1.003
	Coordination	−0.020	0.011	3.279	1	0.07	0.980
B	Strength	0.037	0.015	6.533	1	0.011	1.038
	Muscle endurance	0.053	0.016	11.298	1	0.001	1.054
	Power	0.037	0.016	5.215	1	0.022	1.037
	Cardiorespiratory function	−0.011	0.017	0.437	1	0.508	0.989
	Agility	0.000	0.017	0.000	1	0.996	1.000
	Flexibility	0.008	0.017	0.223	1	0.637	1.008
	Balance	0.021	0.014	2.299	1	0.129	1.022
	Coordination	0.002	0.014	0.024	1	0.876	1.002
C	Strength	−0.008	0.035	0.054	1	0.816	0.992
	Muscle endurance	0.089	0.040	4.901	1	0.027	1.093
	Power	−0.041	0.039	1.139	1	0.286	0.959
	Cardiorespiratory function	0.073	0.035	4.462	1	0.035	1.076
	Agility	0.033	0.035	0.895	1	0.344	1.034
	Flexibility	0.016	0.030	0.261	1	0.609	1.016
	Balance	−0.001	0.025	0.001	1	0.971	0.999
	Coordination	0.011	0.023	0.209	1	0.647	1.011

Table 8. Cont.

Type	Variables	B	SE	Wald	df	p	Exp(B)
D	Strength	0.016	0.010	2.255	1	0.133	1.016
	Muscle endurance	−0.009	0.011	0.743	1	0.389	0.991
	Power	−0.005	0.012	0.204	1	0.651	0.995
	Cardiorespiratory function	−0.003	0.010	0.071	1	0.789	0.997
	Agility	0.002	0.013	0.028	1	0.866	1.002
	Flexibility	0.017	0.011	2.531	1	0.112	1.017
	Balance	−0.012	0.009	1.692	1	0.193	0.988
	Coordination	0.018	0.010	3.062	1	0.08	1.018

4. Discussion

As confirmed in many cases from advanced sports countries, physical factors are essential factors in improving athletic performance [8,9]. Objective and accurate physical examination and evaluation of physical strength related to performance improvement by sport are emphasized. In particular, efforts to explore and apply performance-related physical factors in each sport have been attempted due to the problem of specificity in each event [1–3].

Relative weighs of physical factors in each sport can be assessed quantitatively and this might be used as a useful as baseline data for selecting athletes. Nevertheless, it is not easy to see the effort needed to calculate the relative weights of each physical factor. Therefore, this study aimed to compare the importance of physical factors in each sport and calculate the relative weighs of the various physical factors. In order to achieve the purposes of the study, the sports groups were divided into four types according to the sports physiology perspective: A type: sports that focus on short-term muscular power and short-term muscular endurance, B type: sports that focus on mid-term muscular endurance, C type: sports that focus on long-term cardiorespiratory endurance and D type: sports that focus on agility, coordination capabilities, flexibility and balance.

In the type A case, according to the result of our logistic regression analysis, only the power factor had a statistically significant effect on performance, and the relative weights from the Wald values were high in order power, strength, and coordination. In other words, power has the most relevance in type A sports. This is consistent with the importance of power mentioned in the studies of short-distance runners [10] and weightlifters [11] which are type A sports. Serresse and colleagues said that the ability to exert a sudden burst of force, or power, affects the performance of short-distance track and field athletes [10]. Hakkinen and colleagues explained that strength and power are important factors in weightlifters' performance [11].

The relative weight of coordination was 16 percent, the third highest. In this study, the data of eye-hand coordination tests was used, and eye-hand coordination is the technology that identifies visual information of the eye in the brain which responds to the motion information of the hand [12]. This means how accurate and fast an athlete reacts to visually perceived information, and in another study, it was stated that reaction time and eye-hand coordination are highly relevant [13].

In the type B case, according to the logistic regression analysis results, the factors strength, muscle endurance and power had statistically significant effects on performance, and from the the calculation of relative weights using the corresponding Wald values, the results were high in the order of factors strength, muscle endurance and power. In a related study about Type B sports, Shaharudin and Agrawal mentioned that the ability of muscular function, average power and highest power, including muscular and muscular endurance are the main factors affecting the performance of rowers, which is believed to support the results of this study [14]. Also, Hernandez and colleagues reported power, strength, and balance as the determinant factors [15]. The results of this study show that calculated balance factors had relatively small weights compared to the factors of strength, muscle endurance and power, and they represented the fourth highest calculated point at 9%.

In the type C case, according to the logistic regression analysis results, muscle endurance and cardiorespiratory function factors had statistically significant effects, and from the calculation of relative weights using the corresponding Wald values, the results were in the order of muscle endurance, cardiorespiratory function and power. If one looks at the type C events, most of them are long-distance sports, and the importance of endurance performance such as muscular endurance and cardiorespiratory endurance cannot be denied. On the other hand, if we look at the reason for the power factor weight, which is the third highest, Riechman and colleagues have reported that strength and power of the lower body are important factors for endurance performance, and in particular, it is reported that there is a correlation between aerobic capacity and muscular power [16]. In addition, in a study of biathlon athletes, it was reported that maximum oxygen intake has a high correlation with standing long jump and standing high jump performance, and considering that characteristics of biathlon running on inclined planes, anaerobic capacity is described as an important performance factor as well as aerobic capacity [17], so it is believed that power can also be an important factor.

In the type D case, according to the logistic regression analysis results, none of the physical factors had a statistically significant effect, and there was also no statistically significant effect in the Wald values from the analysis results of fidelity of the logistic regression model. It would seem that physical factors fail to explain performance and it is inappropriate to apply information about the relative weights that are calculated on this basis. It can be inferred that this result was due to the broad classification criteria of the type D sports. In this study, similar sports types were grouped from a physiological standpoint and the criteria are classified in detail according to the degree of muscle endurance, power, cardiorespiratory function in the type A, B and C, but in the case of type D, the criteria for classification are agility, coordination, flexibility, balance etc., which are somewhat unclear. Therefore, for type D, it is deemed necessary to classify the sport type by applying more detailed classification criteria, and we look forward to future studies supplementing our resulyts.

This study was carried out to calculate the relative weights of sport event physical factors which are sorted from a physiological standpoint. Our research team is also aware that the classification of types according to the physiological standpoint in this study will be controversial for some sports experts and because of the special nature of each sport, clustering might seem meaningless. However, it is impossible to subdivide every sport using a consistent standard and apply it to the field. This is because for team sports, it needs to be subdivided for each position to apply, and for weight division of sports, it needs to be divided into each weight. Furthermore, one needs to calculate the physical importance of each individual according to performance management style, and apply the training program that suits that individual. Athletes at a national level or above deserve individualized assessment and training programs, but for when recruiting future talent, the objective evaluation process based on generalized evaluation methods should be prioritized. Therefore, it is believed that the clustering of similar sports type groups is necessary at the national level.

The past studies on clustering of similar sports type groups reported relations between physical factors categorized into combat, team, individual, target, challenge, etc. This is a classification that takes into account those with characteristics similar to the content area presented [18]. In the national-level curriculum this study will therefore have significant implications in that it newly classifies sport type groups from a physiological standpoint and calculates the importance of performance and physical factors. More subdivisions are needed for type D, and we look forward to this in future studies.

The study also used statistical techniques to calculate the degree of importance of the physical factors of each sport. The results produced by statistical techniques are objective but will not be an absolute criterion. In order to calculate more relevant weighing factors for each sport, the content validity, including the Delphi method, which reflects expert opinion, should also be reflected in the results.

5. Conclusions

The conclusions of this study are as follows: First of all, the relative weighs of type A sports are power 30%, strength18%, coordination 16%, agility, 11%, flexibility 10%, cardiorespiratory function 1%, balance 0%. Secondly, the relative weighs of type B sports are muscle endurance 43%, strength 25%, power 20%, balance 9%, cardiorespiratory function 2%, flexibility 1%, agility 0%, coordination 0%. Thirdly, the relative weighs of type C sports are muscle endurance 41%, cardiorespiratory function 37%, power 10%, agility 8%, flexibility 2%, coordination 2%, strength 0%, balance 0%. D sports should be classified by applying more detailed classification criteria.

Author Contributions: K.-H.L. designed and performed the experiments. J.-S.L. and B.-C.L. analysed the data and advanced research, and wrote the manuscript. E.-H.C. contributed to the design and implementation of the research, to perform the experiments and to the analysis of results and to the writing of the manuscript. All authors have read and agreed to the published version of the manuscript.

Funding: This study was funded by the Korean Institute of Sport Science.

Acknowledgments: The authors would like to express heartfelt thanks to the Korean athletes and coaches who participated in the study.

Conflicts of Interest: The authors declare no conflict of interest. Furthermore, the funders had no role in the design of the study; in the collection, analyses, or interpretation of data; in the writing of the manuscript, or in the decision to publish the results.

References

1. Čular, D.; Krstulović, S.; Katić, R.; Primorac, D.; Vučić, D. Predictors of fitness status on success in taekwondo. *Coll. Antropol.* **2013**, *37*, 1267–1274. [PubMed]
2. Leyhr, D.; Kelava, A.; Raabe, J.; Höner, O. Longitudinal motor performance development in early adolescence and its relationship to adult success: An 8-year prospective study of highly talented soccer players. *PLoS ONE* **2018**, *13*, e0196324. [CrossRef] [PubMed]
3. Triplett, A.N.; Ebbing, A.C.; Green, M.R.; Connolly, C.P.; Carrier, D.P.; Pivarnik, J.M. Changes in collegiate ice hockey player anthropometrics and aerobic fitness over 3 decades. *Appl. Physiol. Nutr. Me.* **2018**, *43*, 950–955. [CrossRef] [PubMed]
4. Bale, J. *Landscapes of Modern Sport*; Leicester University Press: Leicester, UK, 1994.
5. Korean Olympic Committee. *Measurement and Evaluation for Selection of Young Athletes in 2016*; Korea Institute of Sport Science: Seoul, Korea, 2016.
6. Ministry of Culture. *Research Task Report on Local Sports Science 2017: From the Development of Physical Training in Each Sport*; Korea Institute of Sport Science: Seoul, Korea, 2017.
7. Kang, M.; Ragan, B.G.; Park, J.H. Issues in outcomes research: An overview of randomization techniques for clinical trials. *J. Athl. Train.* **2008**, *43*, 215–221. [CrossRef] [PubMed]
8. Harriss, D.J.; Atkinson, G. Ethical standards in sport and exercise science research: 2014 update. *Int. J. Sports Med.* **2013**, *34*, 1025–1028. [CrossRef] [PubMed]
9. Vaara, J.P.; Kyröläinen, H.; Niemi, J.; Ohrankämmen, O.; Häkkinen, A.; Kocay, S.; Häkkinen, K. Associations of maximal strength and muscular endurance test scores with cardiorespiratory fitness and body composition. *J. Strength. Cond. Res.* **2012**, *26*, 2078–2086. [CrossRef] [PubMed]
10. Serresse, O.; Ama, P.F.; Simoneau, J.A.; Lortie, G.; Bouchard, C.; Boulay, M.R. Anaerobic performances of sedentary and trained subjects. *Can. J. Sport. Sci.* **1989**, *14*, 46–52. [PubMed]
11. Häkkinen, K.; Mero, A.; Kauhanen, H. Specificity of endurance, sprint and strength training on physical performance capacity in young athletes. *J. Sports. Med. Phys. Fit.* **1989**, *29*, 27–35.
12. Buys, H. The Development of Norms and Protocols in Sports Vision Evaluations. Ph.D. Thesis, University of Johannesburg, Johannesburg, South Africa, 2002.
13. Osman, N.A.A.; Yusof, A.; Thompson, M.W.; Aboodarda, S.J.; Mokhtar, A.H. Effectiveness of an alternate hand wall toss on reaction time among archery, shooting and fencing athletes. *Indones. Malay. World.* **2010**, *38*, 161–180.
14. Shaharudin, S.; Agrawal, S. Muscle synergies during incremental rowing VO2max test of collegiate rowers and untrained subjects. *J. Sports. Med. Phys. Fit.* **2016**, *56*, 980–989.

15. Hernández, L.E.M.; Pérez, A.P.; Alvarado, A.O.; del Villar Morales, A.; Flores, V.H.; Villaseñor, C.P. Isokinetic evaluation of the muscular strength and balance of knee extensor and flexor apparatus of taekwondo athletes. *Gac. Med. Mex.* **2014**, *150*, 272–278.
16. Riechman, S.E.; Zoeller, R.F.; Balasekaran, G.; Goss, F.L.; Robertson, R.J. Prediction of 2000 m indoor rowing performance using a 30 s sprint and maximal oxygen uptake. *J. Sports. Sci.* **2002**, *20*, 681–687. [CrossRef] [PubMed]
17. Rusko, H.; Rahkila, P.; Karvinen, E. Anaerobic threshold, skeletal muscle enzymes and fiber composition in young female cross-country skiers. *Acta. Physiol. Scand.* **1980**, *108*, 263–268. [CrossRef] [PubMed]
18. Lee, G.B.; Kim, H.W. Relative significance of sports talent identification factor: Comparison of Different types of sports. *Kor. J. Meas. Eval. Phys. Edu. Sport. Sci.* **2015**, *17*, 33–46.

Publisher's Note: MDPI stays neutral with regard to jurisdictional claims in published maps and institutional affiliations.

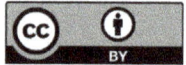

© 2020 by the authors. Licensee MDPI, Basel, Switzerland. This article is an open access article distributed under the terms and conditions of the Creative Commons Attribution (CC BY) license (http://creativecommons.org/licenses/by/4.0/).

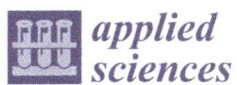

Article

Effect of Mat Pilates on Body Fluid Composition, Pelvic Stabilization, and Muscle Damage during Pregnancy

Ah-Hyun Hyun [1] and Yoo-Jeong Jeon [2],*

[1] Department of Health and Exercise Science, Korea National Sport University, 1239, Yangjae-daero, Songpa-gu, Seoul 05541, Korea; knupe838@knsu.ac.kr
[2] Department of Sports & Health Science, Hanbat National University, Yoo Seong-gu 125, Daejeon 34158, Korea
* Correspondence: jyjong20@hanbat.ac.kr

Received: 26 October 2020; Accepted: 17 December 2020; Published: 20 December 2020

Abstract: In this study, according to the exercise intensity (50–60% of HRmax (Maximum Heart Rate), RPE (Rating of Perceived Exertion: 11–13) proposed by The American Congress of Obstetricians and Gynecologists (ACOG) for pregnant women, mat Pilates exercise is related to body composition, lipid parameters, and pelvic stabilization. The effects on muscle and muscle damage were investigated. The subjects of this study were 16 pregnant women registered at the Cultural Center of Gyeonggi-do C Women's Hospital, and the gestation period was 16 to 24 weeks. The mat Pilates exercise program (twice a week, 60 min per day, total 12 weeks) changed the Pilates exercise program every 6 weeks according to the subject's pain level and physical fitness. Body composition before and after exercise, hip flexion, abduction and dilated lipids, inflammation, muscle damage, and stress hormones were measured through blood biochemical analysis. First, the difference in total body water, intracellular water, and skeletal muscle changes (post-pre) increased significantly in the Pilates exercise (PE) group compared to the control (CON) group, while the extracellular/intracellular water ratio significantly decreased. The effect of Pilates on body composition and lipid profile confirmed that, after testing, total body water (TBW), intracellular water (ICW), and extracellular water (ECW) were significantly greater than pre-test values in both groups (TBW: $z = -2.286$, $p = 0.022$, $r = 0.572$; ICW: $z = -2.818$, $p = 0.005$, $r = 0.705$; ECW: $z = -1.232$, $p = 0.218$, $r = 0.308$), whereas the ECW/ICW ratio decreased significantly only in the PE group ($z = -2.170$, $p = 0.030$, $r = 0.543$); while the increases in TBW and ICW were greater in the PE group than in the CON group, the ECW/ICW ratio decreased significantly in the PE group. Blood tests showed significant increases in body weight (BW), body fat mass (BFM), and percentage of body fat (PBF) in both groups post-test as compared to pre-test (BW: $z = -1.590$, $p = 0.112$, $r = 0.398$; BFM: $z = -0.106$, $p = 0.916$; PBF: $z = -1.643$, $p = 0.100$, $r = 0.411$). There was a slight increase in creatine kinase (CK) and lactate dehydrogenase (LDH), which are indices of muscle damage, and in the difference between the periods within the group, the CK and LDH of the CON group showed a tendency to increase significantly after inspection compared to the previous values (CK: $z = -1.700$, $p = 0.089$, $r = 0.425$, LDH: $z = -2.603$, $p = 0.009$, $r = 0.651$). Aspartate aminotransferase (AST) decreased significantly in the Pilates exercise group compared to that in the control group, and as a result of confirming the difference in the amount of change in C-reactive protein (CRP), there was no significant difference between the two groups, and the PE group showed a tendency to decrease after inspection compared to the previous period even in the difference between the periods in the group. The CON group showed an increasing trend, but no significant difference was found. Cortisol, a stress hormone, also increased significantly after inspection both groups compared to before (CON group: $z = -2.201$, $p = 0.028$; PE group: $z = -2.547$, $p = 0.011$). Therefore, the 12 week Pilates exercise program conducted in this study has a positive effect on body water balance and strengthens the muscles related to pelvic stabilization within the range of reducing muscle damage or causing muscle damage and stress in pregnant women. We think that it has an effective exercise intensity.

Keywords: exercise intensity; body composition; lactate dehydrogenase; stress hormone

Appl. Sci. **2020**, *10*, 9111; doi:10.3390/app10249111   www.mdpi.com/journal/applsci

1. Introduction

In general, pregnancy causes a variety of anatomical, physiological, and mental changes in women [1]. They experience physical changes such as low back pain, pelvic pain, and swelling due to weight gain and body shape change and feel joint pain due to spasms and hormone secretion [2]. In the latter half of pregnancy, there is the additional weight of the fetus and amniotic fluid, and women experience a great deal of physical stress and suffer from insomnia [3,4]. Consequently, failure to adapt to physical changes during pregnancy may lead to gestational depression, and the mother's mental stress has a negative effect on the fetus [5–7]. Therefore, efforts to manage the series of changes caused by pregnancy are essential. Methods such as massage, nutrition, music, and psychological counseling have been suggested to reduce the physical and mental stress of pregnant women, and the American Congress of Obstetricians and Gynecologists (ACOG) recommends physical activities, including stretching [8–10].

Participation in exercise for pregnant women is effective in managing weight, improving constipation and cardiopulmonary function, reducing neck pain, low back pain, and pelvic pain, and preventing cesarean delivery [11–13]. Exercises recommended by the ACOG include walking, swimming, and indoor cycling, and it has been established that most pregnant women choose walking as a physical activity that they can perform without burden [14–17]. However, walking has a risk of falling due to a change in the center of gravity and weight gain during pregnancy and is considered to be functionally insufficient to improve physical strength for childbirth and to reinforce weak muscle strength due to pregnancy. In addition, since the application of exercise programs that do not take into account individual characteristics and pregnancy status may negatively affect the mother or fetus, safe guidelines for exercise programs during pregnancy are essential. In this regard, it has recently been suggested that Pilates exercise is safe for pregnant women and can stimulate the muscles around the core and pelvis, and the ACOG also actively recommends Pilates exercise for pregnant women [18]. Pilates exercise has been suggested to increase muscle strength, flexibility, coordination, and pelvic stability in the form of a combination of aerobic and anaerobic exercise [19–21], it especially improves physical discomfort in pregnant women and is effective for weight control and back pain [22–25].

Previous studies on pregnant women suggested that regular Pilates improves breathing ability, muscle strength, and postural stability and is effective in improving basic physical strength such as cardiopulmonary function through whole-body exercise [25,26]. In addition, resistance exercise using props increases muscle strength and balance ability to prevent falls, increases basal metabolism, and reduces pain and fatigue at the end of pregnancy [25]. However, contradictory studies have reported that Pilates is not effective in improving the core muscles of pregnant women [27,28]. This is probably due to the lack of previous studies demonstrating the effectiveness of Pilates exercise for pregnant women and the lack of various data on the intensity and frequency of appropriate types of exercise for pregnant women [29].

Particularly, since repetitive Pilates movements and excessive muscle use in pregnant women have the potential to cause more muscle damage as well as damage to joints [30], the Pilates exercise program for pregnant women should be carefully selected. Creatine kinase (CK) is an index indicating the degree of muscle damage. The blood CK concentration of pregnant women before 34 weeks is correlated with gestational hypertension [31], and the level is high depending on the amount of activity with high exercise intensity [32,33]. Previous studies have suggested that Pilates exercise using resistance tools directly stimulates the muscles to induce muscle damage and increases CK concentration [30,31], whereas the exercise group in the 12 week yoga exercise group compared unfavorably to the control group. It was suggested that the level of inflammation markers decreased, thereby reducing inflammation [34]. As such, the different results of the CK study are due to the fact that the results of muscle injury vary greatly depending on the intensity of the exercise. In particular, studies on Pilates exercise and CK studies in pregnant women are insufficient, and additional verification is needed. Therefore, it is necessary to first evaluate the exercise experience and physical ability of the pregnant woman before pregnancy, collect the mother's information, and then divide and program the exercise intensity according to the pregnancy week. Therefore, in this study, according to the exercise guidelines proposed by the ACOG (50~60% of the maximum heart rate) and exercise awareness using the Borg Scale (11~13), 12 weeks of Pilates exercise is used [35]. The purpose of this study is to analyze the effects of body composition, lipid variables, and muscle and muscle damage related to pelvic stabilization to confirm the intensity and effect of Pilates exercise during pregnancy.

2. Materials and Methods

2.1. Participants

The subjects of this study were 16 pregnant women registered at the Cultural Center of C Women's Hospital in Gyeonggi-do, South Korea, who did not have specific diseases or receive specific medications, had no pregnancy complications, and were expected to have a normal delivery (Gestination period: 16~24 weeks, PE group: n = 9, CON group: n = 7). Prior to conducting the study, all subjects were fully aware of the prior explanations, and voluntary participation and consent were ascertained before conducting the study.

This study was a cluster-randomized controlled experiment. A total of 16 subjects were recruited to the Pilates exercise group (PE, n = 9; age: 31.78 ± 4.68 years; body weight (BW): 57.97 ± 7.91 kg; height: 160.56 ± 3.78 cm, using the block randomization method; body fat mass (BFM): 18.40 ± 4.92 g; body mass index(BMI): 39.57 ± 4.52; skeletal muscle mass (SMM): 21.10 ± 2.66 g)), and the control group participants (CON, n = 7; age: 32.00 ± 3.46 years; BW: 53.67 ± 5.70 kg; height: 161.29 ± 3.54 cm; BFM: 15.86 ± 3.06 g; BMI: 37.81 ± 3.37; SMM: 20.09 ± 2.00 g) were randomly assigned.

A comparison of the reference values between groups was performed by obtaining Cohen's r values. The research protocol was approved by the Bioethics Committee of Korea National Sports University (1263-201803-BR-001-01).

2.2. Pilates Exercise Protocols

The Pilates exercise program consisted of warm-up, main, and cool-down exercises and was conducted for 60 min per day, twice a week, for 12 weeks. The exercise intensity was set as 50–60% of maximum heart rate, as suggested by the ACOG [23], and the Borg Scale was implemented during the exercise to maintain an RPE(Rating of Perceived Exertion) of 11~13. Depending on the participants' level of pain and physical fitness, the intensity of the Pilates exercise was progressively increased every 6 weeks (Table 1).

2.3. Pelvic Stabilization Muscle Strength Test

To measure the strength of muscles involved in pelvic stabilization, hip flexion (HF), hip abduction (HA), and hip extension (HE) were measured. Considering that the participants were pregnant women, muscle strength was measured after sufficient explanation and 1–2 practice sessions. Approximately 1 min was provided for rest for each area of measurement, and a trained physical therapist made the measurements in a stable position that did not cause any pain. HF was measured using the de Groot active straight leg raising (ASLR) test method, with both hands lowered to the floor and both feet shoulder-width wide in a straight position [36]. The examiner placed a manual muscle strength tester (HOGGAN PROOF Preferred, HOGGAN HEALTH, USA) on the participant's right ankle, and the participant was asked to raise the leg being measured toward the ceiling completely to measure the muscle strength.

Table 1. Pilates exercise program.

Modes	Week	Contents	Time (min)	Reps, Set, and Rest	RPE
Warm-up	1–12	(Breathing · Static Stretching) Neck and Shoulder Stretch, Deep Breathing Leg Stretch	10		9
Main Exercise	1–6 (Level 1)	Torso Twist, Cat Cow, Kneeling Half Push-up Lying One-Leg Circles One-Leg Side Kick, Pelvic Stretch	30	8~12 reps × 3 set 20 s rest between sets	9~11
	7–12 (Level 2)	Spine Stretch, Double-Arm Circles Half Roll Down and Up, One-Leg Side Rotation Lying Leg Scissors, Donkey Kick	30	8~12 reps × 3 set 30 s rest between sets	12~13
Cool-down	1–12	(Breathing · Static Stretching) Neck and Shoulder Stretch Deep Breathing	10		9

To measure HA, the participant was asked to lie down in a lateral decubitus position with the head resting comfortably on one arm and one foot on top of the other, and the examiner placed the manual muscle strength tester on the ankle on the top. Subsequently, the participant was asked to raise the side of the hip joint completely toward the ceiling to measure the HA strength. Lastly, to measure HE, the participant was asked to stand with her legs shoulder-width apart while placing her hands on the wall. The examiner placed the manual muscle strength tester on the participant's right ankle, and the participant was asked to completely raise the right leg posteriorly to measure the HE strength. Three measurements were made for all variables, and the mean of the measurements was used for analysis. The unit of measurement was 0.45 kg, and the margin of error was ±1%.

2.4. Body Composition

BW, total body water (TBW), intracellular water (ICW), extracellular water (ECW), body fat mass (BFM), percent body fat (%BF), and skeletal muscle mass (SMM) were measured using eight-polar bioelectrical impedance analysis (BIA) with multiple impedance frequencies (Inbody 770, Biospace Co., Seoul, Korea). All participants were allowed to limit food intake and empty their bladder 4 h before measurement according to the instructions of the manufacturer. After that, it was measured using a fatness measuring system (Dong-Sahn Jenix, Korea). Each participant stood with her soles in contact with the foot electrodes and grabbed the hand electrodes, wearing light clothing and removing all metal items to ensure accurate body composition measurement.

2.5. Blood Collection and Biochemical Analyses

Blood samples were drawn from the antecubital vein via multiple venipunctures for the determination of Ferritin; HbA1c; cortisol; lipid-related markers, such as total triglycerides (TG), total cholesterol (TC), high-density lipoprotein (HDL), low-density lipoprotein (LDL); and muscle damage markers such as creatine kinase (CK), lactate dehydrogenase (LDH), C-reactive protein (CRP), and aspartate aminotransferase (AST). Blood samples were taken 12 h before and 12 h after the 12week intervention period and frozen at −80 °C to prevent denaturation and ensure stability of all analytes stored in a deep freezer (Nihon Freezer Co., Japan, VT-208) until analysis. All the assays were carried out according to the instructions of the manufacturers.

2.6. Statistical Analysis

SPSS 24.0 was used to analyze the pre- and post-test differences in body composition, strength of muscles involved in pelvic stabilization, and muscle damage markers after Pilates exercise. Due to the small sample size for the measured variables, normal distribution could not be assumed for the variables; therefore, all statistical analyses were conducted through non-parametric tests. For between-group differences, the differences in mean (the post-test mean minus the pre-test mean) obtained through change-score analysis were analyzed through Mann–Whitney U test, and within-group differences were analyzed through Wilcoxon signed-rank test. All statistics are presented as mean and standard deviation, and the level of significance for statistical analysis was set as $\alpha < 0.05$.

3. Results

3.1. Effect of Pilates on the Body Compositions and Lipid Profiles

In this study, confirmed post-test TBW, ICW, and ECW were significantly greater than pre-test values in both groups (TBW: $z = -2.286$, $p = 0.022$, $r = 0.572$; ICW: $z = -2.818$, $p = 0.005$, $r = 0.705$; ECW: $z = -1.232$, $p = 0.218$, $r = 0.308$; Table 2), whereas the ECW/ICW ratio decreased significantly only in the Pilates exercise (PE) group ($z = -2.170$, $p = 0.030$, $r = 0.543$; Table 2). While the increases in TBW and ICW were greater in the PE group than in the control (CON) group, the ECW/ICW ratio decreased significantly in the PE group.

Table 2. Body composition.

	Pilates (n = 9)		CON (n = 7)		Diff (Post-Pre)		
	Pre	Post	Pre	Post	z	p	Cohen's r
BW (kg)	57.98 ± 7.91	64.01 ± 7.76 **	53.67 ± 5.70	58.37 ± 5.65 *	−1.590	0.112	0.398
TBW (L) #	28.97 ± 3.33	31.59 ± 3.50 **	27.63 ± 2.45	29.26 ± 2.84 *	−2.286	0.022	0.572
ICW (L) ##	17.71 ± 2.06	19.54 ± 2.12 **	16.90 ± 1.54	17.99 ± 1.66 *	−2.818	0.005	0.705
ECW (L)	11.26 ± 1.28	12.04 ± 1.39 **	10.73 ± 0.92	11.27 ± 1.18 *	−1.232	0.218	0.308
ECW/ICW ratio #	0.64 ± 0.01	0.62 ± 0.01 *	0.64 ± 0.01	0.63 ± 0.01	−2.170	0.030	0.543
BFM (kg)	18.40 ± 4.92	20.70 ± 5.04 **	15.86 ± 3.06	18.30 ± 3.06 *	−0.106	0.916	0.027
PBF (%)	22.50 ± 3.15	24.84 ± 3.02 **	20.59 ± 1.64	22.41 ± 1.67 *	−1.643	0.100	0.411
SMM (kg) ##	21.10 ± 2.66	23.49 ± 2.76 **	20.09 ± 2.00	21.41 ± 2.18 *	−2.811	0.005	0.703

BW: body weight, TBW: total body water, ICW: intracellular water, ECW: extracellular water, ECW/ICW: ECW to ICW ratio, BFM: body fat mass, PBF: percentage of body fat, SMM: skeletal muscle mass. Diff (post − pre): difference change from pre to post between groups. * $p < 0.05$, ** $p < 0.01$ from pre and post. # $p < 0.05$, ## $p < 0.01$ change (post − pre) between groups. Values are presented as mean ± SD.

Blood tests showed significant increases in BW, BFM, and PBF in both groups post-test as compared to pre-test (BW: $z = -1.590$, $p = 0.112$, $r = 0.398$; BFM: $z = -0.106$, $p = 0.916$; PBF: $z = -1.643$, $p = 0.100$, $r = 0.411$; Table 2). Significant post-test increases in TG, TC, and LDL were also observed when compared to pre-test values (TG: $z = -0.106$, $p = 0.916$, $r = 0.027$; TC: $z = -1.059$, $p = 0.289$, $r = 0.265$; LDL: $z = -1.272$, $p = 0.203$, $r = 0.318$; HbA1a: $z = -0.530$, $p = 0.596$, $r = 0.133$; Table 3). In contrast, ferritin decreased significantly in both groups (Ferritin: $z = -0.530$, $p = 0.596$, $r = 0.133$) (Table 3).

3.2. Effect of Pilates on the Pelvic Stabilization Muscle Strength

In this study, we confirmed pre-test and post-test HF, HA, and HS. When changes in HF, HA, and HS were analyzed, they were found to have increased significantly in the PE group when compared to the CON group (HF: $z = -3.037$, $p = 0.002$, HA: $z = -3.344$, $p = 0.001$, HS: $z = -2.595$, $p = 0.009$; Figure 1A–C). Moreover, in terms of within-group differences, all measurements increased significantly post-test compared to the pre-test measurements in the PE group (HF: $z = -2.371$, $p = 0.018$; HA: $z = -2.670$, $p = 0.008$; HS: $z = -2.192$, $p = 0.028$), whereas only HA decreased significantly post-test in the CON group ($z = -2.375$, $p = 0.018$).

Table 3. Lipid profiles.

	Pilates (n = 9)		CON (n = 7)		Diff (Post-Pre)		
	Pre	Post	Pre	Post	z	p	Cohen's r
TG (kg)	140.67 ± 35.25	201.56 ± 54.24 **	141.00 ± 38.59	205.86 ± 48.46 *	−0.106	0.916	0.027
TC (mg/dL)	220.33 ± 27.00	236.56 ± 25.93 *	222.14 ± 28.54	248.29 ± 38.10 *	−1.059	0.289	0.265
HDL (mg/dL)	92.56 ± 11.67	90.11 ± 12.67	89.57 ± 13.62	85.00 ± 18.91	−0.638	0.524	0.160
LDL (mg/dL)	110.67 ± 26.17	135.78 ± 25.25 *	115.00 ± 18.06	152.00 ± 31.25 *	−1.272	0.203	0.318
HbA1c (%)	4.91 ± 0.18	5.13 ± 0.21 *	4.91 ± 0.15	5.14 ± 0.15 *	−0.108	0.914	0.027
Ferritin (ng/mL)	55.44 ± 49.27	23.11 ± 11.41 *	34.14 ± 6.72	16.57 ± 8.89 *	−0.530	0.596	0.133

Values are means ± SD. Main time effect: * $p < 0.05$ and ** $p < 0.01$ from pre and post. TC: total cholesterol, TG: triglycerides, LDL: low-density lipoprotein, HDL: high-density lipoprotein, HbA1c: hemoglobin A1c. Diff (post − pre): difference change from pre to post between groups. Values are presented as mean ± SD.

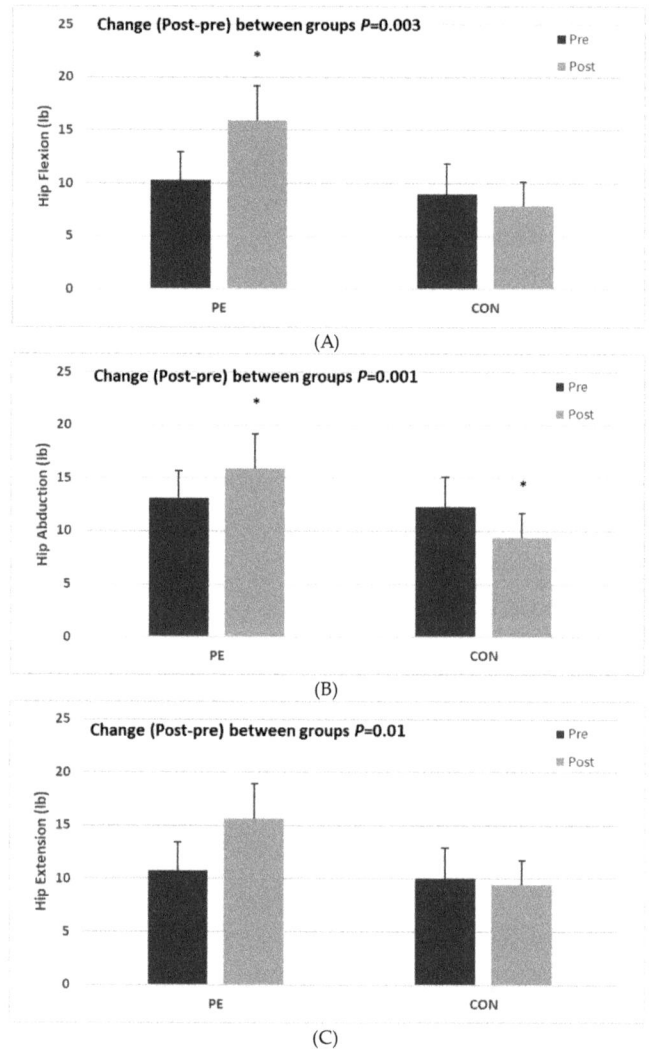

Figure 1. Effect of Pilates exercise on back pain-related muscle strength, (**A**) Hip flexion, (**B**) Hip abduction, and (**C**) Hip extension following 12 weeks of Pilates exercise. Bars represent mean ± SD (PE: n = 9, CON: 7, per group). * $p < 0.05$ from Pre to Post. PE: Pilates exercise group, CON: control group.

3.3. Muscle Damage and Stress Markers

In this study, the difference between CK and lactate dehydrogenase (LDH) changes was found to increase slightly in the PE group compared to that in the CON group (Table 4). In addition, differences in timing within the group indicated a significant post-test increase in CK and LDH for the CON group compared to that in the PE group (CK: $z = -1.700$, $p = 0.089$, $r = 0.425$; LDH: $z = -2.603$, $p = 0.009$, $r = 0.651$). AST changes were shown to have significantly decreased in the PE group compared to in the CON group (AST: $z = -2.566$, $p = 0.010$, $r = 0.642$) and showed a significant post-test increase in terms of timing in the CON group only. The difference in the amount of change in CRP, an indicator of inflammation, was not significant between the two groups (CRP: $z = -1.230$, $p = 0.219$, $r = 0.308$). Even in differences in timing within a group, PE groups tended to decrease after exercise compared to dictionaries, while CON groups tended to increase but with no significant differences (Table 4). The stress hormone cortisol also showed a significant post-test increase in both groups compared to the standard levels (cortisol: $z = -2.547$, $p = 0.011$, $r = 0.636$) (Figure 2), but there was no significant difference in the variation between the two groups.

Table 4. Muscle damage and inflammation marker.

	Pilates (n = 9)		CON (n = 7)		Diff (Post − Pre)		
	Pre	Post	Pre	Post	z	p	Cohen's r
CK (U/L)	34.78 ± 8.66	42.22 ± 13.15	39.57 ± 16.06	59.43 ± 27.72 **	−1.700	0.089	0.425
LDH (U/L) ##	159.00 ± 15.67	159.78 ± 15.09	162.29 ± 21.40	186.57 ± 26.79 **	−2.603	0.009	0.651
AST (U/L) #	20.22 ± 6.32	17.78 ± 5.02	14.71 ± 4.11	16.29 ± 4.03 *	−2.566	0.010	0.642
CRP (mg/L)	0.25 ± 0.20	0.24 ± 0.23	0.10 ± 0.07	0.10 ± 0.06	−1.230	0.219	0.308

Values are means ± SD. Main time effect: * $p < 0.05$ and ** $p < 0.01$ pre- versus post-Pilates period in the between groups. CK: creatine kinase, LDH: lactate dehydrogenase, AST: aspartate aminotransferase, CRP: C-reactive protein. * $p < 0.05$ from pre and post. # $p < 0.05$, ## $p < 0.01$ change (post − pre) between groups. Diff (post − pre): difference change from pre to post between groups. Values are presented as mean ± SD.

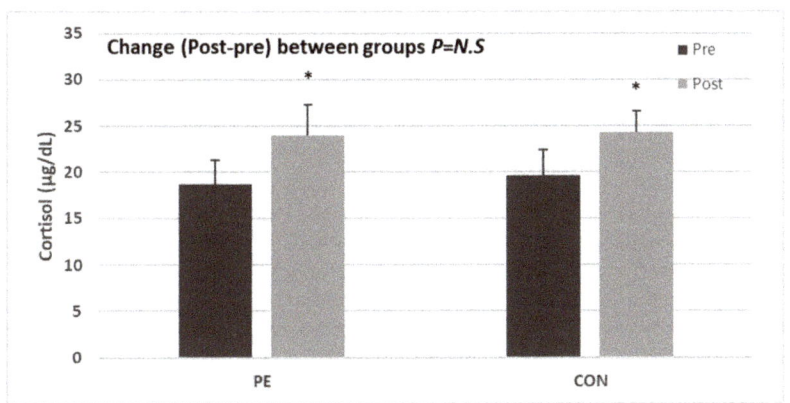

Figure 2. Effect of Pilates exercise on cortisol hormone level, bars represent mean ± SD (PE: n = 9, CON: 7, per group). * $p < 0.05$ from Pre to Post. PE: Pilates exercise group, CON: control group.

4. Discussion

4.1. Effect of Pilates on Body Compositions and Lipid Profiles

In general, as the number of weeks of pregnancy increases, most mothers have an imbalance in body fat and blood lipid metabolism, which can lead to hyperlipidemia and ischemic heart disease in the mother, so continuous management is required during pregnancy. In addition, sudden weight gain after pregnancy causes gestational hypertension and diabetes and negatively affects the microbial environment in the intestine, leading to postpartum obesity [25,37]. Gestational edema, another characteristic that pregnant women experience, not only causes discomfort and pain but also decreases the growth of the fetus in the uterus and is deeply related to gestational hypertension [38].

In general, body hydration increases as the number of gestational weeks increases, and in particular, an increase in ECW causes edema [39]. The ACOG [40] reported an increase in ECW during pregnancy and that ECW and the ECW/ICW ratio are significantly higher in pregnant women with pre-eclampsia. Similarly, in this study, both groups significantly increased post TBW, ICW, and ECW compared to the standard values, while the ECW/ICW ratio decreased significantly only in the PE group.

Interestingly, the difference between TBW and ICW changes in the PE group was found to have increased over that in the CON group, while the ECW/ICW ratio was significantly reduced. These results may be thought to be partially mitigated by the increased rate of ECW that occurs during pregnancy and have shown some consistent results, with prior studies reporting a decrease in edema through Pilates exercise in cancer patients [41]. Moreover, the finding that Pilates exercise led to partial decreases in the ECW/ICW ratio, which increases in pre-eclampsia, suggests that Pilates exercise could be effective in relieving not only edema but also edema-induced gestational hypertension. On the other hand, since the increase in ICW shows a positive correlation with muscle mass [42], as a result of checking the SMM in this study, it was found that all groups significantly increased muscle mass after exercise compared to before (CON group: SMM: $z = -2.371$, $p = 0.018$, PE group: SMM: $z = -2.670$, $p = 0.008$; Table 2), which is thought to be due to the increase in SMM as part of the weight gain. In the difference in the amount of change in SMM, the PE group showed a significant increase compared to the CON group, and the results were consistent with previous studies that reported an increase in skeletal muscle after Pilates exercise [43,44]. In addition, the same result was obtained by a study showing that the group who did Pilates exercise for 8 weeks for pregnant women increased grip strength [45] and that symptoms of urinary incontinence, which are common in pregnant women, were more effectively reduced in the Pilates exercise group than in Kegel exercise one [46].

It is believed that static and dynamic Pilates movements of contraction and relaxation induce skeletal muscle increase, and this is thought to be a result partially supporting the significantly increased ICW level in the PE group presented above. Many previous studies reported that Pilates exercise reduced body fat and had a positive effect on blood lipid metabolism [25,26]. The increased body fat and blood lipid index during pregnancy may be partially reduced through Pilates exercise. In a study related to lipid indicators in pregnant women, Elena Rita [45] suggested that participation in Pilates exercise by overweight and obese pregnant women reduces the risk of diabetes and requires aerobic exercise to prevent weight gain. However, in this study, there was no significant difference in the amount of change (post − pre) between the PE group and the CON group. These results suggest that the subjects of this study were not overweight or obese pregnant women who could benefit from exercise intervention via an advantage in blood index [47] and that there were few statistically significant changes, including those with normal BMI levels. In addition, some studies examining the effect of exercise participation on the prevention of gestational diabetes regardless of obesity have shown contradictory results. The different results of several clinical studies related to pregnant women are probably due to the fact that the subjects participating in this study are pregnant women who have no choice but to show an imbalance in lipid metabolism, which is highly related to increased body fat, unlike the case in the general population. Therefore, in future studies, there seems to be a need for a more randomized trial on the type, intensity, and duration of exercise in preventing GDM (Gestational Diabetes Mellitus) [48].

4.2. Effect of Pilates on the Pelvic Stabilization Muscle Strength

During pregnancy, the anterior tilt of the pelvis disrupts the alignment of the spine and destabilizes the surrounding muscles, resulting in low back pain and pelvic pain [49,50]. Therefore, in order to alleviate the low back pain that occurs in most pregnant women, it is necessary to strengthen the muscles of the back and stabilize the hip joint [25]. Since Pilates exercise is known to induce movement of the core muscles around the waist to improve the function of the muscles related to low back pain [51], it can be predicted that there will be a difference in the amount of change in HF, HA, and HS before and after. According to a previous study, in a randomized clinical trial in pregnant women, after 8 weeks of Pilates exercise, low back pain in pregnant women was significantly reduced, grip strength and lower limb flexibility increased, and spinal curvature was significantly improved [52]. As a result of confirming the difference in the amount of change in HF, HA, and HS before and after exercise in this study, it was found that it was significantly increased in the PE group compared to that in the CON group. These results suggest that the Pilates exercise program consists of movements that stimulate the core muscles related to pelvic stabilization, and as a result, muscle strength is thought to have increased. The results were similar to those of previous studies that reported improvement of hip function and muscle strength after Pilates exercise [53,54]. It is worth noting that the ASLR test was used for pregnant women. It reported a very high correlation with back pain, pelvic pain, and muscle function of load transfer over the pelvic reaction in pregnant women, presented as indicators of indirect confirmation of pain in pregnant women. It has also been reported that the decrease in ASLR is related to the deterioration of pelvic basal muscle function, which is important for childbirth and postpartum recovery [55].

Thus, Pilates is thought to be effective in decreasing or relieving low back pain commonly observed in pregnant women, as it increases the strength of muscles related to pelvic stabilization. However, some previous studies have reported no changes in core muscle strength in pregnant women after Pilates exercise. As mentioned earlier, the exacts effects would differ depending on the type, intensity, and duration of Pilates exercise; therefore, more studies are required to confirm the exact efficacy of Pilates.

4.3. Muscle Damage and Stress Markers

Since an increase in abdominal load due to fetal development causes pelvic pain, muscle stiffness, and a vicious cycle of body imbalance, inflammation and muscle damage are caused, and various methods have been used to reduce inflammation and muscle damage [56,57]. In particular, Pilates exercise is used as rehabilitation to treat or prevent inflammation and muscle damage by repeating muscle contraction and relaxation [56]. However, rather than the general public, the subjects who participated in this study were all pregnant women, and accurate information on the intensity of Pilates exercise is not yet known. Therefore, although in this study the activity of muscles related to body water balance and pelvic stabilization was shown by setting the intensity of Pilates exercise based on ACOG guidelines, the Pilates exercise program and intensity may prevent muscle damage and increased stress due to excessive and repetitive movements. Therefore, the muscle damage index and the stress index confirmed the Pilates efficiency applied in this study.

CK is a biochemical indicator of muscle damage that is present in muscle in large quantities and has a high correlation with the type of exercise and intensity, time, and quantity [32,33]. Furthermore, LDH, a representative muscle damage marker, is a result of muscle damage due to excessive exercise. It is known to increase with exercise intensity [58–60]. Interestingly, in the results of this study, CK and LDH between the periods within the group showed a tendency to increase significantly after the period compared to before (CK: $z = -1.700$, $p = 0.089$, $r = 0.425$; LDH: $z = -2.603$, $p = 0.009$, $r = 0.651$). AST, another indicator of muscle damage, is generally used as an indicator of liver damage, but is known to increase after muscle injury according to some studies [59,60]. As a result of confirming the difference in the amount of AST change in this study, similar to LDH, it was found to be significantly reduced in the PE group compared to in the CON group (Table 4), and in the difference between the periods within the group, only the CON group was significant compared with the before and after. It showed a tendency to increase. Previous studies have shown that these results may differ depending on the type of exercise, the degree of muscle contraction, and physical overload in the muscle damage of the human body [60], whereas these results show that the muscle damage that occurs during pregnancy is partially reduced by Pilates. It is believed that the Pilates program conducted in this study improved muscle strength within the range that did not cause muscle damage.

Changes in body shape during pregnancy and pain such as low back pain induce stress in the tissues of cells, increasing the level of stress hormones along with inflammation [61]. In this study, as a result of confirming the difference in the amount of change in CRP, which is an inflammatory indicator that increases due to non-specific stress in the human body, there was no significant difference between the two groups. The CON group showed an increasing tendency, but there was no significant difference (Table 4). In addition, the stress hormone cortisol also increased significantly after in both groups compared to before (CON group: $z = -2.201$, $p = 0.028$; PE group: $z = -2.547$, $p = 0.011$; Figure 2); there was no significant difference in the amount of change between the two groups. This is believed to be due to the inevitable physiological changes that occur during pregnancy, and since there are various factors that cause inflammation and stress, further research is necessary. Furthermore, the small number of subjects who participated in this study seem to be insufficient to generalize the results. Recently, the fertility rate in South Korea has continued to decline, and there has been great difficulty in securing subjects to participate in studies. If more subjects are selected and studied in the future, it is expected that the effect of Pilates could be confirmed more concretely and scientifically.

5. Conclusions

This study confirmed the effects of 12 weeks of Pilates exercise on body composition, lipid metabolism, and pelvic stabilization-related muscle and muscle damage in pregnant women. Pilates exercise has been shown to improve body water balance and increase skeletal muscle. In addition, HF, HA, and HS, which affect muscles related to low back pain and pelvic stabilization, were improved through Pilates, while the index of muscle damage that could be increased by pregnancy was decreased. Therefore, Pilates exercise at the intensity conducted in this study is considered to be an effective and safe exercise that can strengthen the muscles related to pelvic stabilization within a range that does not cause muscle damage and stress in pregnant women.

6. Ethics Approval and Informed Consent

The research protocol was approved by the Bioethics Committee of Korea National Sports University (1263-201803-BR-001-01).

Author Contributions: Conceptualization, A.-H.H.; data curation, A.-H.H.; formal analysis, A.-H.H.; writing—original draft, A.-H.H.; project administration, Y.-J.J.; supervision, Y.-J.J.; validation, Y.-J.J.; writing—review and editing, Y.-J.J. All authors acknowledged responsibility for the full content of the submitted manuscript and approved their submission. All authors have read and agreed to the published version of the manuscript.

Funding: This research received no external funding.

Conflicts of Interest: The authors declare no conflict of interest.

References

1. Dastenaei, B.M.; Aein, F.; Safdari, F.; Karimiankakolaki, Z. Designing an intervention program over the effects of Pilates on pregnancy outcomes among the pregnant women: A protocol study. *Int. J. Surg. Protoc.* **2020**, *24*, 27–30. [CrossRef] [PubMed]
2. Santos-Rocha, R.; Branco, M.; Aguiar, L.; Vieira, F.; Veloso, A.P. Biomechanical Adaptations of Gait in Pregnancy: Implications for Physical Activity and Exercise. In *Exercise and Sporting Activity During Pregnancy*; Springer: Cham, Switzerland, 2019; pp. 95–134. [CrossRef]
3. Güder, D.S.; Yalvaç, M.; Vural, G. The effect of pregnancy Pilates-assisted childbirth preparation training on childbirth fear and neonatal outcomes: A quasi-experimental/quantitative research. *Qual. Quant.* **2018**, *52*, 2667–2679. [CrossRef]

4. Barakat, R.; Pelaez, M.; Cordero, Y.; Perales, M.; Lopez, C.; Coteron, J.; Mottola, M.F. Exercise during pregnancy protects against hypertension and macrosomia: Randomized clinical trial. *Am. J. Obs. Gynecol.* **2016**, *214*, 649.e1–649.e8. [CrossRef] [PubMed]
5. Coll, C.D.V.N.; Domingues, M.R.; Stein, A.; Da Silva, B.G.C.; Bassani, D.G.; Hartwig, F.P.; Da Silva, I.C.M.; Da Silveira, M.F.; Da Silva, S.G.; Bertoldi, A.D. Efficacy of regular exercise during pregnancy on the prevention of postpartum depression: The PAMELA randomized clinical trial. *JAMA Netw. Open* **2019**, *2*, e186861. [CrossRef] [PubMed]
6. Virgara, R.; Maher, C.; Van Kessel, G. The comorbidity of low back pelvic pain and risk of depression and anxiety in pregnancy in primiparous women. *BMC Pregnancy Childbirth* **2018**, *18*, 288. [CrossRef] [PubMed]
7. Cakmak, B.; Inanir, A.; Nacar, M.C.; Filiz, B. The effect of maternity support belts on postural balance in pregnancy. *PM&R* **2014**, *6*, 624–628. [CrossRef]
8. O'Hair, B.C.M.; Armstrong, M.K.; Rutherford, H.J. The potential utility for massage therapy during pregnancy to decrease stress and tobacco use. *Int. J. Massage Bodyw. Res. Educ. Pract.* **2018**, *11*, 15–19. [CrossRef]
9. Mparmpakas, D.; Goumenou, A.; Zachariades, E.; Pados, G.; Gidron, Y.; Karteris, E. Immune system function, stress, exercise and nutrition profile can affect pregnancy outcome: Lessons from a Mediterranean cohort. *Exp. Med.* **2013**, *5*, 411–418. [CrossRef]
10. Van Willenswaard, K.C.; Lynn, F.; McNeill, J.; McQueen, K.; Dennis, C.-L.; Lobel, M.; Alderdice, F. Music interventions to reduce stress and anxiety in pregnancy: A systematic review and meta-analysis. *BMC Psychiatry* **2017**, *17*, 271. [CrossRef]
11. Schmidt, F.M.D.; Fiorini, G.P.; Ramires, V.R.R. Psychoanalytic psychotherapy and the pregnant therapist: A literature review. *Res. Psychother. Psychopathol. Process. Outcome* **2015**, *18*. [CrossRef]
12. Khafagy, G.M.; Gamal, M.G.; El-Rafie, M.M. Effect of aerobic exercise during pregnancy on antenatal depression. *Int. J. Womens Health* **2016**, *8*, 53–57. [CrossRef] [PubMed]
13. Davenport, M.H.; Marchand, A.-A.; Mottola, M.F.; Poitras, V.J.; E Gray, C.; Garcia, A.J.; Barrowman, N.; Sobierajski, F.; James, M.; Meah, V.L.; et al. Exercise for the prevention and treatment of low back, pelvic girdle and lumbopelvic pain during pregnancy: A systematic review and meta-analysis. *Br. J. Sports Med.* **2019**, *53*, 90–98. [CrossRef] [PubMed]
14. Fieril, K.P.; Glantz, A.; Olsén, M.F. The efficacy of moderate-to-vigorous resistance exercise during pregnancy: A randomized controlled trial. *Acta Obs. Gynecol. Scand.* **2015**, *94*, 35–42. [CrossRef] [PubMed]
15. Perales, M.; Santos-Lozano, A.; Ruiz, J.R.; Lucia, A.; Barakat, R. Benefits of aerobic or resistance training during pregnancy on maternal health and perinatal outcomes: A systematic review. *Early Hum. Dev.* **2016**, *94*, 43–48. [CrossRef] [PubMed]
16. Nascimento, S.L.; Surita, F.G.; Godoy, A.C.; Kasawara, K.T.; Morais, S.S. Physical activity patterns and factors related to exercise during pregnancy: A cross sectional study. *PLoS ONE* **2015**, *10*, e0128953. [CrossRef]
17. Muller, A.; Hammill, H.V.; Hermann, C. The effects of Pilates and progressive muscle relaxation therapy on maternal stress and anxiety: A literature review. *Int. J. Humanit. Soc. Sci.* **2016**, *6*, 195–203.
18. Hyun, A.-H.; Cho, J.-Y. Effects of 12-weeks Pilates mat exercise on body composition, delivery confidence, and neck disability index in pregnant women. *Sports Sci.* **2019**, *36*, 43–55. [CrossRef]
19. Wells, C.; Kolt, G.S.; Bialocerkowski, A. Defining Pilates exercise: A systematic review. *Complement. Med.* **2012**, *20*, 253–262. [CrossRef]
20. Patti, A.; Bianco, A.; Paoli, A.; Messina, G.; Montalto, M.-A.; Bellafiore, M.; Battaglia, G.; Iovane, A.; Palma, A. Effects of Pilates exercise programs in people with chronic low back pain: A systematic review. *Medicine* **2015**, *94*, e383. [CrossRef]
21. Cruz-Ferreira, A.; Fernandes, J.; Kuo, Y.-L.; Bernardo, L.M.; Fernandes, O.; Laranjo, L.; Silva, A. Does Pilates-based exercise improve postural alignment in adult women? *Women Health* **2013**, *53*, 597–611. [CrossRef]
22. Panhan, A.C.; Gonçalves, M.; Eltz, G.D.; Villalba, M.M.; Cardozo, A.C.; Bérzin, F. Neuromuscular efficiency of the multifidus muscle in pilates practitioners and non-practitioners. *Complement. Med.* **2018**, *40*, 61–63. [CrossRef] [PubMed]
23. Fayh, A.; Brodt, G.A.; Souza, C.; Loss, J.F. Pilates instruction affects stability and muscle recruitment during the long stretch exercise. *J. Bodyw. Mov. Ther.* **2018**, *22*, 471–475. [CrossRef] [PubMed]
24. Zhou, L.; Xiao, X. The role of gut microbiota in the effects of maternal obesity during pregnancy on offspring metabolism. *Biosci. Rep.* **2018**, *27*, 38. [CrossRef] [PubMed]

25. Mazzarino, M.; Kerr, D.; Morris, M.E. Pilates program design and health benefits for pregnant women: A practitioners' survey. *J. Bodyw. Mov. Ther.* **2018**, *22*, 411–417. [CrossRef] [PubMed]
26. Martin, A.C.; Alvares,, R.F.; Nascimento, T.R.; Paranaiba, S.S.W.; Da Silva-Morais, T.K. Pilates for pregnant women: A healthy alternative. *J. Womens Health Care* **2017**, *6*, 2167. [CrossRef]
27. Bo, K.; Herbert, R.D. There is not yet strong evidence that exercise regimens other than pelvic floor muscle training can reduce stress urinary incontinence in women: A systematic review. *J. Physiother.* **2013**, *59*, 159–168. [CrossRef]
28. Coleman, T.J.; Nygaard, I.E.; Holder, D.N.; Egger, M.J.; Hitchcock, R. Intra-abdominal pressure during Pilates: Unlikely to cause pelvic floor harm. *Int. Urogynecol. J.* **2015**, *26*, 1123–1130. [CrossRef]
29. Mazzarino, M.; Kerr, D.; Wajswelner, H.; Morris, M.E. Pilates Method for Women's Health: Systematic Review of Randomized Controlled Trials. *Arch. Phys. Med. Rehabil.* **2015**, *96*, 2231–2242. [CrossRef]
30. Kim, H.-J.; Kim, J.; Kim, C.S. The effects of Pilates exercise on lipid metabolism and inflammatory cytokines mRNA expression in female undergraduates. *J. Exerc. Nutr. Biochem.* **2014**, *18*, 267–275. [CrossRef]
31. Horjus, D.L.; Bokslag, A.; Hutten, B.A.; Born, B.-J.H.V.D.; Middeldorp, S.; Vrijkotte, T.G. Creatine kinase is associated with blood pressure during pregnancy. *J. Hypertens.* **2019**, *37*, 1467–1474. [CrossRef]
32. Pedersen, E.S.; Tengesdal, S.; Radtke, M.; Langlo, K.A.R.; Radke, M.; Rise, K.A.L. Major increase in creatine kinase after intensive exercise. *Tidsskrift for den Norske Laegeforening: Tidsskrift for Praktisk Medicin, ny Raekke* **2019**, *139*. [CrossRef]
33. Dos Santos, J.M.; Filho, L.F.S.; Carvalho, V.O.; Wichi, R.B.; De Oliveira, E.D. Hemodynamic and creatine kinase changes after a 12-week equipment-based Pilates. A training program in hypertensive women. *J. Bodyw. Mov. Ther.* **2020**, *24*, 496–502. [CrossRef] [PubMed]
34. Ha, M.-S.; Baek, Y.-H.; Kim, J.-W.; Kim, D.-Y. Effects of yoga exercise on maximum oxygen uptake, cortisol level, and creatine kinase myocardial bond activity in female patients with skeletal muscle pain syndrome. *J. Phys. Sci.* **2015**, *27*, 1451–1453. [CrossRef] [PubMed]
35. ACOG. Physical activity and exercise during pregnancy and the postpartum period: ACOG Committee Opinion No. 650. *Obstet. Gynecol.* **2015**, *126*, e1326–e1327. [CrossRef] [PubMed]
36. De Groot, M.; Pool-Goudzwaard, A.; Spoor, C.; Snijders, C. The active straight leg raising test (ASLR) in pregnant women: Differences in muscle activity and force between patients and healthy subjects. *Man Ther.* **2008**, *13*, 68–74. [CrossRef]
37. Amirsasan, R.; Dolgarisharaf, R. Pilates training preventive effects of metabolic syndrome in sedentary overweight females. *Int. J. Sport Stud.* **2015**, *5*, 596–602.
38. Levario-Carrillo, M.; Avitia, M.; Tufiño-Olivares, E.; Trevizo, E.; Corral-Terrazas, M.; Reza-López, S. Body composition of patients with hypertensive complications during pregnancy. *Hypertens. Pregnancy* **2006**, *25*, 259–269. [CrossRef]
39. Duvekot, J.J.; Peeters, L.L. Maternal cardiovascular hemodynamic adaptation to pregnancy. *Obs. Gynecol. Surv.* **1994**, *49*, S1–S14. [CrossRef]
40. Staelens, A.S.; Vonck, S.; Molenberghs, G.; Malbrain, M.L.; Gyselaers, W. Maternal body fluid composition in uncomplicated pregnancies and preeclampsia: A bioelectrical impedance analysis. *Eur. J. Obs. Gynecol. Reprod. Biol.* **2016**, *204*, 69–73. [CrossRef]
41. Ergun, M.; Eyigor, S.; Karaca, B.; Kisim, A.; Uslu, R. Effects of exercise on angiogenesis and apoptosis-related molecules, quality of life, fatigue and depression in breast cancer patients. *Eur. J. Cancer Care* **2013**, *22*, 626–637. [CrossRef]
42. Yoshida, T.; Yamada, Y.; Tanaka, F.; Yamagishi, T.; Shibata, S.; Kawakami, Y. Intracellular-to-total water ratio explains the variability of muscle strength dependence on the size of the lower leg in the elderly. *Exp. Gerontol.* **2018**, *113*, 120–127. [CrossRef] [PubMed]
43. Lee, H.T.; Oh, H.O.; Han, H.S.; Jin, K.Y.; Roh, H.L. Effect of mat pilates exercise on postural alignment and body composition of middle-aged women. *J. Phys. Sci.* **2016**, *28*, 1691–1695. [CrossRef] [PubMed]
44. Queiroz, L.C.S.; Bertolini, S.M.M.G.; Bennemann, R.M.; Silva, E.S. The effect Mat Pilates practice on muscle mass in elderly women. *Rev. Rene* **2016**, *17*, 618. [CrossRef]
45. Magro-Malosso, E.R.; Saccone, G.; Di Mascio, D.; Di Tommaso, M.; Berghella, V. Exercise during pregnancy and risk of preterm birth in overweight and obese women: A systematic review and meta-analysis of randomized controlled trials. *Acta Obs. Gynecol. Scand.* **2017**, *96*, 263–273. [CrossRef]

46. Pavithralochani, V.; Thangavignesh, R.; Saranya, P.; Ramanathan, K. Efficacy of Kegel's Exercise vs Pilates in Subject with Urinary Incontinence during Pregnancy. *Res. J. Pharm. Technol.* **2019**, *12*, 5943. [CrossRef]
47. Du, M.; Ouyang, Y.-Q.; Nie, X.; Huang, Y.; Redding, S.R. Effects of physical exercise during pregnancy on maternal and infant outcomes in overweight and obese pregnant women: A meta-analysis. *Birth* **2018**, *46*, 211–221. [CrossRef]
48. Fatemeh, N.; Sepidarkish, M.; Shirvani, M.A.; Habibipour, P.; Tabari, N.S.M. The effect of exercise on the prevention of gestational diabetes in obese and overweight pregnant women: A systematic review and meta-analysis. *Diabetol. Metab. Syndr.* **2019**, *11*, 72.
49. Bogaert, J.; Stack, M.; Partington, S.; Marceca, J.; Tremback-Ball, A. The effects of stabilization exercise on low back pain and pelvic girdle pain in pregnant women. *Ann. Phys. Rehabil. Med.* **2018**, *61*, e157–e158. [CrossRef]
50. Pascoal, G.A.; Stuge, B.; Mota, P.; Hilde, G.; Bø, K. Therapeutic Exercise Regarding Musculoskeletal Health of the Pregnant Exerciser and Athlete. In *Exercise and Sporting Activity During Pregnancy*; Springer Science and Business Media LLC: Berlin, Germany, 2019; pp. 309–326.
51. Rodríguez-Díaz, L.; Ruiz-Frutos, C.; Vázquez-Lara, J.M.; Ramírez-Rodrigo, J.; Villaverde-Gutiérrez, C.; Torres-Luque, G. Effectiveness of a physical activity programme based on the Pilates method in pregnancy and labour. *Enferm. Clín.* **2017**, *27*, 271–277. [CrossRef]
52. Oktaviani, I. Pilates workouts can reduce pain in pregnant women. *Complement. Clin. Pract.* **2018**, *31*, 349–351. [CrossRef]
53. Phrompaet, S.; Paungmali, A.; Pirunsan, U.; Sitilertpisan, P. Effects of Pilates training on lumbo-pelvic stability and flexibility. *Asian J. Sports Med.* **2011**, *2*, 16–22. [CrossRef] [PubMed]
54. Silva, G.B.; Morgan, M.M.; De Carvalho, W.R.G.; Da Silva, E.F.; De Freitas, W.Z.; Da Silva, F.F.; De Souza, R.A. Electromyographic activity of rectus abdominis muscles during dynamic Pilates abdominal exercises. *J. Bodyw. Mov. Ther.* **2015**, *19*, 629–635. [CrossRef] [PubMed]
55. O'Sullivan, P.B.; Beales, D.J.; Beetham, J.A.; Cripps, J.; Graf, F.; Lin, I.B.; Tucker, B.; Avery, A. Altered motor control strategies in subjects with sacroiliac joint pain during the active straight-leg-raise test. *Spine* **2002**, *27*, E1–E8. [CrossRef] [PubMed]
56. Gaillard, R.; Rifas-Shiman, S.L.; Perng, W.; Oken, E.; Gillman, M.W. Maternal inflammation during pregnancy and childhood adiposity. *Obesity* **2016**, *24*, 1320–1327. [CrossRef]
57. Lindsay, K.L.; Buss, C.; Wadhwa, P.D.; Entringer, S. *The Interactive Effects of Maternal Stress and Diet in Pregnancy on Markers of Inflammation*; Institute for Clinical and Translational Science: Iowa City, IA, USA, 2018.
58. Withee, E.D.; Tippens, K.M.; Dehen, R.; Tibbitts, D.; Hanes, D.; Zwickey, H. Effects of Methylsulfonylmethane (MSM) on exercise-induced oxidative stress, muscle damage, and pain following a half-marathon: A double-blind, randomized, placebo-controlled trial. *J. Int. Soc. Sports Nutr.* **2017**, *14*, 24. [CrossRef]
59. Liu, Y.; Zhao, P.; Cheng, M.; Yu, L.; Cheng, Z.; Fan, L.; Chen, C. AST to ALT ratio and arterial stiffness in non-fatty liver Japanese population: a secondary analysis based on a cross-sectional study. *Lipids Health Dis.* **2018**, *17*, 275. [CrossRef]
60. Pal, S.; Chaki, B.; Chattopadhyay, S.; Bandyopadhyay, A. High-Intensity exercise induced oxidative stress and skeletal muscle damage in postpubertal boys and girls: A comparative study. *J. Strength Cond. Res.* **2018**, *32*, 1045–1052. [CrossRef]
61. Mannaerts, D.; Faes, E.; Cos, P.; Briedé, J.J.; Gyselaers, W.; Cornette, J.; Gorbanev, Y.; Bogaerts, A.; Spaanderman, M.; Van Craenenbroeck, E.; et al. Oxidative stress in healthy pregnancy and preeclampsia is linked to chronic inflammation, iron status and vascular function. *PLoS ONE* **2018**, *13*, e0202919. [CrossRef]

Publisher's Note: MDPI stays neutral with regard to jurisdictional claims in published maps and institutional affiliations.

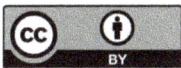

© 2020 by the authors. Licensee MDPI, Basel, Switzerland. This article is an open access article distributed under the terms and conditions of the Creative Commons Attribution (CC BY) license (http://creativecommons.org/licenses/by/4.0/).

Article

Relative Hand Grip and Back Muscle Strength, but Not Mean Muscle Strength, as Risk Factors for Incident Metabolic Syndrome and Its Metabolic Components: 16 Years of Follow-Up in a Population-Based Cohort Study

Yoo Jeong Jeon [1,†], Seung Ku Lee [2,†] and Chol Shin [2,3,4,*]

1. Department of Sports & Health Science, Hanbat National University, Daejeon 34158, Korea; jyjong20@hanbat.ac.kr
2. Institute of Human Genomic Study, College of Medicine, Korea University, Seoul 02841, Korea; leeseungku@korea.ac.kr
3. Division of Pulmonary Sleep and Critical Care Medicine, Department of Internal Medicine, Korea University Ansan Hospital, Ansan 15355, Korea
4. Transdisciplinary Major in Learning Health Systems, Department of Healthcare Sciences, Graduate School, Korea University, Seoul 02841, Korea
* Correspondence: chol-shin@korea.ac.kr; Tel.: +82-31-412-5603
† These authors contributed equally to this work.

Abstract: Muscle strength is associated with health outcomes and can be considered an important disease predictor. There are several studies examining the relationship between hand grip strength (HGS) and metabolic syndrome (MetS). However, no results have been reported for long term longitudinal studies. In this study, we investigated the relationship between mean HGS, back muscle strength (BMS), relative HGS and BMS, and MetS. A total of 2538 non-MetS subjects aged 40–69 years (1215 women and 1323 men) in the Korean Genome and Epidemiology Study (KoGES) Ansan cohort were followed for 16 years. The relationships between incident MetS (iMetS) and muscle strength were estimated using Cox proportional hazard regression models after adjusting for the confounding factors. Increases in standard deviation (SD) and the lower quartile groups for relative HGS and BMS were significantly associated with iMetS in men and women. Moreover, increases in SD and high quintile groups (decreased HGS group) for the delta change in the mean and relative HGS were significantly associated with iMetS in men only. In addition, SD increases for the relative HGS and BMS were significantly associated with iMetS components in men and women. The present study suggests that lower relative HGS and BMS are associated with high risk for the future development of MetS.

Keywords: metabolic syndrome; handgrip strength; back muscle strength; relative muscle strength; physical activity; public health

1. Introduction

Metabolic syndrome (MetS) is a risk factor for cardiovascular disease morbidity and type 2 diabetes mellitus, which can lead to serious disabilities and mortality [1]. Therefore, MetS has become one of the major public health problems worldwide. MetS, also termed insulin resistance syndrome, the deadly quartet, and syndrome X syndrome, is defined as having three or more of five cardiovascular risk factors, including central obesity, hyperglycemia, decreased high density lipoprotein (HDL), elevated triglyceride (TG), and elevated blood pressure [2]. The criteria for MetS usually utilize the three popular definitions provided by the World Health Organization (WHO), the National Cholesterol Education Program (NCEP) Adult Treatment Panel III, and the International Diabetes Federation [3]. MetS is rapidly increasing in Korean society (from 24.9% in 1998 to 29.2% in

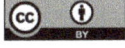

2009, and 31.3% in 2007), especially in those in their 50s and older, with a high prevalence rate of more than 40% [4].

Muscle mass and strength generally increase in adolescents and young people and decrease naturally throughout middle and old age [5]. Handgrip strength (HGS) is a very useful tool because it is an easy and comfortable method for measuring muscle strength [6]. Although muscle mass and muscle strength are highly correlated, muscle strength decreases faster than muscle mass with age [7]. HGS may be a critical important disease predictor because HGS is associated with health outcomes, including type 2 diabetes mellitus (T2DM) [8], hypertension (HTN) [9], mortality [10], and cognitive impairment [11].

The use of a relative method for muscle strength is recommended when investigating the association between disease states, because body composition and body size are highly correlated with muscle strength [12,13]. Relative muscle strength is defined by four popular measuring methods, including body mass index (BMI), body weight, waist circumference (WC), and the waist–hip ratio (WHR) [14,15].

Until recently, most studies of HGS, relative HGS, and MetS have reported cross-sectional findings [4,16–25], with one follow-up investigation reported [26]. Moreover, adolescent studies have shown that weight relative HGS is associated with MetS [22]. In the median 4-year follow-up survey, weight relative HGS showed significant risk rates in the first and second quartiles for incident MetS (iMetS) in comparison with the high quartile group (1.76 times and 1.67 times for men and 1.28 times and 1.3 times for women, respectively) [26]. In addition, the results of various muscle strength measurements, such as upper body strength/weight and skeleton mass index (SMI), showed significant association with iMetS [27,28]. Cardiorespiratory fitness is inversely associated with iMetS [29]. To sum up these results, although direct comparison is difficult, the above findings confirm that muscle mass and MetS are related regardless of the muscle mass measurement method or area. Nevertheless, there is no comparison of the effects of HGS, body mass index (BMI), body weight, and WC relative to HGS on metabolic syndrome. Additionally, there were no reported effects of iMetS due to muscle mass changes during the follow-up period.

Back muscle strength (BMS) decreases with age, similar to HSG, and influences quality of life in older adults [30]. Moreover, the correlation coefficient of HGS and BMS is higher in men (0.67) than in women (0.55) [31]. However, there have been no reports of a relationship between back muscle strength and incident metabolic syndrome. Therefore, this study aimed to assess the relationship between HGS, BMS, BMI-, weight-, WC-relative HGS and BMS, HGS delta change, and iMetS in a 16-year, longitudinal large cohort.

2. Materials and Methods

2.1. Study Participants and Population

Participants were selected among participants from the Korean Genome and Epidemiology Study (KoGES), an ongoing prospective population-based study among the Ansan cohort of middle-aged and older adults in Korea. The Ansan cohort was initiated in 2001 and has been followed biennially during scheduled site visits for 16 years. At baseline, the initial cohort of 5012 participants aged 40 to 69 years were randomly recruited from Ansan city (2518 men and 2494 women). Data collected from the cohort included questionnaires, anthropometric measurements, blood tests, and clinical examinations by trained interviewers and examiners.

For the present study, 1186 out of 5012 participants were excluded at baseline (HGS and BMS (N = 351), body mass index (BMI; N = 1), WC (N = 7), cardiovascular disease (CVD; N = 82), and MetS (N = 743)). During the 16-year study period, 1288 out of 3826 participants were lost to follow-up due to a lack of participation. Finally, 2538 participants remained eligible for this investigation (Figure 1). The follow-up rate at the ninth examination was 50.6%. This study protocol was conducted according to the guidelines of the Declaration of Helsinki and approved by Institutional Review Board of the Korea University Ansan Hospital, and written informed consent was obtained from all study participants.

We obtained the delta change in HGS in baseline and at the eighth follow-up.

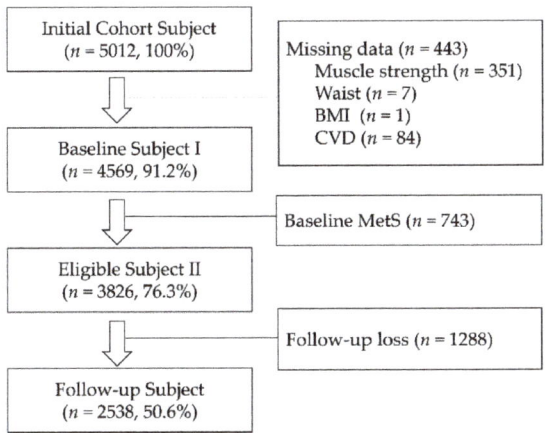

Figure 1. Participant flowchart.

2.2. Muscle Strength

HGS and BMS were measured at baseline using a digital grip dynamometer (Grip-D T.K.K.5401 and T.K.K.5102, TAKEI Science Instruments Co., Ltd., Nigata, Japan). The HGS was measured three or two times in each hand at resting intervals of one-minute. To measure BMS, the participants stood upright and were positioned with their hands on the knob while the values were measured three times by straightening the waist at resting intervals of one-minute. The average muscle strength was used for this study. Body mass index (BMI), body weight, and WC are well-known factors used for relative muscle strength [4,14–25]. Relative muscle strength was calculated as the muscle strength divided by BMI, body weight, and WC for analysis independent of body composition. For further analysis, muscle strength was divided into quartiles or quintiles according to gender. In each case, the highest quintile group was fixed as the reference group for relative muscle strength. For handgrip delta change analysis, we calculated the difference between eighth follow-up examination and baseline. Middle group of quintiles was fixed as the reference group, which is a group where the muscle strength does not change.

2.3. Covariates

Study participants completed questionnaires including demographic information, medical conditions, family history of diseases, and lifestyle. Briefly, BMI was calculated as body weight (kg) divided by height squared (m^2). Family history of diseases were defined as a positive parental history. Metabolic equivalent (MET) values were evaluated based on a compendium of leisure-time physical activity (LPA). Alcohol consumption was calculated using questionnaires, including type of drink, amount, and frequency. Smoking status was categorized as never, past, and current smoker. Blood test was measured using an ADVIA 1650 Auto Analyzer (Siemens Medical Solutions, Tarrytown, NY, USA).

2.4. Definitions of Metabolic Syndrome

MetS was defined according to the NCEP Adult Treatment Panel III [32]. MetS was defined with three of five criteria as follows: WC ($\geq$90 cm for men and $\geq$80 cm for women, abdominal obesity based on Asia–Pacific criteria [33]), TG ($\geq$150 mg/dL), high density lipoprotein (HDL) cholesterol (<40 mg/dL and <50 mg/dL for gender, respectively), presence of HTN (systolic/diastolic blood pressure (SBP/DBP, $\geq$130/85 mmHg and/or the use of antihypertensive agents), and high fasting blood glucose ($\geq$100 mg/dL or the use of antidiabetic agents).

2.5. Statistical Analysis

Baseline characteristics were demonstrated using generalized linear models for continuous variables and chi-square tests for categorical variables. To assess the risk of iMetS, we were used Cox proportional hazard regression models (HRs), 95% confidence intervals (CIs), and p values. The iMetS, according to the increase in the HGS, was shown as a linear trend p. Sensitivity analysis for adjusted Cox hazard ratios demonstrated a one standard deviation (SD) increase in mean HGS, BMS, and relative muscle strength, stratified by follow-up time, gender and age subgroups. The covariates adjusted for in multivariate models were as follows: age, family history of hypertension (yes, no), family history of T2DM (yes, no), job (homemaker, white collar, or blue collar), income (Korean Won (KRW) <1,000,000, 1,000,000≤ or KRW < 2,000,000, KRW 2,000,000≤ or <4,000,000, or KRW 4,000,000≤), education (<12 year and ≥12 year), marriage status (yes, no), smoker (never smoker, ex-smoker, or current smoker), alcohol consumption (g/day), exercise (METs), and menopause (yes, no). Statistical analyses were performed using SAS software (SAS 9.4, SAS Institute, Cary, NC, USA). Statistically significant was defined using a two-tailed $p < 0.05$.

3. Results

3.1. Demographic and Clinical Characteristics of the Study Participants According to Gender

The demographic and clinical characteristics of participants in this study are shown in Table S1. The gender ratio of this study included 47.9% women and 52.1% men in 2538 total subjects. The mean ages were 47.9 ± 7.0 for women and 47.8 ± 6.8 for men ($p = 0.727$). Men constituted higher percentages of ex- or current smokers than women (35.4% vs. 1.0% and 42.8% vs. 1.9%, respectively) ($p < 0.001$). Most women were homemakers (65.8%), followed by blue collar workers (30.0%), whereas most men were blue collar workers (69.7%), followed by white collar workers (23.7%) ($p < 0.001$). The average monthly income of the family was at a higher percentage of KRW 2 to 4 million (43.2% for women and 48.6% for men) and a lower percentage of KRW 1 million (15.1% for women and 7.3% for men) ($p < 0.001$). Men had a higher level of education than women (32.0% vs. 11.3%) ($p < 0.001$). Married status was higher in men than women (90.3% for women and 97.2% for men) ($p < 0.001$). In total, 19.4% of women had experienced menopause. Height, body weight, and alcohol consumption level were significantly higher in men than in women ($p < 0.001$). In five metabolic component factors, WC, TG, SBP, and DBP levels were significantly higher in men than in women ($p < 0.001$). HDL-cholesterol was significantly higher in women than in men ($p < 0.001$). Mean HGS, BMS, BMI-, Weight-, and WC-relative muscle strength levels were higher in men than in women ($p < 0.001$). Family history of DM (FHD, 15.8% for women and 13.3% for men), family history of HTN (FHH, 20.9% for women and 20.0% for men), BMI (24.4 ± 2.8 for women and 24.5 ± 2.7 for men), and exercise (127.0 ± 198.0 for women and 125.3 ± 198.7 for men) were not different between women and men.

3.2. Characteristics of Study Participants in Normal and Incident Metabolic Syndrome According to Gender

The baseline characteristics of the study participants in normal and iMetS, according to gender, are shown in Table 1. Men were significantly more likely to have experienced iMetS than women (41.4% vs. 36.4%) ($p < 0.001$).

In women, age was significantly higher in the iMetS than in the normal group (50.5 ± 7.9 vs. 46.4 ± 5.9) ($p < 0.001$). KRW 1 million of average family monthly income and menopause status in iMetS were higher in percentage (19.9% vs. 12.4% and 26.7% vs. 15.3%, respectively) ($p \leq 0.005$). The BMI and body weight level were higher in the iMetS than in the normal group. In contrast, married status in iMetS was lower by a few percentage points (87.8% vs. 91.7%), and the height level was higher in the normal group than in the iMetS group. In five metabolic component factors, WC, TG, SBP, and DBP levels were significantly higher in iMetS than in the normal group ($p < 0.001$). On the contrary, HDL-cholesterol was significantly higher in the normal group than in iMetS ($p < 0.001$).

BMI-relative, weight-, and WC-relative muscle strength levels were higher in iMetS than in the normal group ($p < 0.001$). In contrast, mean HGS and BMS were not significant between iMetS and normal group. Smoking (1.0% for normal vs. 0.9% for iMetS for ex-smokers and 1.6% for normal vs. 2.5% for iMetS for current smokers); family history of T2DM (14.5% for normal and 18.1% for iMetS); family history of HTN (20.1% for normal and 22.4% for iMetS),;job (30.5% for normal and 29.2% for iMetS in blue collar workers, 4.7% for normal and 3.2% for iMetS in white collar workers, 64.8% for normal and 67.6% for iMetS in homemakers); education (12.4% for normal and 9.3% for iMetS); alcohol consumption (1.3 ± 4.7 for normal and 1.9 ± 6.4 for iMetS); exercise (127.3 ± 200.3 for normal and 126.5 ± 194.3 for iMetS) were not different between the iMetS and normal groups.

Table 1. Demographic and clinical characteristics in baseline according to non-MetS and incident MetS.

		Women (n = 1215)			Men (n = 1323)		
		Normal (n = 773, 63.6%)	iMetS (n = 442, 36.4%)		Normal (n = 775, 58.6%)	iMetS (n = 548, 41.4%)	
		General Characteristics					
Age (year)		46.4 ± 5.9	50.5 ± 7.9	<0.001	47.5 ± 6.5	48.2 ± 7.3	0.062
Smoker	Ex-smoker	8 (1.0%)	4 (0.9%)	0.504	291 (37.5%)	178 (32.5%)	<0.001
	Current smoker	12 (1.6%)	11 (2.5%)		291 (37.5%)	275 (50.2%)	
Family history of T2DM	Yes	112 (14.5%)	80 (18.1%)	0.097	91 (11.7%)	85 (15.5%)	0.047
Family history of hypertension	Yes	155 (20.1%)	99 (22.4%)	0.332	132 (17.0%)	132 (24.1%)	0.002
Job	Blue color	236 (30.5%)	129 (29.2%)	0.363	543 (70.1%)	379 (69.2%)	0.594
	White color	36 (4.7%)	14 (3.2%)		185 (23.9%)	128 (23.4%)	
	Housekeeper	501 (64.8%)	299 (67.6%)		47 (6.1%)	41 (7.5%)	
Income (KRW)	<1 million	96 (12.4%)	88 (19.9%)	0.005	56 (7.2%)	41 (7.5%)	0.515
	1–2	238 (30.8%)	133 (30.1%)		213 (27.5%)	154 (28.1%)	
	2–4	347 (44.9%)	178 (40.3%)		388 (50.1%)	255 (46.5%)	
	4≤	92 (11.9%)	43 (9.7%)		118 (15.2%)	98 (17.9%)	
Education	<12 year	96 (12.4%)	41 (9.3%)	0.096	258 (33.3%)	165 (30.1%)	0.222
Marry Status	Yes	709 (91.7%)	388 (87.8%)	0.026	754 (97.3%)	532 (97.1%)	0.820
Menopause Status	Yes	118 (15.3%)	118 (26.7%)	<0.001	NA	NA	
Body Mass Index (kg/m^2)		23.6 ± 2.5	25.8 ± 2.8	<0.001	23.9 ± 2.6	25.4 ± 2.5	<0.001
Height (cm)		155.7 ± 5.1	154.5 ± 4.9	<0.001	167.8 ± 5.5	167.9 ± 5.8	0.635
Weight (kg)		57.3 ± 6.7	61.6 ± 7.2	<0.001	67.4 ± 8.4	71.6 ± 9.1	<0.001
Alcohol consumption (g/day)		1.3 ± 4.7	1.9 ± 6.4	0.072	17.0 ± 25.2	22.6 ± 30.2	<0.001
Leisure physical activity (Met)		127.3 ± 200.3	126.5 ± 194.3	0.945	124.0 ± 187.9	127.1 ± 213.1	0.781
		Metabolic Components					
Waist circumference (cm)		73.6 ± 6.2	79.5 ± 6.6	<0.001	80.9 ± 6.7	85.4 ± 6.6	<0.001
HDL-cholesterol (mg/dL)		54.9 ± 11.9	49.8 ± 10.7	<0.001	49.6 ± 10.7	44.6 ± 8.9	<0.001
Triglycerides (mg/dL)		100.0 ± 52.0	133.1 ± 75.0	<0.001	132.4 ± 70.1	188.1 ± 109.2	<0.001
Systolic Blood Pressure (mmHg)		107.0 ± 13.8	118.7 ± 15.9	<0.001	114.0 ± 13.8	120.3 ± 15.7	<0.001
Diastolic Blood Pressure (mmHg)		70.8 ± 9.0	78.2 ± 9.9	<0.001	77.9 ± 10.0	82.0 ± 10.8	<0.001
		Muscle Strength					
		Hand grip Strength (HGS)					
Mean HGS (kg)		22.0 ± 3.8	21.4 ± 3.8	<0.001	35.4 ± 5.5	35.0 ± 5.8	0.216
BMI-relative Mean HGS		0.94 ± 0.19	0.84 ± 0.16	<0.001	1.49 ± 0.26	1.39 ± 0.24	<0.001
Weight-relative Mean HGS		0.39 ± 0.07	0.35 ± 0.06	<0.001	0.53 ± 0.09	0.49 ± 0.08	<0.001
WC-relative Mean HGS		0.30 ± 0.06	0.27 ± 0.05	<0.001	0.44 ± 0.08	0.41 ± 0.07	<0.001
		Back Muscle Strength (BMS)					
Mean BMS (kg)		42.9 ± 12.3	42.5 ± 11.8	0.653	83.6 ± 19.2	84.3 ± 19.2	0.536
BMI-relative Mean BMS		1.83 ± 0.55	1.66 ± 0.46	<0.001	3.52 ± 0.82	3.34 ± 0.78	<0.001
Weight-relative Mean BMS		0.76 ± 0.22	0.69 ± 0.19	<0.001	1.25 ± 0.29	1.19 ± 0.28	<0.001
WC-relative Mean BMS		0.59 ± 0.17	0.54 ± 0.15	<0.001	1.04 ± 0.24	0.99 ± 0.23	<0.001

Abbreviation: iMetS, incident metabolic syndrome; T2DM, type 2 diabetes mellitus; KRW, Korean Won; BMI, body mass index; WC, waist circumference.

In men, current smoking, a family history of HTN, and a family history of T2DM were higher by percentage in iMetS than in the normal group (50.2% for iMetS vs. 37.5% for normal group, 24.1% for iMetS vs. 17.0% for normal group, and 11.7% for normal and 15.5%

for iMetS, respectively) ($p \leq 0.002$). The BMI and body weight levels were significantly higher in iMetS than in the normal group (25.4 ± 2.5 for iMetS vs. 23.9 ± 2.6% for normal group, and 71.6 ± 9.1 for iMetS vs. 67.4 ± 8.4 for the normal group, respectively, $p < 0.001$). For five metabolic component factors, WC, TG, SBP, and DBP levels were significantly higher in iMetS than in the normal group ($p < 0.001$). In contrast, HDL-cholesterol was significantly higher in the normal group than in iMetS ($p < 0.001$). BMI-, weight-, and WC-relative muscle strength mean and maximum levels were higher in iMetS than in the normal group ($p < 0.001$). In contrast, mean and maximum HGS and BMS were not significantly different between iMetS and normal group. Age (47.5 ± 6.5 vs. 48.2 ± 7.3, $p = 0.062$); job (70.1% for normal and 69.2% for iMetS in blue collar workers, 23.9% for normal and 23.4% for iMetS in white collar workers, 6.1% for normal and 7.5% for iMetS in homemakers, $p = 0.594$); income (27.5% for normal and 28.1% for iMetS in KRW 1–2 million, 50.1% for normal and 46.5% for iMetS in KRW 2–4 million, 15.2% for normal and 17.9% for iMetS in more than KRW 4 million, $p = 0.515$); more than 12 years of education (33.3% for normal and 30.3% for iMetS, $p = 0.222$); married status (97.3% for normal and 97.1% for iMetS, $p = 0.820$); height (167.8 ± 5.5 for normal and 167.9 ± 5.8 for iMetS, $p = 0.635$); and exercise (124.0 ± 187.9 for normal and 127.1 ± 213.1 for iMetS, $p = 0.781$) were not different between the iMetS and normal groups.

Table S2 shows the sex-adjusted correlation coefficient of relative HGS and metabolic components. BMI, Weight, and WC-relative HGS and BMS showed a higher correlation with metabolic components than means HGS. In particular, relative HGS showed higher correlation than relative BMS.

3.3. Cox Proportional Hazard Ratios for Incident Metabolic Syndrome According to Inverse One Standard Deviation Increase in Mean Hand Grip Strength, Back Muscle Strength, and Relative Muscle Strength in Gender

The MetS risk of inverse one SD increase in muscle strength and relative muscle strength was shown in Table 2, adjusted for the confounding factors.

Table 2. Adjusted hazard ratio (HR) of incident metabolic syndrome associated with inverse one standard deviation increase in mean hand grip strength, back muscle strength, and relative muscle strength according to gender.

	HGS		BMS	
	Univariate HR (95% CI) p	Multivariate HR (95% CI) p *	Univariate HR (95% CI) p	Multivariate HR (95% CI) p *
Women				
Mean (kg)	1.176 (1.066–1.296) 0.001	1.042 (0.938–1.157) 0.445	1.045 (0.951–1.149) 0.355	0.932 (0.845–1.028) 0.161
BMI-relative	1.680 (1.514–1.864) < 0.001	1.494 (1.337–1.671) < 0.001	1.352 (1.224–1.494) < 0.001	1.192 (1.072–1.324) 0.001
Weight-relative	1.618 (1.461–1.792) < 0.001	1.454 (1.306–1.620) < 0.001	1.297 (1.175–1.432) < 0.001	1.158 (1.044–1.283) 0.005
WC-relative	1.662 (1.501–1.841) < 0.001	1.447 (1.293–1.620) < 0.001	1.314 (1.190–1.451) < 0.001	1.135 (1.022–1.261) 0.019
Men				
Mean HGS (kg)	1.076 (0.984–1.176) 0.107	1.078 (0.982–1.182) 0.114	0.982 (0.903–1.069) 0.679	0.987 (0.905–1.076) 0.766
BMI-relative	1.454 (1.324–1.596) < 0.001	1.470 (1.335–1.618) < 0.001	1.203 (1.106–1.309) < 0.001	1.212 (1.113–1.320) < 0.001
Weight-relative	1.465 (1.338–1.604) < 0.001	1.472 (1.342–1.614) < 0.001	1.207 (1.110–1.313) < 0.001	1.212 (1.114–1.317) < 0.001
WC-relative	1.422 (1.298–1.559) < 0.001	1.431 (1.302–1.574) < 0.001	1.187 (1.091–1.292) < 0.001	1.190 (1.092–1.297) < 0.001

Abbreviation: HGS, handgrip strength; BMC, back muscle strength; HR, hazard ratio; CI, confidence interval; BMI, body mass index; WC, waist circumference. * Adjusted for baseline muscle strength plus age; family history of DM (yes, no); family history of hypertension (yes, no); job (homemaker, white collar, or blue collar); income (KRW < 1,000,000, KRW 1,000,000≤ or <2,000,000, KRW 2,000,000≤ or <4,000,000, or KRW 4,000,000≤); education (<12 years and ≥12 years); married status (yes, no); smoker (never smoker, ex-smoker, or current smoker); alcohol consumption (g/day); and leisure physical activity (METs). Women added menopause (yes, no).

In univariate analysis, the HR per inverse one SD increase in BMI-, weight-, and WC-relative HGS and BMS was associated with a lower risk of iMetS in women and men (HR = 1.187–0.168, $p < 0.001$). However, the HGS and BMS in both women and men were not associated with iMetS. After adjusting for confounders, the HR per inverse one SD increase in BMI-, weight-, and WC-relative HGS was associated with a lower risk of iMetS in women and men (HR = 0.135–0.494, $p < 0.005$). However, HGS and BMS were not associated with iMetS in both women and men. For sensitivity analyses, we calculated the HR for inverse one standard deviation increase in mean HGS, BMS, and relative muscle strength, stratified by follow-up time (second, sixth, and ninth follow-up) and gender subgroups (Table S3). We were able to confirm that a similar trend was maintained during the follow-up period.

3.4. Cox Proportional Hazard Ratios for Incident Metabolic Syndrome According to Quartile Groups of Mean Hand Grip Strength, Back Muscle Strength, and Relative Muscle Strength by Gender

Participants were divided into quartile groups based on gender-specific HGS and BMC, and relative HGS and BMC (Table 3 and Table S4). In univariate analysis, HGS and BMS was not associated with iMetS in both women and men. However, BMI-, weight-, and WC-relative HGS and BMS were shown to have higher HR rates for iMetS in women and men (HR = 1.718–3.858, $p \leq 0.001$ in women and HR = 1.377–2.515, $p \leq 0.015$ for men), excluding the third quartile of the BMS of men. After adjusting for confounders, HGS and BMS was also not associated with iMetS in both women and men. However, the first, second, and third quartile of BMI-, weight-, and WC-relative HGS and BMS was shown to have higher HR values for iMetS in women and men (HR = 1.459–2.821, $p \leq 0.001$ for women and HR = 1.368–2.821, $p \leq 0.024$ for men), excluding the third quartile of the BMS of men. Additionally, the p value for linear trend was shown to be significant ($p < 0.001$).

Table 3. Adjusted hazard ratio (HR) of incident metabolic syndrome associated with quartile group of mean hand grip strength, back muscle strength, and relative muscle strength according to gender.

Muscle Strength	Group	HGS		BMS	
		Women HR (95% CI) p *	Men HR (95% CI) p *	Women HR (95% CI) p *	Men HR (95% CI) p *
Mean (kg)	Q4	Reference	Reference	Reference	Reference
	Q3	0.880 (0.669–1.159) 0.363	1.032 (0.805–1.323) 0.801	1.135 (0.877–1.469) 0.336	0.897 (0.706–1.139) 0.372
	Q2	0.896 (0.685–1.173) 0.426	1.117 (0.875–1.426) 0.375	0.907 (0.688–1.197) 0.491	1.141 (0.903–1.441) 0.268
	Q1	0.897 (0.674–1.194) 0.456	1.173 (0.914–1.505) 0.211	0.895 (0.676–1.185) 0.439	0.968 (0.757–1.238) 0.794
p value for linear trend		0.506	0.166	0.224	0.72
BMI-relative	Q4	Reference	Reference	Reference	Reference
	Q3	1.801 (1.293–2.511) 0.001	1.369 (1.042–1.799) 0.024	1.787 (1.334–2.393) < 0.001	1.188 (0.921–1.531) 0.185
	Q2	2.209 (1.597–3.057) < 0.001	1.553 (1.188–2.030) 0.001	1.631 (1.213–2.193) 0.001	1.551 (1.215–1.980) < 0.001
	Q1	2.821 (2.028–3.923) < 0.001	2.401 (1.854–3.110) < 0.001	1.579 (1.163–2.143) 0.003	1.596 (1.247–2.041) < 0.001
p value for linear trend		<0.001	<0.001	0.009	<0.001
Weight-relative	Q4	Reference	Reference	Reference	Reference
	Q3	1.868 (1.350–2.585) < 0.001	1.486 (1.129–1.955) 0.005	1.649 (1.236–2.200) 0.001	1.193 (0.925–1.538) 0.174
	Q2	2.166 (1.572–2.986) < 0.001	1.858 (1.420–2.431) < 0.001	1.601 (1.197–2.141) 0.002	1.484 (1.165–1.890) 0.001
	Q1	2.700 (1.962–3.717) < 0.001	2.514 (1.940–3.258) < 0.001	1.531 (1.134–2.067) 0.005	1.642 (1.291–2.089) < 0.001
p value for linear trend		<0.001	<0.001	0.01	<0.001
WC-relative	Q4	Reference	Reference	Reference	Reference
	Q3	1.694 (1.229–2.335) 0.001	1.517 (1.156–1.991) 0.003	1.670 (1.258–2.217) < 0.001	1.006 (0.780–1.299) 0.962
	Q2	2.109 (1.536–2.896) < 0.001	1.743 (1.333–2.279) < 0.001	1.459 (1.092–1.950) 0.011	1.368 (1.076–1.739) 0.011
	Q1	2.242 (1.613–3.115) < 0.001	2.315 (1.783–3.006) < 0.001	1.485 (1.100–2.004) 0.010	1.460 (1.144–1.862) 0.002
p value for linear trend		<0.001	<0.001	0.03	<0.001

Abbreviation: HGS, hand grip strength; BMS, back muscle strength; HR, hazard ratio; CI, confidence interval; BMI, body mass index; WC, waist circumference. * Adjusted for baseline muscle strength plus age; family history of diabetes (yes, no); family history of hypertension (yes, no); job (homemaker, white collar, or blue collar); income (KRW < 1,000,000, KRW 1,000,000≤ or <2,000,000, KRW 2,000,000≤ or <4,000,000, or KRW 4,000,000≤); education (<12 year and ≥12 year), married status (yes, no); smoker (never smoker, ex-smoker, or current smoker); alcohol consumption (g/day); and leisure physical activity (METs). Women added menopause (yes, no).

3.5. Cox Proportional Hazard Ratios for Incident Metabolic Syndrome According to Delta Change of Mean Hand Grip Strength and Relative Hand Grip Strength in Gender

We obtained the delta change in HGS in baseline and at the which we used to confirm risk of iMetS (Tables 4 and 5).

Table 4. Adjusted hazard ratio (HR) of incident metabolic syndrome associated with invers one standard deviation increase in mean hand grip strength delta change and relative muscle strength according to gender.

Standardized Delta Change of HGS	Women		Men	
	HR (95% CI) p *	HR (95% CI) p §	HR (95% CI) p *	HR (95% CI) p §
Δ Mean (kg)	0.971 (0.865–1.091) 0.624	0.918 (0.816–1.031) 0.150	1.048 (0.946–1.160) 0.370	1.058 (0.953–1.176) 0.290
Δ BMI-relative	1.131 (1.009–1.269) 0.035	1.034 (0.916–1.168) 0.585	1.173 (1.060–1.297) 0.002	1.148 (1.033–1.276) 0.010
Δ Weight-relative	1.127 (1.003–1.267) 0.045	1.025 (0.907–1.159) 0.692	1.216 (1.099–1.345) < 0.001	1.174 (1.057–1.304) 0.003
Δ WC-relative	1.160 (1.033–1.302) 0.012	1.064 (0.942–1.201) 0.318	1.158 (1.046–1.283) 0.005	1.160 (1.041–1.291) 0.007

Abbreviation: HGS, hand grip strength; BMS, back muscle strength; HR, hazard ratio; CI, confidence interval; BMI, body mass index; WC, waist circumference. * Adjusted for baseline muscle strength. § Adjusted for baseline muscle strength plus age; family history of DM (yes, no); family history of hypertension (yes, no); job (homemaker, white collar, or blue collar); income (KRW < 1,000,000, KRW 1,000,000≤ or <2,000,000, KRW 2,000,000≤ or <4,000,000, or KRW 4,000,000≤); education (<12 years and ≥12 years); married status (yes, no); smoker (never smoker, ex-smoker, or current smoker); alcohol consumption (g/day); and leisure physical activity (METs). Women added menopause.

Table 5. Adjusted hazard ratio (HR) of incident metabolic syndrome associated with quintiles group of mean hand grip strength, back muscle strength, and relative muscle strength according to gender.

Standardized Delta Change in HGS		Women		Men	
		HR (95% CI) p *	HR (95% CI) p §	HR (95% CI) p *	HR (95% CI) p §
Δ Mean (kg)	Q1	1.105 (0.799–1.529) 0.545	1.181 (0.849–1.643) 0.323	1.425 (1.035–1.960) 0.030	1.349 (0.973–1.870) 0.073
	Q2	0.762 (0.536–1.082) 0.128	0.749 (0.526–1.068) 0.110	1.389 (1.011–1.907) 0.043	1.192 (0.864–1.646) 0.285
	Q3	Reference	Reference	Reference	Reference
	Q4	0.927 (0.661–1.301) 0.662	0.970 (0.689–1.365) 0.861	1.333 (0.967–1.837) 0.080	1.325 (0.959–1.832) 0.089
	Q5	0.864 (0.612–1.221) 0.408	0.776 (0.547–1.100) 0.155	1.560 (1.136–2.142) 0.006	1.500 (1.080–2.085) 0.016
Δ BMI-relative	Q1	0.938 (0.658–1.337) 0.725	1.184 (0.825–1.699) 0.359	1.057 (0.769–1.454) 0.732	1.102 (0.798–1.523) 0.556
	Q2	1.105 (0.784–1.559) 0.567	1.117 (0.789–1.581) 0.533	1.082 (0.789–1.485) 0.625	1.155 (0.840–1.589) 0.376
	Q3	Reference	Reference	Reference	Reference
	Q4	1.417 (1.006–1.997) 0.046	1.332 (0.942–1.885) 0.105	1.342 (0.986–1.826) 0.061	1.335 (0.978–1.821) 0.069
	Q5	1.305 (0.913–1.865) 0.144	1.258 (0.874–1.811) 0.217	1.504 (1.101–2.054) 0.010	1.502 (1.091–2.067) 0.013
Δ Weight-relative	Q1	0.842 (0.592–1.197) 0.337	1.028 (0.719–1.472) 0.878	1.066 (0.775–1.467) 0.693	1.157 (0.838–1.598) 0.376
	Q2	1.005 (0.715–1.413) 0.977	0.993 (0.705–1.399) 0.966	1.057 (0.768–1.454) 0.734	1.132 (0.821–1.560) 0.450
	Q3	Reference	Reference	Reference	Reference
	Q4	1.228 (0.872–1.730) 0.240	1.131 (0.796–1.606) 0.493	1.522 (1.119–2.069) 0.007	1.486 (1.089–2.029) 0.013
	Q5	1.313 (0.923–1.866) 0.130	0.869 (0.612–1.234) 0.433	1.531 (1.117–2.099) 0.008	1.530 (1.107–2.114) 0.010
Δ WC-relative	Q1	0.719 (0.510–1.015) 0.061	0.836 (0.594–1.175) 0.303	1.130 (0.824–1.550) 0.448	1.044 (0.756–1.443) 0.792
	Q2	0.812 (0.579–1.139) 0.227	Reference	1.100 (0.801–1.510) 0.557	1.028 (0.744–1.421) 0.866
	Q3	Reference	1.160 (0.831–1.617) 0.383	Reference	Reference
	Q4	1.134 (0.817–1.574) 0.452	1.007 (0.710–1.428) 0.968	1.378 (1.010–1.881) 0.043	1.292 (0.944–1.768) 0.109
	Q5	1.108 (0.785–1.564) 0.560	1.181 (0.849–1.643) 0.323	1.524 (1.114–2.085) 0.008	1.445 (1.048–1.992) 0.025

Abbreviation: HGS, hand grip strength; BMS, back muscle strength; HR, hazard ratio; CI, confidence interval; BMI, body mass index; WC, waist circumference. * Adjusted for baseline muscle strength. § Adjusted for baseline muscle strength plus age; family history of DM (yes, no); family history of hypertension (yes, no); job (homemaker, white collar, or blue collar); income (KRW< 1,000,000, KRW 1,000,000 ≤or <2,000,000, KRW 2,000,000≤ or <4,000,000, or KRW 4,000,000≤); education (<12 years and ≥12 years); married status (yes, no); smoker (never smoker, ex-smoker, or current smoker); alcohol consumption (g/day); leisure physical activity (METs); and BMI. Women added menopause.

The MetS risk of increase in normalized delta change in muscle strength and relative muscle strength was shown in Table 4. After the adjustment of baseline muscle strength, the HRs per invers one SD increase in delta change in BMI-, weight-, and WC-relative HGS and BMS were associated with a high risk of iMetS in women and men (HR = 1.131–1.216, $p \leq 0.005$). However, the delta changes in HGS in both women and men were not associated with iMetS. In the full model, the HR per one SD increase in delta change in BMI-, weight-, and WC-relative HGS were associated with a high risk of iMetS in only men (HR = 1.148–1.174, $p \leq 0.010$). However, women were not associated with iMetS.

The participants were divided into quintile groups based on gender-specific HGS and relative HGS. The middle (third) quintile group was fixed as the reference group. The first quintiles group is the group with increased HGS during the follow-up period, whereas the last quintile group is that with decreased HGS (Table 5). After the adjustment of baseline muscle strength, the fourth quintile of BMI-relative HGS was associated with iMetS in women.

However, the other groups were not associated with iMetS in women. In men, the first, second, and fifth delta changes in mean HGS, and fifth delta changes in BMI- and WC-relative HGS, and fourth and fifth delta changes in weight-relative HGS were associated with iMetS. In the full model, the fifth delta change in HGS and BMI-, and WC-relative HGS, and the fourth and fifth delta changes in weight-HGS were also associated with iMetS (HR = 1.486–1.530, $p \leq 0.025$). Based on the comparison of the differences between baseline and the eighth follow-up muscle strength and LPA, HGS and relative HGS were significantly reduced in women ($p < 0.001$) and there was no difference in LPA. On the other hand, men showed significant increases in HGS, relative HGS, and LPA ($p < 0.05$; Supplementary Table S5). Similarly, we analyzed the effect of vigorous-LPA [34] and these delta changes on incident metabolic syndrome, but the results were not significant (data not shown).

3.6. Cox Proportional Hazard Ratios for Incident Metabolic Syndrome Components According to Mean Hand Grip Strength, Back Muscle Strength, and Relative Muscle Strength in Gender

We showed HR per one SD increase, 95% CIs, and p values for each one SD increase in muscle strength and relative muscle strength in the incidence of each MetS component adjusted for the confounding factors (Table 6 and Table S6).

Table 6. Adjusted hazard ratio (HR) of incident metabolic syndrome components associated with one standard deviation increase in mean hand grip strength, back muscle strength, and relative muscle strength according to gender.

	WC	HDL	TG	HTN	DM
	HR (95% CI) p *	HR (95% CI) p *	HR (95% CI) p *	HR (95% CI) p *	HR (95% CI) p *
	Women				
HGS (kg)	1.040 (0.913–1.185) 0.554	0.902 (0.796–1.021) 0.103	0.924 (0.835–1.022) 0.124	1.046 (0.940–1.163) 0.409	0.818 (0.702–0.953) 0.010
BMI-relative HGS	0.579 (0.503–0.667) <0.001	0.875 (0.773–0.990) 0.034	0.829 (0.747–0.919) <0.001	0.826 (0.739–0.923) 0.001	0.650 (0.552–0.765) <0.001
Weight-relative HGS	0.530 (0.462–0.608) <0.001	0.880 (0.778–0.995) 0.042	0.846 (0.765–0.937) 0.001	0.833 (0.748–0.928) 0.001	0.693 (0.592–0.811) <0.001
WC-relative HGS	0.647 (0.562–0.745) <0.001	0.861 (0.759–0.976) 0.020	0.833 (0.748–0.927) 0.001	0.841 (0.751–0.942) 0.003	0.655 (0.556–0.772) <0.001
BMS (kg)	1.088 (0.962–1.231) 0.180	0.924 (0.819–1.043) 0.202	0.957 (0.869–1.054) 0.373	1.028 (0.932–1.134) 0.579	0.916 (0.792–1.059) 0.235
BMI-relative BMS	0.740 (0.646–0.849) <0.001	0.901 (0.798–1.018) 0.094	0.879 (0.797–0.970) 0.010	0.893 (0.804–0.991) 0.033	0.772 (0.660–0.904) 0.001
Weight-relative BMS	0.711 (0.621–0.813) <0.001	0.907 (0.804–1.024) 0.114	0.900 (0.817–0.993) 0.035	0.905 (0.817–1.003) 0.056	0.820 (0.705–0.955) 0.011
WC-relative BMS	0.820 (0.717–0.938) 0.004	0.900 (0.796–1.018) 0.094	0.892 (0.808–0.986) 0.026	0.911 (0.820–1.012) 0.082	0.800 (0.684–0.935) 0.005
	Men				
HGS (kg)	1.073 (0.805–1.430) 0.632	0.963 (0.875–1.060) 0.441	1.007 (0.907–1.119) 0.891	0.927 (0.843–1.018) 0.114	0.925 (0.824–1.037) 0.182
BMI-relative HGS	0.416 (0.302–0.572) <0.001	0.813 (0.739–0.894) <0.001	0.870 (0.787–0.962) 0.007	0.793 (0.723–0.869) <0.001	0.689 (0.612–0.775) <0.001
Weight-relative HGS	0.322 (0.237–0.437) <0.001	0.826 (0.754–0.905) <0.001	0.861 (0.781–0.949) 0.003	0.780 (0.712–0.854) <0.001	0.691 (0.617–0.774) <0.001
WC-relative HGS	0.448 (0.329–0.610) <0.001	0.826 (0.751–0.909) <0.001	0.863 (0.780–0.954) 0.004	0.812 (0.740–0.891) <0.001	0.700 (0.622–0.787) <0.001
BMS (kg)	1.268 (0.967–1.663) 0.086	1.054 (0.963–1.153) 0.251	1.015 (0.919–1.120) 0.772	0.942 (0.861–1.031) 0.196	1.093 (0.982–1.216) 0.103
BMI-relative BMS	0.665 (0.502–0.882) 0.005	0.941 (0.862–1.027) 0.174	0.924 (0.840–1.015) 0.100	0.847 (0.776–0.923) <0.001	0.890 (0.802–0.988) 0.028
Weight-relative BMS	0.560 (0.421–0.745) <0.001	0.954 (0.876–1.040) 0.290	0.917 (0.836–1.005) 0.065	0.841 (0.771–0.917) <0.001	0.894 (0.807–0.991) 0.033
WC-relative BMS	0.698 (0.527–0.925) 0.012	0.953 (0.872–1.041) 0.287	0.916 (0.832–1.008) 0.071	0.859 (0.787–0.938) 0.001	0.904 (0.813–1.004) 0.059

Abbreviation: HR, hazard ratio; CI, confidence interval; WC, waist circumference; HDL, high density lipoprotein; TG, triglyceride; HTN, hypertension; DM, diabetes mellitus; HGS, hand grip strength; BMS, back muscle strength. * Adjusted for baseline muscle strength plus age; family history of DM (yes, no); family history of hypertension (yes, no); job (homemaker, white collar, or blue collar); income (KRW < 1,000,000, KRW 1,000,000 $\leq$ or <2,000,000, KRW 2,000,000$\leq$ or <4,000,000, or KRW 4,000,000$\leq$); education (<12 years and $\geq$12 years); married status (yes, no); smoker (never smoker, ex-smoker, or current smoker); alcohol consumption (g/day); leisure physical activity (METs); and BMI. Women added menopause.

In univariate analysis, the HR per one SD increase for incident WC, incident dyslipidemia (HDL-cholesterol and TG), incident HTN, and incident DM in women and men was associated with a lower risk in BMI-, weight-, and WC-relative HGS and BMS (HR = 0.492–0.666, $p < 0.001$ for women, and HR = 0.334–0.698, $p \leq 0.011$ for men in incident WC; HR = 0.863–0.892, $p \leq 0.044$ for women, and HR = 0.803–0.818, $p < 0.001$ for men in incident HDL-cholesterol; HR = 0.806–0.875, $p \leq 0.005$ for women, and HR = 0.879–0.900, $p \leq 0.032$ for men in incident TG; HR = 0.739–0.836, $p < 0.001$ for women, and HR = 0.788–0.877, $p \leq 0.003$ for men in incident HTN; HR = 0.610–0.769, $p < 0.001$ for women, and HR = 0.687–0.891, $p \leq 0.029$ for men in incident DM), excluding HSG and BMS in both women and men, weight-relative HGS of women, and relative BMS of men.

After adjusting for confounders, the HR for all the metabolic components was not associated with HGS and BMS in both men and women. The HR for incident WC, incident dyslipidemia (HDL-cholesterol and TG), incident HTN, and incident DM in women and men was associated with a lower risk in BMI-, weight-, and WC-relative HGS (HR = 0.530–0.647, $p < 0.001$ for women, and HR = 0.322–0.448, $p < 0.001$ for men in incident WC; HR = 0.861–0.880, $p \leq 0.042$ for women, and HR = 0.813–0.826, $p < 0.001$ for men in incident HDL-cholesterol; HR = 0.829–0.846, $p \leq 0.001$ for women, and HR = 0.870–0.863, $p \leq 0.007$ for men in incident TG; HR = 0.826–0.841, $p \leq 0.003$ for women, and HR = 0.780–0.812, $p < 0.001$ for men in incident HTN; HR = 0.650–0.693, $p < 0.001$ for women, and HR = 0.689–0.700, $p < 0.001$ for men in incident DM). The HR for incident WC, HTN, and DM in women and men was associated with a lower risk in BMI-, weight-, and WC-relative BMS (HR = 0.711–0.820, $p \leq 0.004$ for women, and HR = 0.560–0.698, $p \leq 0.012$ for men in incident WC; HR = 0.893, $p = 0.033$ for women, and HR = 0.841–0.859, $p \leq 0.001$ for men in incident HTN; HR = 0.772–0.820, $p \leq 0.011$ for women, and HR = 0.890–0.894, $p \leq 0.033$ for men in incident DM), excluding weight- and WC-relative BMS for women, and WC-relative BMS for men. The HR for incident TG in women was only associated with a lower risk in BMI-, weight-, and WC-relative BMS (HR = 0.879–0.900, $p \leq 0.035$).

4. Discussion

In this study, we studied relationship between mean and relative HGS and BMS and iMetS using a 16-year follow-up of the population-based cohort. The present study revealed that BMI-, weight-, and WC-relative HGS and BMS at baseline were independently associated with iMetS in men and women. In addition, the changes in muscle strength over 16 years was significant in iMetS in men. Unfortunately, baseline LPA and these changes were not associated with iMetS. The results of changes in muscle strength and LPA that had not been previously demonstrated were shown here. Additionally, we showed that iMetS components were strongly associated with a one standard deviation increase in relative HGS and BMS both in women and men.

Muscle strength can be measured in various areas, such as the knee, elbow, hand, leg, and back [15,35,36]. Additionally, it can be measured by an isokinetic dynamometer, cardiorespiratory fitness, dual-energy X-ray absorptiometry (DEX), and bioelectrical impedance analysis (BIA) [37]. Several studies have been reported, varying by the measurement site and measurement method, but there are few studies compared to those for HGS due to problems such as the measurement difficulty, high test cost, and challenges in validation [37,38]. Therefore, HGS is being used to research muscle strength in clinical and epidemiological studies [8]. Body composition and body size-independent measurements for muscle strength are important. The use of a relative method is recommended when investigating the relationship between diseases such as T2DM, HTN, MetS, and dementia [8–11]. Therefore, BMI-, weight-, and WC-relative muscle strength are frequently used methods for normalizing muscle strength [15].

The relevance of MetS components, iMetS, and HGS has also been reported in previous reports. Lower HGS was associated with incident T2DM [15,39,40], and meta-analysis results using the results of 10 observational cohort studies also demonstrated its relevance to DM [8]. Weak HGS is associated with HTN [9,41]. The results of HGS and MetS showed contradictory results. In women, all results showed no association results [17,18]. Some of the results showed significant results in men [24]. Weight- [16,20,21,23] and BMI-relative [4,17–19] HGS were consistently associated with MetS both men and women. In addition, weight-relative HGS was associated with iMetS in both men and women [26]. In our results, BMI-, weight-, and WC-relative HGS were related to iMetS. The mean HGS was not significant. Moreover, sarcopenia is the age-related loss of skeletal muscle mass, quality, and strength [42]. The results of the meta-analysis using the results of 13 observational studies also demonstrated its relevance to MetS (2.01 fold) [43]. The development of MetS by HGS change has not been reported. Our results show that the decrease in HGS in men was significantly associated with iMetS.

Unfortunately, LPA was not relevant to the iMetS in our results. These results can be explained through previous reports that aerobic exercise does not significantly affect HGS. Therefore, resistance exercise is needed to improvement HGS [44,45]. In addition, in a four-year follow-up study, iMetS did not differ by moderate-LPA, but was only 0.36-fold lower in groups with a vigorous LPA of more than 7.5 METs per week for more than 60 min [34]. Another study showed an association with a 0.54-fold increase in MetS of more than 990 MET-minutes per week [46]. The baseline average leisure activity of the subjects in this study was 127.0 MET-minutes per week for women and 125.3 MET-minutes per week for men, showing very low LPA compared to previous studies. The difference between baseline and eighth follow-up HGS and relative HGS were significantly reduced in women. LPA was not different in women. On the other hand, men showed significant increases in HGS, relative HGS, and LPA. In our results, men showed high iMetS and decreased HGS. It is thought that increased or maintained LPA offset the effects of iMetS on HGS, while decreased LPA reduces HGS, increasing iMetS.

As the pace of aging increases, interest in dementia is also increasing. A recent meta-analysis has shown that MetS groups have 2.95-fold higher progression from MCI to dementia than in normal groups [47]. Therefore, the prevention of MetS is considered an important preventive factor for chronic diseases as well as the dementia of aging. In addition, HGS is used for the diagnosis of sarcopenia and frailty [48]. Sarcopenia is emerging as a large problem in old age. Only persistent LPA can maintain or increase muscles, which is essential for improving the quality of health, life, and living in aging [18,42].

MetS is not a disease. It is clustering of risk factors. MetS is a public problem because it leads to cardiovascular disease morbidity, T2DM, serious disabilities, and mortality [10]. Interpretation is also very complex and not fully elucidated because the development of MetS is a combination of five components [49]. Recent GWAS results have given us a partial understanding of their varying pathophysiology [50]. The relevant genes included genes related to T2DM (APOC1, FADS2, NEU2, SLC18A1, CMIP, PABPC4, etc.); HTN (blood pressure; NEU2, CMIP, CELF1, JMJD1C, ARID1A, CEP68, etc.); lipid regulation (ZPR1, CETP, LPL, CD300LG, TRIB1, ANGPTL4, etc.), and obesity (APOC1, FTO, BAZ1B, CELF1, PABPC4, PCCB, etc.). The analysis contained most genes traditionally thought to be the cause of metabolic syndrome [49,51]. Moreover, results of pathway analysis using these significant genes showed involvement of immunity pathway [51], inflammation [52], endosomal/vacuolar and ER-phagosome [53], and regulation of lipids and lipoprotein [54].

Recently, gender difference was confirmed in the longitudinal study [26]. However, our results did not show the relative HGS of genders and baseline and the interaction of BMS. Interestingly, in the delta change of relative HGS, women were not significant in DM development, but men showed significance with iMetS. As a result, it is thought that in-depth research between genders will be needed.

This study had some limitations. First, this study was limited to Koreans and, due to ethnic differences, it is difficult to generalize the results of our research. Second, a more accurate measurement of exercise is needed because the amount of exercise was calculated by the questionnaires. Third, muscle mass, muscle strength, and function may be different in various outcomes, so more research on this is needed.

5. Conclusions

The results of this study show that BMI-, weight-, WC-relative HGS and BMS are more sensitive indicators for iMetS than mean HGS and BMS. From the results of this study, it is possible to elucidate, to some extent, the relationship between the development of MetS through HGS and BMS. Studies are needed to confirm the exact mechanism and the associations of relative HGS and BMS with MetS. Nevertheless, our results suggest that relative HGS and BMS can be conveniently used as the simplest predictive method for screening and preventing subjects at risk of metabolic syndrome.

Supplementary Materials: The following are available online at https://www.mdpi.com/article/10.3390/app11115198/s1, Table S1. Baseline characteristics according to gender; Table S2. Sex adjusted partial correlation coefficient of relative hand grip strength and metabolic components. Table S3. Sensitivity analysis for adjusted Cox hazard ratios for one standard deviation of relative hand grip strength and back muscle strength stratified by follow up time, gender and age subgroups; Table S4. Univariate hazard ratio (HR) of incident metabolic syndrome associated with quartile group of mean hand grip strength, back muscle strength, and relative muscle strength according to gender; Table S5. Change in handgrip, relative handgrip, and leisure physical activity at baseline and eighth follow-up; Table S6. Univariate hazard ratio (HR) of incident metabolic syndrome components associated with one standard deviation increase in mean hand grip strength, back muscle strength, and relative muscle strength according to gender.

Author Contributions: Conceptualization, Y.J.J., S.K.L.; data curation, S.K.L.; funding acquisition, C.S.; methodology, S.K.L. project administration, C.S.; supervision, C.S.; validation, S.K.L.; writing—original draft, Y.J.J., S.K.L.; writing—review and editing, Y.J.J. and S.K.L. All authors have read and agreed to the published version of the manuscript.

Funding: This research was supported by a research funds of Korea Centers for Disease Control and Prevention (2001-347-6111-221, 2002-347-6111-221, 2003-347-6111-221, 2004-E71001-00, 2005-E71001-00, 2006-E71005-00, 2007-E71001-00, 2008-E71001-00, 2009-E71002-00, 2010-E71001-00, 2011-E71004-00, 2012-E71005-00, 2013-E71005-00, 2014-E71003-00, 2015-P71001-00, 2016-E71003-00, 2017-E71001-00, 2018-E7101-00) and Korea University.

Institutional Review Board Statement: The study was conducted according to the guidelines of the Declaration of Helsinki and approved by the Institutional Review Board (or Ethics Committee) of the Korea University Ansan Hospital.

Informed Consent Statement: Informed consent was obtained from all subjects involved in the study.

Acknowledgments: The authors thank the participants and support staff who participated in the study.

Conflicts of Interest: The authors declare no conflict of interest.

References

1. Lee, W.J.; Peng, L.N.; Chiou, S.T.; Chen, L.K. Relative Handgrip Strength Is a Simple Indicator of Cardiometabolic Risk among Middle-Aged and Older People: A Nationwide Population-Based Study in Taiwan. *PLoS ONE* **2016**, *11*, e0160876. [CrossRef] [PubMed]
2. National Cholesterol Education Program Expert Panel on Detection, Evaluation and Treatment of High Blood Cholesterol in Adults. Third Report of the National Cholesterol Education Program (NCEP) Expert Panel on Detection, Evaluation, and Treatment of High Blood Cholesterol in Adults (Adult Treatment Panel III) final report. *Circulation* **2002**, *106*, 3143–3421. [CrossRef]
3. Sarafidis, P.A.; Nilsson, P.M. The metabolic syndrome: A glance at its history. *J. Hypertens.* **2006**, *24*, 621–626. [CrossRef]
4. Lim, S.; Shin, H.; Song, J.H.; Kwak, S.H.; Kang, S.M.; Won Yoon, J.; Choi, S.H.; Cho, S.I.; Park, K.S.; Lee, H.K.; et al. Increasing prevalence of metabolic syndrome in Korea: The Korean National Health and Nutrition Examination Survey for 1998–2007. *Diabetes Care* **2011**, *34*, 1323–1328. [CrossRef] [PubMed]
5. Kim, C.R.; Jeon, Y.J.; Kim, M.C.; Jeong, T.; Koo, W.R. Reference values for hand grip strength in the South Korean population. *PLoS ONE* **2018**, *13*, e0195485. [CrossRef] [PubMed]
6. Bohannon, R.W. Grip Strength: An Indispensable Biomarker for Older Adults. *Clin. Interv. Aging* **2019**, *14*, 1681–1691. [CrossRef] [PubMed]
7. Barbat-Artigas, S.; Plouffe, S.; Pion, C.H.; Aubertin-Leheudre, M. Toward a sex-specific relationship between muscle strength and appendicular lean body mass index? *J. Cachexia Sarcopenia Muscle* **2013**, *4*, 137–144. [CrossRef]

8. Kunutsor, S.K.; Isiozor, N.M.; Khan, H.; Laukkanen, J.A. Handgrip strength-A risk indicator for type 2 diabetes: Systematic review and meta-analysis of observational cohort studies. *Diabetes Metab. Res. Rev.* **2021**, *37*, e3365. [CrossRef]
9. Ji, C.; Zheng, L.; Zhang, R.; Wu, Q.; Zhao, Y. Handgrip strength is positively related to blood pressure and hypertension risk: Results from the National Health and nutrition examination survey. *Lipids Health Dis.* **2018**, *17*, 86. [CrossRef] [PubMed]
10. Lakka, H.M.; Laaksonen, D.E.; Lakka, T.A.; Niskanen, L.K.; Kumpusalo, E.; Tuomilehto, J.; Salonen, J.T. The metabolic syndrome and total and cardiovascular disease mortality in middle-aged men. *JAMA* **2002**, *288*, 2709–2716. [CrossRef]
11. Vancampfort, D.; Stubbs, B.; Firth, J.; Smith, L.; Swinnen, N.; Koyanagi, A. Associations between handgrip strength and mild cognitive impairment in middle-aged and older adults in six low- and middle-income countries. *Int. J. Geriatr. Psychiatry* **2019**, *34*, 609–616. [CrossRef]
12. Crewther, B.T.; Gill, N.; Weatherby, R.P.; Lowe, T. A comparison of ratio and allometric scaling methods for normalizing power and strength in elite rugby union players. *J. Sports Sci.* **2009**, *27*, 1575–1580. [CrossRef]
13. Maranhao Neto, G.A.; Oliveira, A.J.; Pedreiro, R.C.; Pereira-Junior, P.P.; Machado, S.; Marques Neto, S.; Farinatti, P.T. Normalizing handgrip strength in older adults: An allometric approach. *Arch. Gerontol. Geriatr.* **2017**, *70*, 230–234. [CrossRef]
14. Choquette, S.; Bouchard, D.R.; Doyon, C.Y.; Senechal, M.; Brochu, M.; Dionne, I.J. Relative strength as a determinant of mobility in elders 67-84 years of age. a nuage study: Nutrition as a determinant of successful aging. *J. Nutr. Health Aging* **2010**, *14*, 190–195. [CrossRef]
15. Jeon, Y.J.; Lee, S.K.; Shin, C. Normalized Hand Grip and Back Muscle Strength as Risk Factors for Incident Type 2 Diabetes Mellitus: 16 Years of Follow-Up in a Population-Based Cohort Study. *Diabetes Metab. Syndr. Obes.* **2021**, *14*, 741–750. [CrossRef]
16. Kawamoto, R.; Ninomiya, D.; Kasai, Y.; Kusunoki, T.; Ohtsuka, N.; Kumagi, T.; Abe, M. Handgrip strength is associated with metabolic syndrome among middle-aged and elderly community-dwelling persons. *Clin. Exp. Hypertens* **2016**, *38*, 245–251. [CrossRef] [PubMed]
17. Byeon, J.Y.; Lee, M.K.; Yu, M.S.; Kang, M.J.; Lee, D.H.; Kim, K.C.; Im, J.A.; Kim, S.H.; Jeon, J.Y. Lower Relative Handgrip Strength is Significantly Associated with a Higher Prevalence of the Metabolic Syndrome in Adults. *Metab. Syndr. Relat. Disord.* **2019**, *17*, 280–288. [CrossRef]
18. Chun, S.W.; Kim, W.; Choi, K.H. Comparison between grip strength and grip strength divided by body weight in their relationship with metabolic syndrome and quality of life in the elderly. *PLoS ONE* **2019**, *14*, e0222040. [CrossRef] [PubMed]
19. Hong, S. Association of Relative Handgrip Strength and Metabolic Syndrome in Korean Older Adults: Korea National Health and Nutrition Examination Survey VII-1. *J. Obes. Metab. Syndr.* **2019**, *28*, 53–60. [CrossRef] [PubMed]
20. Wu, H.; Liu, M.; Chi, V.T.Q.; Wang, J.; Zhang, Q.; Liu, L.; Meng, G.; Yao, Z.; Bao, X.; Gu, Y.; et al. Handgrip strength is inversely associated with metabolic syndrome and its separate components in middle aged and older adults: A large-scale population-based study. *Metabolism* **2019**, *93*, 61–67. [CrossRef]
21. Ji, C.; Xia, Y.; Tong, S.; Wu, Q.; Zhao, Y. Association of handgrip strength with the prevalence of metabolic syndrome in US adults: The national health and nutrition examination survey. *Aging* **2020**, *12*, 7818–7829. [CrossRef]
22. Kang, Y.; Park, S.; Kim, S.; Koh, H. Handgrip Strength among Korean Adolescents with Metabolic Syndrome in 2014–2015. *J. Clin. Densitom.* **2020**, *23*, 271–277. [CrossRef] [PubMed]
23. Choi, E.Y. Relationship of Handgrip Strength to Metabolic Syndrome among Korean Adolescents 10–18 Years of Age: Results from the Korean National Health and Nutrition Examination Survey 2014–18. *Metab. Syndr. Relat. Disord.* **2021**, *19*, 93–99. [CrossRef] [PubMed]
24. Lopez-Lopez, J.P.; Cohen, D.D.; Ney-Salazar, D.; Martinez, D.; Otero, J.; Gomez-Arbelaez, D.; Camacho, P.A.; Sanchez-Vallejo, G.; Arcos, E.; Narvaez, C.; et al. The prediction of Metabolic Syndrome alterations is improved by combining waist circumference and handgrip strength measurements compared to either alone. *Cardiovasc. Diabetol.* **2021**, *20*, 68. [CrossRef] [PubMed]
25. Song, P.; Han, P.; Zhao, Y.; Zhang, Y.; Wang, L.; Tao, Z.; Jiang, Z.; Shen, S.; Wu, Y.; Wu, J.; et al. Muscle mass rather than muscle strength or physical performance is associated with metabolic syndrome in community-dwelling older Chinese adults. *BMC Geriatr.* **2021**, *21*, 191. [CrossRef] [PubMed]
26. Shen, C.; Lu, J.; Xu, Z.; Xu, Y.; Yang, Y. Association between handgrip strength and the risk of new-onset metabolic syndrome: A population-based cohort study. *BMJ Open* **2020**, *10*, e041384. [CrossRef] [PubMed]
27. McCowan, T.C.; Ferris, E.J.; Baker, M.L.; Robbins, K.V.; Reifsteck, J.E.; Fleisher, H.L.; Barnes, R.W. Human percutaneous laser angioplasty. *J. Ark Med. Soc.* **1986**, *82*, 594–596.
28. Jurca, R.; Lamonte, M.J.; Barlow, C.E.; Kampert, J.B.; Church, T.S.; Blair, S.N. Association of muscular strength with incidence of metabolic syndrome in men. *Med. Sci. Sports Exerc.* **2005**, *37*, 1849–1855. [CrossRef]
29. LaMonte, M.J.; Barlow, C.E.; Jurca, R.; Kampert, J.B.; Church, T.S.; Blair, S.N. Cardiorespiratory fitness is inversely associated with the incidence of metabolic syndrome: A prospective study of men and women. *Circulation* **2005**, *112*, 505–512. [CrossRef]
30. Kasukawa, Y.; Miyakoshi, N.; Hongo, M.; Ishikawa, Y.; Kudo, D.; Suzuki, M.; Mizutani, T.; Kimura, R.; Ono, Y.; Shimada, Y. Age-related changes in muscle strength and spinal kyphosis angles in an elderly Japanese population. *Clin. Interv. Aging* **2017**, *12*, 413–420. [CrossRef]
31. Toyoda, H.; Hoshino, M.; Ohyama, S.; Terai, H.; Suzuki, A.; Yamada, K.; Takahashi, S.; Hayashi, K.; Tamai, K.; Hori, Y.; et al. The association of back muscle strength and sarcopenia-related parameters in the patients with spinal disorders. *Eur. Spine J.* **2019**, *28*, 241–249. [CrossRef] [PubMed]

32. Expert Panel on Detection, Evaluation, and Treatment of High Blood Cholesterol in Adults. Executive Summary of the Third Report of the National Cholesterol Education Program (NCEP) Expert Panel on Detection, Evaluation, and Treatment of High Blood Cholesterol in Adults (Adult Treatment Panel III). *JAMA* **2001**, *285*, 2486–2497. [CrossRef] [PubMed]
33. WHO Expert Consultation. Appropriate body-mass index for Asian populations and its implications for policy and intervention strategies. *Lancet* **2004**, *363*, 157–163. [CrossRef]
34. Laaksonen, D.E.; Lakka, H.M.; Salonen, J.T.; Niskanen, L.K.; Rauramaa, R.; Lakka, T.A. Low levels of leisure-time physical activity and cardiorespiratory fitness predict development of the metabolic syndrome. *Diabetes Care* **2002**, *25*, 1612–1618. [CrossRef] [PubMed]
35. Frontera, W.R.; Hughes, V.A.; Fielding, R.A.; Fiatarone, M.A.; Evans, W.J.; Roubenoff, R. Aging of skeletal muscle: A 12-yr longitudinal study. *J. Appl. Physiol.* **2000**, *88*, 1321–1326. [CrossRef] [PubMed]
36. Miyatake, N.; Wada, J.; Saito, T.; Nishikawa, H.; Matsumoto, S.; Miyachi, M.; Makino, H.; Numata, T. Comparison of muscle strength between Japanese men with and without metabolic syndrome. *Acta Med. Okayama* **2007**, *61*, 99–102. [CrossRef]
37. Lee, S.Y.; Ahn, S.; Kim, Y.J.; Ji, M.J.; Kim, K.M.; Choi, S.H.; Jang, H.C.; Lim, S. Comparison between Dual-Energy X-ray Absorptiometry and Bioelectrical Impedance Analyses for Accuracy in Measuring Whole Body Muscle Mass and Appendicular Skeletal Muscle Mass. *Nutrients* **2018**, *10*, 738. [CrossRef]
38. Beaudart, C.; Rolland, Y.; Cruz-Jentoft, A.J.; Bauer, J.M.; Sieber, C.; Cooper, C.; Al-Daghri, N.; Araujo de Carvalho, I.; Bautmans, I.; Bernabei, R.; et al. Assessment of Muscle Function and Physical Performance in Daily Clinical Practice: A position paper endorsed by the European Society for Clinical and Economic Aspects of Osteoporosis, Osteoarthritis and Musculoskeletal Diseases (ESCEO). *Calcif. Tissue Int.* **2019**, *105*, 1–14. [CrossRef]
39. Cuthbertson, D.J.; Bell, J.A.; Ng, S.Y.; Kemp, G.J.; Kivimaki, M.; Hamer, M. Dynapenic obesity and the risk of incident Type 2 diabetes: The English Longitudinal Study of Ageing. *Diabet. Med.* **2016**, *33*, 1052–1059. [CrossRef]
40. Larsen, B.A.; Wassel, C.L.; Kritchevsky, S.B.; Strotmeyer, E.S.; Criqui, M.H.; Kanaya, A.M.; Fried, L.F.; Schwartz, A.V.; Harris, T.B.; Ix, J.H.; et al. Association of Muscle Mass, Area, and Strength with Incident Diabetes in Older Adults: The Health ABC Study. *J. Clin. Endocrinol. Metab.* **2016**, *101*, 1847–1855. [CrossRef]
41. Bai, T.; Fang, F.; Li, F.; Ren, Y.; Hu, J.; Cao, J. Sarcopenia is associated with hypertension in older adults: A systematic review and meta-analysis. *BMC Geriatr.* **2020**, *20*, 279. [CrossRef]
42. Morley, J.E.; Baumgartner, R.N.; Roubenoff, R.; Mayer, J.; Nair, K.S. Sarcopenia. *J. Lab. Clin. Med.* **2001**, *137*, 231–243. [CrossRef] [PubMed]
43. Zhang, H.; Lin, S.; Gao, T.; Zhong, F.; Cai, J.; Sun, Y.; Ma, A. Association between Sarcopenia and Metabolic Syndrome in Middle-Aged and Older Non-Obese Adults: A Systematic Review and Meta-Analysis. *Nutrients* **2018**, *10*, 364. [CrossRef] [PubMed]
44. Artero, E.G.; Lee, D.C.; Lavie, C.J.; Espana-Romero, V.; Sui, X.; Church, T.S.; Blair, S.N. Effects of muscular strength on cardiovascular risk factors and prognosis. *J. Cardiopulm Rehabil. Prev.* **2012**, *32*, 351–358. [CrossRef] [PubMed]
45. Tieland, M.; Verdijk, L.B.; de Groot, L.C.; van Loon, L.J. Handgrip strength does not represent an appropriate measure to evaluate changes in muscle strength during an exercise intervention program in frail older people. *Int. J. Sport Nutr. Exerc. Metab.* **2015**, *25*, 27–36. [CrossRef] [PubMed]
46. Cho, E.R.; Shin, A.; Kim, J.; Jee, S.H.; Sung, J. Leisure-time physical activity is associated with a reduced risk for metabolic syndrome. *Ann. Epidemiol.* **2009**, *19*, 784–792. [CrossRef]
47. Pal, K.; Mukadam, N.; Petersen, I.; Cooper, C. Mild cognitive impairment and progression to dementia in people with diabetes, prediabetes and metabolic syndrome: A systematic review and meta-analysis. *Soc. Psychiatry Psychiatr. Epidemiol.* **2018**, *53*, 1149–1160. [CrossRef]
48. Sousa-Santos, A.R.; Amaral, T.F. Differences in handgrip strength protocols to identify sarcopenia and frailty—A systematic review. *BMC Geriatr.* **2017**, *17*, 238. [CrossRef]
49. Cornier, M.A.; Dabelea, D.; Hernandez, T.L.; Lindstrom, R.C.; Steig, A.J.; Stob, N.R.; van Pelt, R.E.; Wang, H.; Eckel, R.H. The metabolic syndrome. *Endocr. Rev.* **2008**, *29*, 777–822. [CrossRef]
50. Lind, L. Genome-Wide Association Study of the Metabolic Syndrome in UK Biobank. *Metab. Syndr. Relat. Disord.* **2019**, *17*, 505–511. [CrossRef]
51. Misselbeck, K.; Parolo, S.; Lorenzini, F.; Savoca, V.; Leonardelli, L.; Bora, P.; Morine, M.J.; Mione, M.C.; Domenici, E.; Priami, C. A network-based approach to identify deregulated pathways and drug effects in metabolic syndrome. *Nat. Commun.* **2019**, *10*, 5215. [CrossRef] [PubMed]
52. Zmora, N.; Bashiardes, S.; Levy, M.; Elinav, E. The Role of the Immune System in Metabolic Health and Disease. *Cell Metab.* **2017**, *25*, 506–521. [CrossRef] [PubMed]
53. Dingjan, I.; Linders, P.T.A.; Verboogen, D.R.J.; Revelo, N.H.; Ter Beest, M.; van den Bogaart, G. Endosomal and Phagosomal SNAREs. *Physiol. Rev.* **2018**, *98*, 1465–1492. [CrossRef] [PubMed]
54. Iqbal, J.; Al Qarni, A.; Hawwari, A.; Alghanem, A.F.; Ahmed, G. Metabolic Syndrome, Dyslipidemia and Regulation of Lipoprotein Metabolism. *Curr. Diabetes Rev.* **2018**, *14*, 427–433. [CrossRef] [PubMed]

MDPI
St. Alban-Anlage 66
4052 Basel
Switzerland
Tel. +41 61 683 77 34
Fax +41 61 302 89 18
www.mdpi.com

Applied Sciences Editorial Office
E-mail: applsci@mdpi.com
www.mdpi.com/journal/applsci

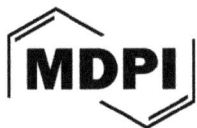

www.ingramcontent.com/pod-product-compliance
Lightning Source LLC
LaVergne TN
LVHW070410100526
838202LV00014B/1426